INTERVENTIONAL CARDIOLOGY CLINICS

www.interventional.theclinics.com

Editor-in-Chief

MARVIN H. ENG

Peripheral Vascular Disease and Interventions

April 2025 • Volume 14 • Number 2

Editors

Dmitriy N. Feldman
Andrew J.P. Klein

ELSEVIER

1600 John F. Kennedy Boulevard • Suite 1800 • Philadelphia, Pennsylvania, 19103-2899

http://www.theclinics.com

INTERVENTIONAL CARDIOLOGY CLINICS Volume 14, Number 2
April 2025 ISSN 2211-7458, ISBN-13: 978-0-443-34417-6

Editor: Joanna Gascoine
Developmental Editor: Akshay Samson

Interventional Cardiology Clinics (ISSN 2211-7458) is published quarterly by Elsevier Inc., 360 Park Avenue South, New York, NY 10010-1710. Months of issue are January, April, July, and October. Subscription prices are USD 224 per year for US individuals, USD 100 per year for US students, USD 224 per year for Canadian individuals, USD 100 per year for Canadian students, USD 317 per year for international individuals, and USD 150 per year for international students. For institutional access pricing please contact Customer Service via the contact information below. To receive student/resident rate, orders must be accompanied by name of affiliated institution, date of term, and the *signature* of program/residency coordinator on institution letterhead. Orders will be billed at individual rate until proof of status is received. Foreign air speed delivery is included in all *Clinics* subscription prices. All prices are subject to change without notice. Orders, claims, and journal inquiries: Please visit our Support Hub page https://service.elsevier.com for assistance.

Reprints. For copies of 100 or more of articles in this publication, please contact the Commercial Reprints Department, Elsevier Inc., 360 Park Avenue South, New York, NY 10010-1710. Tel.: 212-633-3874; Fax: 212-633-3820; E-mail: reprints@elsevier.com.

Printed in the United States of America.

CONTRIBUTORS

CONSULTING EDITOR

MARVIN H. ENG, MD
Structural Heart Program Medical Director,
Structural Heart Disease Fellowship Director,
Director of Cardiovascular Quality, Banner
University Medical Center, Phoenix,
Arizona, USA

EDITORS

DMITRIY N. FELDMAN, MD, FACC, FSCAI,
FSVM
Professor of Medicine, Cardiovascular
Medicine, Director, Greenberg Division of
Cardiology, Department of Medicine,
Endovascular Service of Interventional Cardiac
and Endovascular Laboratory, Weill Cornell
Medical College, New York–Presbyterian
Hospital, New York, New York

ANDREW J.P. KLEIN, MD, FACC, FSVM,
FSCAI
Interventional Cardiologist, Interventional
Cardiology, Vascular and Endovascular
Medicine, Piedmont Heart Institute, Piedmont
Healthcare, Atlanta, Georgia

AUTHORS

ASMAA AHMED, MD
Resident, Department of Internal Medicine,
Rochester General Hospital, Rochester,
New York

KHAWAJA HASSAN AKHTAR, MD
Fellow, Department of Cardiovascular
Diseases, University of Oklahoma Health
Sciences Center, Oklahoma City, Oklahoma
City, US

ZAFAR ALI, MD
Clinical Assistant Professor, Department of
Cardiovascular Medicine, University of Kansas
School of Medicine, Kansas City, Kansas

ELISSA ALTIN, MD, PhD
Associate Professor of Medicine
(Cardiovascular Medicine), Section of
Cardiovascular Medicine, Department of
Internal Medicine, Yale University School of
Medicine, West Haven VA Medical Center,
West Haven, Connecticut

EHRIN J. ARMSTRONG, MD, MSc, MAS,
FACC, FSCAI, FSVM
Interventional Cardiology and Vascular
Intervention, Director of Clinical Research,
Advanced Heart and Vein Center, Denver,
Colorado

SAHEJ ARORA, MD
Resident, Department of Internal Medicine,
Rochester General Hospital, Rochester,
New York

ROBERT R. ATTARAN, MD, FSCAI, FACC,
DABVLM
Associate Professor, Section of Cardiovascular
Medicine, Yale School of Medicine, New
Haven, Connecticut

GOLSA BABAPOUR, MD
Postdoctoral Fellow, Section of Cardiovascular
Medicine, Yale School of Medicine, New
Haven, Connecticut

JU YOUNG BAE, MD
Cardiology Fellow, Section of Cardiovascular
Medicine, Department of Internal Medicine,
Yale New Haven Health Bridgeport Hospital,
Bridgeport, Connecticut

YULANKA CASTRO-DOMINGUEZ, MD,
FACC, FSCAI, FSVM, RPVI
Clinical Assistant Professor of Medicine,
Harrington Heart & Vascular Institute,
University Hospitals, Case Western Reserve
University School of Medicine, Cleveland,
Ohio

DEBBIE L. COHEN, MD
Professor of Medicine, Renal, Electrolytes, and Hypertension, Director, Division of Renal, Electrolyte and Hypertension, Hospital of the University of Pennsylvania, Philadelphia, Pennsylvania

GHASSAN DAHER, MD
Physician, Harrington Heart and Vascular Institute, University Hospitals Cleveland Medical Center, Cleveland, Ohio

ISLAM Y. ELGENDY, MD, FACC, FAHA, FSCAI, FSVM, FESC
Assistant Professor, Division of Cardiovascular Medicine, Gill Heart Institute, University of Kentucky, Lexington, Kentucky

DMITRIY N. FELDMAN, MD, FACC, FSCAI, FSVM
Cardiovascular Medicine, Director, Greenberg Division of Cardiology, Associate Professor, Department of Medicine, Endovascular Service of Interventional Cardiac and Endovascular Laboratory, Weill Cornell Medical College, New York–Presbyterian Hospital, New York, New York

DMITRIY N. FELDMAN, MD
Associate Professor of Medicine, Cardiovascular Medicine, Director, Division of Cardiology, Endovascular Service of Interventional Cardiac and Endovascular Laboratory, Weill Cornell Medical College, New York Presbyterian Hospital, New York, New York

BRIAN FULTON, MD
Assistant Professor of Clinical Medicine, Division of Cardiovascular Medicine, Hospital of the University of Pennsylvania, Philadelphia, Pennsylvania; Director of Structural Heart Interventions, Chester County Hospital, West Chester, Pennsylvania

JON C. GEORGE, MD, FSCAI
Interventional Cardiology and Endovascular Medicine, Medical Director, ReVascMedProfessionals, Thomas Jefferson University Hospital, Philadelphia, Pennsylvania

KAMAL GUPTA, MD
Professor, Department of Cardiovascular Medicine, University of Kansas School of Medicine, Kansas City, Kansas

JORGE ANTONIO GUTIERREZ, MD, MHS
Associate Professor, Department of Medicine, Division of Cardiology, Durham Veterans Administration Medical Center, Duke University Health System, Durham, North Carolina

AAKRITI JAIN, MD
Resident, Department of Internal Medicine, Rochester General Hospital, Rochester, New York

ADAM P. JOHNSON, MD, MPH
Assistant Professor, Department of Surgery, Division of Vascular and Endovascular Surgery, Duke University Health System, Durham Veterans Administration Medical Center, Durham, North Carolina

HILLARY JOHNSTON-COX, MD, PhD
Cardiologist, Northwell Health, Manhasset, New York

WILLIAM SCHUYLER JONES, MD
Assistant Professor of Medicine, Division of Cardiology, Duke University Medical Center, Durham, North Carolina

AMAN KANSAL, MD
Fellow, Division of Cardiology, Duke University Medical Center, Durham, North Carolina

TAKEHIKO KIDO, MD
Department of Medicine, Division of Cardiology, Columbia University Irving Medical Center and Columbia University Vagelos College, Investigator, Clinical Trials Center, Cardiovascular Research Foundation, New York, New York

LUKE KIM, MD
Associate Professor of Medicine, Weill Cornell Medical College, New York, New York

ANDREW J.P. KLEIN, MD, FACC, FSVM, FSCAI
Interventional Cardiologist, Interventional Cardiology, Vascular and Endovascular Medicine, Piedmont Heart Institute, Piedmont Healthcare, Atlanta, Georgia

TAISEI KOBAYASHI, MD
Assistant Professor of Clinical Medicine, Division of Cardiovascular Medicine, Hospital of the University of Pennsylvania, Director,

Cardiac Catheterization Laboratory, Corporal Michael J. Crescenz VA Medical Center, Philadelphia, Pennsylvania

FAISAL LATIF, MD, FSCAI, FACC
Clinical Associate Professor of Medicine, University of Oklahoma Health Sciences Center, Director, Cardiac Catheterization Laboratory, SSM Health St. Anthony Hospital, Oklahoma City, Oklahoma

JUN LI, MD, FACC, FSCAI
Interventional Cardiologist, Harrington Heart and Vascular Institute, University Hospitals Cleveland Medical Center, Co-Director, Vascular Center, Co-Director, Pulmonary Embolism Response Team, University Hospitals Harrington Heart & Vascular Institute, Cleveland, Ohio; Assistant Professor of Medicine, Case Western Reserve University School of Medicine, Parma, Ohio

CARLOS MENA-HURTADO, MD, FSCAI, FACC, RPVI
Associate Professor, Section of Cardiovascular Medicine, Yale School of Medicine, New Haven, Connecticut

ADAVID C. METZGER, MD
Interventional Cardiologist, OhioHealth Vascular Institute, Columbus, Ohio

SAMANTHA D. MINC, MD, MPH
Associate Professor, Department of Surgery, Division of Vascular and Endovascular Surgery, Duke University Health System, Durham, North Carolina; Department of Surgery, Division of Vascular Surgery, West Virginia University School of Medicine, Morgantown, West Virginia

JAY MOHAN, DO, FACC, FSCAI, FASE, RPVI
Program Director, Cardiology Fellowship, Department of Cardiovascular Medicine, Michigan State University McLaren Macomb-Oakland Medical Center, Mount Clemens, Michigan

NAUMAN NAEEM, MD
Resident, Department of Internal Medicine, Rochester General Hospital, Rochester, New York

CASSIUS IYAD OCHOA CHAAR, MD, MPH, MS, RPVI
Associate Professor Surgery (Vascular), Division of Vascular Surgery and Endovascular

Therapy, Department of Surgery, Yale School of Medicine, New Haven, Connecticut

SAHIL A. PARIKH, MD, FACC, FSCAI
Director of Endovascular Services, Associate Professor, Department of Medicine, Division of Cardiology, Columbia University Irving Medical Center and Columbia University Vagelos College; Clinical Trials Center, Cardiovascular Research Foundation, New York, New York

JACQUELINE POWERS, BS
Clinical Research Fellow, Advanced Heart and Vein Center, Denver, Colorado

JACOB RICCI, MS
Graduate Assistant, Division of Cardiovascular Medicine, University of Florida College of Medicine, Gainesville, Florida

JENNIFER A. RYMER, MD, MBA, MHS
Associate Professor of Medicine, Division of Cardiology, Duke University Medical Center, Durham, North Carolina

SANJUM S. SETHI, MD, MPH
Assistant Professor of Medicine, Division of Cardiology, Columbia University, Columbia University Medical Center, Director, Pulmonary Embolism Response Team, Columbia Interventional Cardiovascular Care, New York, New York

KHANJAN B. SHAH, MD
Interventional Cardiologist, Division of Cardiovascular Disease, University of Florida College of Medicine, Gainesville, Florida

DANIEL J. SNYDER, MD
Postdoctoral Fellow in Cardiovascular Diseases, Department of Medicine, Division of Cardiology, Columbia University Irving Medical Center and Columbia University Vagelos College, Clinical Trials Center, Cardiovascular Research Foundation, New York, New York

RAJESH V. SWAMINATHAN, MD
Associate Professor, Department of Medicine, Division of Cardiology, Duke University Health System, Durham Veterans Administration Medical Center, Duke Clinical Research Institute, Duke University School of Medicine, Durham, North Carolina

JOSE D. TAFUR, MD
Interventional Cardiologist, Department of
Cardiovascular Diseases, John Ochsner Heart
& Vascular Center, Ochsner Medical Center,
The Ochsner Clinical School, Univ of
Queensland, New Orleans, Louisiana

ANTHONY TETA, MD
Cardiovascular Medicine Fellow, Department
of Cardiovascular Medicine, McLaren
Macomb Medical Center, Mount Clemens,
Michigan

MONICA TUNG, MD
Fellow, Division of Cardiovascular Medicine,
Hospital of the University of Pennsylvania,
Philadelphia, Pennsylvania

SATAWART UPADHYAY, MD
Resident Physician, Department of Medicine,
University Hospitals, Cleveland, Ohio

VINCENT VARGHESE, DO
Interventional Cardiology and Endovascular
Medicine, Medical Co-Director,

ReVascMedProfessionals, Philadelphia,
Pennsylvania

**CHRISTOPHER J. WHITE, MD, MACC,
MSCAI, FAHA, FESC, FACP**
Professor and Chair, Department of
Cardiovascular Diseases, John Ochsner Heart
& Vascular Center, Ochsner Medical Center,
The Ochsner Clinical School, Univ of
Queensland, Department of Cardiology,
Ochsner Medical Center, New Orleans,
Louisiana; Professor and Chairman of
Medicine and Cardiology, Medical Director,
Value Based Care, System Chair for
Cardiovascular Diseases

ROBERT S. ZILINYI, MD
Postdoctoral Fellow in Cardiovascular
Diseases, Department of Medicine, Division of
Cardiology, Columbia University Irving
Medical Center and Columbia University
Vagelos College, Clinical Trials Center,
Cardiovascular Research Foundation,
New York, New York

CONTENTS

> Peripheral artery disease (PAD) is a highly prevalent subset of cardiovascular disease associated with significant limb-related and concomitant atherosclerotic complications, resulting in high morbidity and mortality. Consequently, appropriate identification and timely initiation of guideline-directed medical therapy is crucial. Despite its widespread prevalence, PAD remains underdiagnosed and undertreated, posing a substantial public health challenge. This review delves into the evidence-based nonpharmacological and pharmacologic treatment strategies for PAD, underscoring the necessity of a multidisciplinary approach.

> Vascular access requires a deliberate and thoughtful approach. Optimal femoral access involves understanding anatomic, fluoroscopic, and ultrasound principles. Combining all 3 approaches optimizes femoral access and minimizes complications, with ultrasound guidance showing the most promising results for procedural success and safety. Transradial access for PCI and peripheral interventions offers benefits like reduced complications, shorter hospital stays, and improved safety. However, challenges include equipment limitations, radial spasm, and procedural complexity. Lower extremity interventions carry risks of access site complications. Prevention involves careful access technique, imaging, and timely management, including endovascular or surgical interventions for severe cases.

> Peripheral arterial disease affects more than 10 million individuals in the United States and over 200 million people worldwide. In the past, the majority of patients were treated with open bypass surgery, but an increasing number are now treated with minimally invasive peripheral endovascular intervention (PVI). To be successful, operators are reliant on the quality of the imaging data obtained during the case. This article reviews the data supporting the use of intravascular imaging in PVI, focusing specifically on lower extremity arterial interventions.

> A great majority of abdominal aortic aneurysm are treated with endovascular aortic repair (EVAR) in current practice. EVAR has lower peri-procedural

The femoropopliteal segment is a common anatomic location for peripheral artery disease. The clinical presentation of occlusive disease of the femoropopliteal segment can range from symptomatic or severe claudication if in isolation, or acute or chornic limb threatening ischemia often in the setting of multilevel disease. Patients can be treated with various therapies to improve symptoms and restore perfusion, including medical, exercise, endovascular, and open surgical therapies. The current literature is rapidly evolving on the best management algorithms and strategies based on patient presentation, severity of occlusive disease, and desired therapy goals. This paper summarizes current literature on available medical, endovascular, and surgical therapies for treating peripheral artery occlusive disease of the femoropopliteal segment.

Chronic limb-threatening ischemia (CLTI) is the end-stage presentation of peripheral artery disease and requires comprehensive care. Despite advancements in treatments, providing timely and equitable care remains challenging. Ongoing research and interdisciplinary collaboration are vital for improving outcomes. Implementing strategies that combine appropriate diagnostics, advanced and innovative revascularization techniques, guideline-directed medical therapies, and efforts to tackle socioeconomic disparities can better address patient needs and enhance quality and quantity of life. This multifaceted approach offers promise for improved long-term outcomes in CLTI patients.

Acute limb ischemia (ALI) is characterized by a sudden decrease in limb perfusion that threatens the viability of the limb. ALI can result from various causes including arterial embolism, thrombosis, or trauma. The diagnosis is predominantly clinical, guided by the "6 Ps" mnemonic—pain, pallor, pulse deficit, paralysis, paresthesia, and poikilothermia—and confirmed through imaging modalities if needed. Treatment decisions are informed by the Rutherford classification, ranging from viable to irreversibly damaged limbs. Early diagnosis and timely intervention are critical for improving limb salvage and reducing amputation rates.

Chronic venous insufficiency is common and is associated with progressive leg discomfort, heaviness, edema, discoloration and ulceration, and venous obstruction, reflux, or both. Venous insufficiency and varicose veins are widespread and are common in Western countries. Risk factors include age, female gender, positive family history, pregnancy and parity, obesity, prolonged standing, and history of deep vein thrombosis. Chronic venous disease is the leading etiology of leg ulcers, which are associated with poor quality of life. Compression, pharmacologic therapy, and catheter-based techniques have shown promise for deep vein recanalization, closure of incompetent superficial veins, and elimination of varicose veins.

Acute iliofemoral deep vein thrombosis (DVT) is associated with higher rates of severe chronic symptoms and complications, and in rare cases with acute limb ischemia. Early detection is a key to provide prompt treatment, including endovascular intervention, in selected patients. When iliofemoral DVT is related to external compression of the left iliac vein by the right common iliac artery is termed May-Thurner syndrome. Approximately, 20% to 50% of patients with chronic DVT will develop post-thrombotic syndrome, a collection of symptoms including lower extremity edema, skin changes, vein dilation, pain, fatigue, and ulcer formation.

PERIPHERAL VASCULAR DISEASE AND INTERVENTIONS

THE CLINICS ARE NOW AVAILABLE ONLINE!

ISSUES OF RELATED INTEREST

Cardiology Clinics
https://www.cardiology.theclinics.com/
Cardiac Electrophysiology Clinics
http://www.cardiacep.theclinics.com/
Heart Failure Clinics
https://www.heartfailure.theclinics.com/

Access your subscription at:
www.theclinics.com

FOREWORD

Peripheral Vascular Interventions

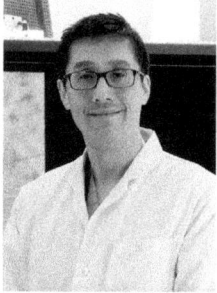

Marvin H. Eng, MD
Consulting Editor

Interventional Cardiology Clinics is pleased to present this issue of peripheral arterial interventions. This issue brings forth the state-of-the-art in both arterial and venous interventions from leaders at the top of the field.

The combined vascular tree composes the majority of the cardio**vascular** system, and with all of the focus on the heart, the periphery deserves more attention. This issue provides a primer for everything necessary for interventional management of peripheral artery disease, starting with medical therapy and vascular access. Furthermore, the issue covers treating atherosclerotic disease from cerebrovascular disease to below-the-knee arterial insufficiency. Covering a broad spectrum of disease, the issue discusses the treatment of aneurysmal disease of the abdominal aorta, chronic venous disease, and acute arterial thrombosis. This issue encompasses all these issues, covering nearly all of the interventional techniques for revascularization, including the use of intravascular imaging.

This issue of *Interventional Cardiology Clinics* was edited by Drs. Dmitriy N. Feldman and Andrew J.P. Klein, stewards of excellence in interventional cardiology. We congratulate them on a comprehensive issue that will be a tremendous foundation of knowledge for anyone searching for excellence in peripheral vascular interventions.

Marvin H. Eng, MD
Banner University Medical Center
1111 East McDowell Road
Phoenix, AZ 85006, USA

E-mail address:
engm@email.arizona.edu

Intervent Cardiol Clin 14 (2025) xiii
https://doi.org/10.1016/j.iccl.2025.01.002
2211-7458/25/© 2025 Published by Elsevier Inc.

PREFACE

Peripheral Arterial and Venous Disease: A "Head-to-Toe" Vascular Journey

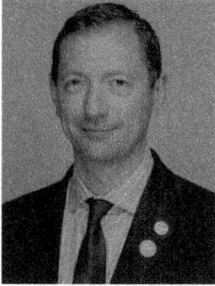

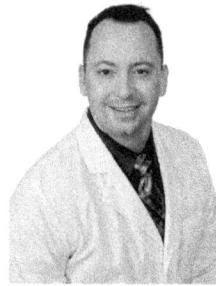

Dmitriy N. Feldman, MD, FACC, FSCAI, FSVM   **Andrew J.P. Klein, MD, FACC, FSVM, FSCAI**
Editors

Vascular and endovascular medicine has evolved tremendously in the last decade, from novel antiplatelet and antithrombotic pharmacotherapies to innovative endovascular devices and surgical revascularization techniques. Newer data from randomized and nonrandomized multicenter clinical trials have contributed to our understanding, management strategies, and treatment algorithms of peripheral arterial and venous disease. Multidisciplinary guidelines, expert consensus documents, and appropriate use criteria have helped to shape our day-to-day vascular therapies and have provided clinicians with evidence-based tools to guide diagnosis and treatment of complex vascular disorders. This collection of the state-of-the-art review articles in this issue provides a thorough overview from "head to toe" of indications, techniques, and outcomes associated with contemporary catheter-based arterial and venous revascularization.

We start our endovascular journey with an overview by Altin and J.Y. Bae of the evidence-based nonpharmacologic and pharmacologic treatment strategies for *Peripheral Arterial Disease (PAD)*, underscoring the necessity of a multidisciplinary vascular approach. Kansal, Jones, Sethi, and Rymer describe vascular access techniques, imaging, and timely management of complications, including endovascular or surgical interventions. Next, Snyder, Zilinyi, Kido, and Parikh teach us about the use of intravascular imaging in vascular interventions, focusing particularly on lower-extremity arterial interventions. The readers learn about recent trends in current usage of intravascular imaging in the United States as well as recent consensus statements and expert opinion documents that have been published. Adjunct intravascular imaging for PAD to guide interventions is of particular interest given data suggesting improved outcomes, similar to the coronary space. Gupta, Kim, and Ali review the evolving technology and techniques that allow more patients to be treated for abdominal aortic aneurysms with EVAR compared with traditional open surgical repair. Latif, Metzger, and Akhtar provide us with a focused overview of data for carcinoembryonic antigen carotid artery stenting (CAS) for treatment of symptomatic and asymptomatic carotid disease, focusing on clinical characteristics, symptomatic status, anatomical characteristics, and institutional local expertise. This is of particular interest given recent reimbursement changes in the United States for CAS. Shah, White, and Tafur teach us about renal artery interventions for uncontrolled hypertension, ischemic nephropathy, and cardiac destabilization syndromes and mesenteric artery interventions for symptomatic chronic mesenteric ischemia. Tung, Kobayashi, Swaminathan, Cohen, Feldman, and Fulton take us on a tour of

Intervent Cardiol Clin 14 (2025) xv–xvi
https://doi.org/10.1016/j.iccl.2025.01.001

transcatheter renal denervation targeting sympathetic nervous system overactivity, which offers an additive benefit to medications for patients with uncontrolled hypertension as well as for patients who are not able or unwilling to be treated with medications.

Klein, Johnston-Cox, and Ricci go over the evaluation and characterization of iliac arterial disease as well as the associated interventional procedures focusing on techniques, device choice, potential complications, and postprocedural care. Johnson, Swaminathan, Minc, and Gutierrez summarize the current literature on available medical, endovascular, and surgical therapies for treating femoropopliteal PAD. Daher, Upadhyay, and Li dive into the complexity of the chronic limb-threatening ischemia, and how to implement strategies that combine appropriate diagnostics, advanced and innovative revascularization techniques, and guideline-directed medical therapies. Elgendy, Ahmed, Naeem, Jain, Arora, and Elkholy describe how to manage acute limb ischemia and recent advancements in diagnostic imaging and therapeutic modalities, as well as techniques for timely intervention to improve patient outcomes. Attaran, Babapour, Mena-Hurtado, and Chaar educate us about chronic venous insufficiency, associated with venous obstruction and reflux, which lead to chronic inflammation and debilitating symptoms. The authors review the evidence for compression and pharmacologic therapy, catheter-based techniques for deep vein recanalization, closure of incompetent superficial veins, and elimination of varicose veins. And finally, Teta, Mohan, Castro-Dominguez, Varghese, George, Powers, and Armstrong teach us about the diagnosis and management option for acute iliofemoral deep vein thrombosis (DVT), chronic DVT, and May-Thurner Syndrome.

We hope that our readers will enjoy this comprehensive state-of-the-art "head-to-toe" review of the indications, techniques, and outcomes associated with contemporary medical, surgical, and catheter-based arterial and venous revascularization.

Dmitriy N. Feldman, MD, FACC, FSCAI, FSVM
Greenberg Division of Cardiology
Department of Medicine
Interventional Cardiology and
Endovascular Laboratory
New York-Presbyterian Hospital
Weill Cornell Medicine
520 East 70th Street
New York, NY 10021, USA

Andrew J.P. Klein, MD, FACC, FSVM, FSCAI
Piedmont Heart Institute
Piedmont Healthcare
Suite 2065
95 Collier Road
Atlanta, GA 30309, USA

E-mail addresses:
dnf9001@med.cornell.edu (D.N. Feldman)
Andrew.Klein@piedmont.org (A.J.P. Klein)

Optimal Medical Therapy in Peripheral Artery Disease

Ju Young Bae, MD[a], Elissa Altin, MD, PhD[b,c],*

KEYWORDS

- Antiplatelet therapy • Atherosclerosis • Guideline-directed medical therapy
- Peripheral artery disease • Peripheral vascular disease • Supervised exercise therapy

KEY POINTS

- Patient counseling and risk factor identification are crucial in preventing major adverse limb events and improving high mortality rates in patients with peripheral artery disease.
- Structured exercise therapy is a vital nonpharmacological approach to managing peripheral artery disease, as it enhances quality of life, walking performance, and overall functional status.
- Early detection of peripheral artery disease allows timley initiation of guideline-based medical therapies to significantly reduce the risk of major adverse cardiovascular and limb events.

INTRODUCTION

Peripheral artery disease (PAD) is a form of cardiovascular disease affecting the peripheral vasculature, impacting over 10 million Americans aged over 40 years and 200 million individuals globally.[1] PAD is associated with a number of modifiable and nonmodifiable risk factors that significantly increase the likelihood of major adverse cardiovascular events (MACE) and major adverse limb events (MALE). Despite the availability of numerous evidence-based therapies, persistent social and health disparities pose substantial barriers to the timely detection and comprehensive management of PAD. In this dedicated issue on vascular disorders, we comprehensively review strategies to mitigate PAD risk factors and explore evidence-based nonpharmacological and pharmacologic approaches for PAD treatment.

DISCUSSION

Addressing Risk Factors in Peripheral Artery Disease

Blood pressure optimization

Hypertension is identified as the predominant risk factor in 30% to 80% of patients at the time of initial PAD diagnosis.[2] Despite its strong association, blood pressure treatment rates in this subgroup remain lower at approximately 80% compared to over 90% among those with other cardiovascular diseases.[3] In addition to its epidemiologic significance, hypertension contributes to the pathogenesis of atherosclerosis and may account for the observed longitudinal decline in ankle-brachial index among adults aged over 65 years.[4] The 2024 guidelines from the American College of Cardiology/American Heart Association (ACC/AHA) for the management of PAD recommend a target systolic blood pressure of less than 130/80 mm Hg in

[a] Section of Cardiovascular Medicine, Department of Internal Medicine, Yale New Haven Health Bridgeport Hospital, 256 Grant Street, Bridgeport, CT 06610, USA; [b] Section of Cardiovascular Medicine, Department of Internal Medicine, Yale University School of Medicine, New Haven, CT, USA; [c] West Haven VA Medical Center, West Haven, CT, USA
* Corresponding author. Yale New Haven Hospital, 20 York Street, New Haven, CT, 06510.
E-mail address: elissa.altin@yale.edu
Twitter: sallyjybaeMD (J.Y.B.); sealtin1 (E.A.)

Intervent Cardiol Clin 14 (2025) 137–148
https://doi.org/10.1016/j.iccl.2024.11.002
2211-7458/25/© 2024 Elsevier Inc. All rights reserved, including for text and data mining, AI training, and similar technologies.

Abbreviations	
ACC/AHA	American College of Cardiology/American Heart Association
ACE	angiotensin-converting enzyme
ACEi	angiotensin-converting enzyme inhibitor
ALI	acute limb ischemia
ARB	angiotensin receptor blockers
CI	confidence interval
CKD	chronic kidney disease
CLTI	chronic limb-threatening ischemia
COX-1	cyclooxygenase 1
FDA	US Food and Drug Administration
GLP-1	glucagon-like peptide-1
HMG-CoA	hydroxymethylglutaryl-CoA
ISR	in-stent restenosis
LDL	low-density lipoprotein
LDL-C	low-density lipoprotein cholesterol
MACE	major adverse cardiovascular events
MALE	major adverse limb events
PAD	peripheral artery disease
PCSK9	proprotein convertase subtilisin/kexin type 9
PO	per os
SET	supervised exercise therapy
SGLT-2	sodium-glucose cotransporter-2
SPRINT	Systolic Blood Pressure Intervention Trial
SubQ	subcutaneous
UTI	urinary tract infection

individuals with concurrent PAD and hypertension as a class I recommendation.[5] This is in alignment with the 2017 ACC/AHA recommendation for the management of blood pressure in patients with PAD.[6]

There is variability in perspectives on optimal blood pressure targets concerning MACE and MALE, such as acute limb ischemia (ALI), peripheral

revascularization, and amputation. The Systolic Blood Pressure Intervention Trial (SPRINT), a randomized prospective study, evaluated the outcomes of intensive blood pressure control (systolic blood pressure <120 mm Hg) versus standard treatment (systolic blood pressure <140 mm Hg) in patients with cardiovascular risk factors. The trial demonstrated lower rates of both fatal and nonfatal MACE and all-cause mortality in a small subset of the patients with PAD subjected to intensive blood pressure management.[7] A post hoc analysis of the SPRINT trial by Frary and colleagues[8] further demonstrated greater absolute risk reduction of efficacy outcomes as well as greater absolute risk increase on safety outcomes in the intensive treatment group. This was further supported by the Appropriate Blood-Pressure Control in Diabetes trial, which revealed that among patients with PAD and diabetes mellitus, intensive blood pressure control to a mean of 128/75 mm Hg was associated with reduced MACE compared to standard average blood pressure goal of 137/81 mm Hg.[9] The 2024 ACC/AHA guideline recommends the use of angiotensin-converting enzyme (ACE) inhibitors or angiotensin-receptor blockers as the first line for hypertension management in those with concomitant PAD.[5] This is a class I recommendation and is driven from multiple trials that have shown significant reduction in the risk of MACE, including minimizing the risk of major amputation.[10-14] Current guidelines do not specify a target blood pressure range for patients with PAD.[5] However, evidence suggests that patients at the extremes blood pressure (defined as systolic blood pressure <120 mm Hg or >160 mm Hg) are at an increased risk for PAD ischemic events.[15,16] This underscores the importance of optimizing blood pressure to mitigate risk in the PAD population with the caveat of the need to maintain normotension to avoid possible complications associated with low-flow states.

Chronic kidney disease

Chronic kidney disease (CKD) is associated with an increased risk for PAD and was shown to affect 24% of individuals with CKD stage 3 or higher, a 6 fold increase compared to those with normal creatinine clearance.[17-19] It is believed that chronic systemic inflammation, prothrombotic state, and hypoalbuminemia increase the risk of PAD.[20] While individuals with both PAD and CKD are at increased risk for MACE, they were not found to be at elevated risk for MALE, hospitalization for ALI, or major amputation.[21,22] Conversely, patients with end-stage renal disease and PAD were found to have a higher risk for amputation and a higher likelihood of readmission after revascularization compared to those with CKD and PAD.[23] Risk modification for patients with PAD and CKD should focus on treatment of intermittent claudication, and amputation prevention. The 2024 KDIGO (kidney disease improving global outcomes) guidelines suggest the use of low-dose aspirin (or antiplatelet therapy if aspirin intolerant) for secondary prevention in patients with CKD and ischemic cardiovascular disease.[24] However, data from the Clopidogrel for Reduction of Events During Observation trial indicated that patients with CKD may not experience the same benefits from clopidogrel use as those with normal creatinine clearance, due to increased platelet reactivity causing resistance.[25]

Diabetes

Diabetes is an important independent risk factor of PAD and is over twice as prevalent in diabetics compared with nondiabetics.[26] As with other modifiable risk factors, diabetes is associated with a higher risk of all-cause death, MACE, and MALE outcomes, including the risk for chronic limb-threatening ischemia (CLTI) and lower extremity amputation.[27,28] Around 50% of patients with CLTI have been found to have diabetes.[29] A 1% rise in hemoglobin A1c has been linked to a 30% higher risk of PAD during follow-up, highlighting the potential for rapid disease progression associated with poor glycemic control.[30] Multiple studies have demonstrated the efficacy of glucagon-like peptide-1 (GLP-1) agonists as well as sodium-glucose cotransporter-2 (SGLT-2) inhibitors to reduce MACE in patients with cardiovascular conditions including PAD. Specifically, the liraglutide and cardiovascular outcomes in type 2 diabetes and semaglutide and cardiovascular outcomes in patients with type 2 diabetes trials showed significant reductions in MACE with liraglutide and semaglutide, respectively.[31,32] Similarly, the empagliflozin reduced mortality and hospitalization for heart failure across the spectrum of cardiovascular risk and canagliflozin and cardiovascular and renal events in type 2 diabetes trials found significant reduction in MACE in patients with PAD with empagliflozin and canagliflozin.[33,34] Despite initial concerns about increased lower extremity amputations with canagliflozin, subsequent studies did not replicate these findings, and the US Food and Drug Administration (FDA) removed the black box warning in 2020, further supporting the use of these agents to reduce MACE in patients

with PAD and type 2 diabetes and is currently a class I recommendation by ACC/AHA.[5,34]

Smoking cessation

Cigarette smoking is a strong risk factor for PAD, increasing the risk by 2 to 4 fold, with an attributable risk exceeding 40%.[35] The 2024 ACC/AHA guidelines recommend smoking cessation or the maintenance of smoking cessation for individuals with PAD, whether they use cigarettes or other forms of tobacco.[5] The association between PAD and cigarette use has been well recognized since 1911, when Erb, a German neurologist, described a dose-dependent relationship between intermittent claudication and smoking, noting a higher incidence of PAD in smokers compared to nonsmokers.[36] Tobacco use promotes atherosclerotic plaque formation through adverse effects on endothelial tissue, smooth muscle cells, lipid regulation, coagulation pathways, and platelet function.[37] Smoking cessation not only prevents disease progression but also reduces potential complications. A retrospective study by Armstrong and colleagues[38] reviewed patients undergoing diagnostic and therapeutic angiography for CLTI or symptomatic PAD, despite receiving medical therapy, to evaluate the impact of smoking cessation on clinical outcomes. The study found that smoking cessation in this cohort was associated with lower all-cause mortality and improved amputation-free survival compared to active smokers. Additionally, smoking cessation improved claudication, walking distance, and the patency of bypass grafts. Patient counseling combined with early referral to a smoking cessation program, where pharmacologic therapy is provided, has been shown to improve smoking cessation rates by 21%, compared to only 7% with standard counseling alone.[39] Currently, 3 FDA-approved agents for smoking cessation—varenicline, bupropion, and nicotine replacement therapy—are available.[39] Lastly, with the increase in the use of electronic cigarettes and cannabis, future longitudinal studies are needed to evaluate the effect of these substances on the long-term risks for PAD, as current data are sparse.

Nonpharmacologic Management of Peripheral Artery Disease
Role of exercise training

Supervised exercise therapy (SET) is an essential part of PAD management for those with chronic symptomatic disease and individuals with chronic PAD postrevascularization.[40] The 2024 ACC/AHA guidelines recommend SET as an initial treatment strategy for individuals with intermittent claudication before any invasive approach.[5] SET is typically conducted in hospitals or cardiac rehabilitation settings and involves intermittent treadmill walking, with rest periods triggered by moderate-to-severe pain. The recommended session schedule is 30 to 60 minutes per session, at least 3 times a week for a minimum of 12 weeks.[41] The benefits of exercise therapy for PAD date back to 1966, when 6 months of unsupervised walking improved pain onset times in patients with intermittent claudication.[42] Although the precise mechanisms by which SET enhances functional performance are not fully understood, it is thought to involve multiple factors, including improved endothelial and mitochondrial function, angiogenesis, reduced inflammation, and increased muscle fiber strength.[43] Robust evidence consistently demonstrates that SET enhances walking performance, exercise tolerance, quality of life, and functional status in those with chronic symptomatic PAD.[44] While higher baseline functional performance is linked to reduced mortality, direct evidence connecting SET to mortality outcomes is lacking. Furthermore, despite approval for reimbursement by the Centers for Medicare and Medicaid Services in 2017, utilization of this service remains low. Only 1.3% of Medicare beneficiaries diagnosed with intermittent claudication participated in SET between 2017 and 2018.[45] Future studies are needed to better understand the reasons for this underutilization but identified barriers include interference with work schedule, limited number of sites offering SET, copay requirements, among others.[46]

Pharmacologic Management of Peripheral Artery Disease
Lipid-lowering therapy
Statins are competitive inhibitors of hydroxymethylglutaryl-CoA (HMG-CoA) reductase, the enzyme responsible for converting HMG-CoA to mevalonate, thereby reducing hepatic cholesterol synthesis. This reduction facilitates the upregulation of hepatic low-density lipoprotein (LDL) receptors, enhancing the uptake of LDL cholesterol from the bloodstream.[47] Multiple studies have highlighted the benefits of statins in reducing MACE in PAD. Specifically, a reduction in LDL cholesterol by 1 mmol/L (38.7 mg/dL) is associated with a 22% relative risk reduction in MACE.[48,49] Statins have also proven to improve MALE outcomes specifically associated with lower rates of amputation, and death.[50] Furthermore, an observational study by Kumbhani and colleagues[51] demonstrated a 14% relative risk

reduction of primary composite endpoint, which included progression of claudication, CLTI, peripheral vascular intervention, and amputation at 4 years in patients on statin therapy. In patients with an established diagnosis of PAD, the high-intensity statin should be initiated with the goal reduction in low-density lipoprotein cholesterol (LDL-C) level by 50% or greater to less than 70 mg/dL. If LDL-C remains greater than 70 mg/dL despite maximum statin therapy, it is reasonable to add ezetimibe or proprotein convertase subtilisin/kexin type 9 (PCSK9) inhibitors (class IIa recommendation).[5]

The addition of PCSK9-inhibitors such as evolocumab or alirocumab in patients with LDL-C greater than 70 mg/dL on high-intensity statin therapy has been shown to lower MACE and MALE.[5] PCSK9 is a proprotein that targets degradation of hepatic LDL receptors. PCSK9 inhibitor is a monoclonal antibody against this proprotein to inhibit the binding of PCSK9 and LDL receptor to increase the expression of LDL receptor on the cell membrane and increase hepatic uptake of LDL-C.[52] Subgroup analysis of PAD from Further Cardiovascular Outcomes Research with PCSK9 Inhibition in Subjects with Elevated Risk trial demonstrated lower occurrence of MACE (hazard ratio [HR] 0.79, 95% confidence interval [CI]: 0.66–0.94, P=.0098) and MALE (HR 0.63, CI: 0.39–1.03, P = .063) compared to standard therapy alone.[53] Evaluation of Cardiovascular Outcomes After an Acute Coronary Syndrome During Treatment With Alirocumab trial showed lower MACE (22.8% vs 23.9%) and MALE (HR 0.59, 95% CI: 0.40–0.86) with the addition of alirocumab compared to the control group.[54]

The 2024 ACC/AHA guidelines for the management of PAD give a class IIa recommendation for the addition of ezetimibe in patients with PAD on maximum tolerated statin therapy with LDL-C level greater than 70 mg/dL.[5] Ezetimibe is a selective inhibitor of intestinal cholesterol absorption by blocking the niemann-pick-c1-like protein in the jejunal brush border.[55] Subgroup analysis of the Improved Reduction of Outcomes: Vytorin Efficacy International trial evaluated the effectiveness of simvastatin monotherapy versus simvastatin combined with ezetimibe in patients with cardiovascular disease, including PAD in individuals with LDL-C levels below 125 mg/dL. The trial demonstrated a significantly lower rate of cardiovascular events at 7 years in the dual therapy group (32.7% vs 34.7%) in the control group.[56] However, there is currently no study to support the role of ezetimibe in preventing MALE.

Antiplatelet therapy
While cardiovascular risk reduction through blood pressure and diabetes optimization, smoking cessation, lipid control, and preventive foot care are the mainstay treatments for individuals with asymptomatic PAD, antiplatelet and antithrombotic therapy are cornerstones in the management of symptomatic PAD.

For individuals without recent revascularization therapy, either monotherapy with aspirin 75 to 325 mg once daily or clopidogrel 75 mg once daily, or combination therapy with aspirin 81 mg once daily and rivaroxaban 2.5 mg 2 times daily is recommended (Class I recommendation).[5] While low-dose aspirin has traditionally been used as monotherapy to reduce MACE by 12% in the PAD population, the Clopidogrel versus Aspirin in Patients with Risk of Ischemic Events trial has demonstrated improved efficacy in MACE prevention by 23.8% in the clopidogrel group compared to aspirin group with comparable bleeding risk.[57,58] A randomized control trial by Bonaca and colleagues[59] showed that patients on ticagrelor with aspirin were found to have lower limb events with an absolute risk reduction of 0.3% and less need for revascularization. However, the risk of bleeding was increased. Ticagrelor was compared to clopidogrel in the Ticagrelor versus Clopidogrel in Symptomatic Peripheral Artery Disease trial, which failed to show superiority in the prevention of MACE and showed a similar risk of major bleeding.[60]

Vorapaxar is a reversible antagonist for protease-activated receptor-1, which inhibits thrombin-mediated activation of platelets. The Preventing Heart Attack and Stroke in Patients With Atherosclerosis trial assessed the efficacy of vorapaxar as a secondary prevention for patients with established atherosclerosis including PAD. While patients on vorapaxar were found to have reduced ALI and peripheral vascular intervention, it did not significantly reduce MACE, and patients were at an increased risk of bleeding.[61]

Antithrombotic therapy
The Cardiovascular Outcomes for People Using Anticoagulation Strategies trial compared the efficacy of low-dose rivaroxaban and aspirin with aspirin monotherapy in individuals with PAD with at least 1 high-risk comorbidity or high-risk presentation showed reduced risk of MACE by 24%, 46% in MALE, and total mortality by 18% in dual therapy compared to aspirin monotherapy.[62,63]

For patients following endovascular or surgical revascularization, there is most evidence for dual agent therapy with low-dose aspirin and rivaroxaban 2.5 mg 2 times daily. The Vascular Outcomes Study of ASA Along with Rivaroxaban in Endovascular or Surgical Limb Revascularization for PAD trial showed 2.6% absolute risk reduction in ALI, major amputation in the rivaroxaban and aspirin combination therapy group compared with aspirin monotherapy cohort.[64]

Peripheral vasodilators
Cilostazol is a phosphodiesterase III inhibitor with multiple pharmacokinetic profiles of vasodilation and antiplatelet properties.[65] Cilostazol is recommended for improving claudication symptoms, increasing pain-free walking distance, and enhancing the quality of life, but has not been shown to reduce MACE.[66–68] It has demonstrated additional benefits in prevention of in-stent restenosis (ISR) and target lesion revascularization with both bare metal stents and paclitaxel-eluting stents in patients after femoropopliteal endovascular therapy.[69–71] The 2024 ACC/AHA guidelines recommend the use of cilostazol to improve leg symptoms and increase walking distance (class I) and those following endovascular therapy to reduce ISR (class IIb).[5]

Pentoxifylline is a methylxanthine derivative and nonselective phosphodiesterase inhibitor used for intermittent claudication by decreasing blood viscosity. A meta-analysis by the Cochrane group reviewed 24 studies that showed significant interstudy variability and concluded the indetermined effectiveness of pentoxifylline in intermittent claudication.[72] A randomized control study also failed to show any significant difference in maximal walking distance between placebo and pentoxifylline.[73] Furthermore, there are no studies to suggest a reduction of MACE of MALE. The 2024 ACC/AHA guide does not recommend the use of pentoxifylline in the management of claudication (class III recommendation).[5] A list of pharmacologic therapies of PAD has been summarized in Table 1.

Miscellaneous
Novel experimental strategies, such as gene therapy, remain investigational, aiming to stimulate angiogenesis and arteriogenesis by modifying genetic expression, especially in patients with CLTI who are poor candidates for endovascular or surgical interventions.[74]

Summary
Despite the low cost of PAD screening, many patients remain underdiagnosed and subsequently undertreated. Individuals with PAD face elevated risks of cardiovascular events and diminished quality of life, necessitating proactive

Table 1
Summary of pharmacologic therapies for peripheral artery disease

Medication	Indication	Dosage	Mechanism of Action	Common Adverse Effects	ACC/AHA Recommendation
Lipid Lowering Therapy					
Statins (atorvastatin and rosuvastatin)	Asymptomatic and symptomatic PAD	Atorvastatin 40–80 mg daily Rosuvastatin 20–40 mg daily	HMG-CoA reductase inhibitor	Headache, hoarseness, back pain, difficulty urination, and myalgia	Class I
Ezetimibe	Patients with PAD on maximally tolerated statin therapy and LDL-C >70 mg/dL	Ezetimibe 10 mg daily	Selective inhibition of cholesterol and phytosterol absorption by small intestine	Upper respiratory tract infection, diarrhea, joint pain, sinusitis, and pain in arm or leg	Class IIA
PCSK9 inhibitors (evolocumab and alirocumab)	Patients with PAD on maximally tolerated statin therapy and LDL-C >70 mg/dL	Evolocumab 140 mg every 2 wk or 420 mg monthly (subQ) Alirocumab 75 mg every 2 wk or 300 mg monthly (subQ)	Monoclonal antibody against PCSK9 to inhibit the binding of PCSK9 and LDL receptor	Injection site reaction, nasopharyngitis, headache, upper respiratory tract infection, musculoskeletal pain, back pain, elevated blood pressure, diarrhea, myalgia, and elevated liver enzymes	Class IIA

Antiplatelet and Anticoagulation Therapy

Drug	Indication	Dose	Mechanism	Side effects	Class
Clopidogrel	Symptomatic PAD, no recent revascularization	Clopidogrel 75 mg daily	P2Y12 inhibitor	Bleeding, bruising, and itching	Class I
Aspirin	Symptomatic PAD, no recent revascularization	Aspirin 75–325 mg daily	Irreversible inhibitor of COX-1	Dyspepsia, bleeding, and bruising	Class I
Rivaroxaban	Symptomatic PAD, no recent or recent revascularization (endovascular or surgical)	Aspirin 81 mg daily + rivaroxaban 2.5 mg 2 times daily	Factor Xa inhibitor	Bleeding, bruising, headaches, dizziness, bowel or bladder dysfunction, and back pain	Class I

Peripheral Vasodilators

Drug	Indication	Dose	Mechanism	Side effects	Class
Cilostazol	Chronic symptomatic PAD	Cilostazol 100 mg 2 times daily	Phosphodiesterase III inhibitor	Headache, diarrhea, dizziness, and palpitations	Class I
Pentoxifylline	Chronic symptomatic PAD	Pentoxifylline 400 mg 3 times daily	Nonspecific phosphodiesterase inhibitor	Headache, dizziness, nausea, vomiting, diarrhea, and bloating	Class III

Antihypertensive Therapy

Drug	Indication	Dose	Mechanism	Side effects	Class
ACE inhibitors/angiotensin-receptor blockers	Hypertension and PAD	Dose to target blood pressure goal <130/80 mm Hg	ACE inhibitor (blockade of angiotensin II) ARB Competitive antagonism of angiotensin II receptors	Dry cough (ACEi), dizziness, acute renal injury, and hyperkalemia	Class I

(continued on next page)

Table 1
(continued)

Medication	Indication	Dosage	Mechanism of Action	Common Adverse Effects	ACC/AHA Recommendation
Smoking Cessation Therapy					
Varenicline	Active cigarette use	Days 1–3: 0.5 mg daily Days 4–7: 0.5 mg 2 times daily Day 8 to end of treatment: 1 mg PO 2 times daily (total of 12 wk)	Partial agonist for nicotinic acetylcholine receptors and serotonergic agonist	Nausea, headache, vomiting, drowsiness, constipation, unusual dreams, change in taste, and insomnia	Class I
Bupropion	Active cigarette use	150 mg daily for 3 d then increase to 150 mg 2 times daily	Norepinephrine–dopamine reuptake inhibitor and nicotinic receptor antagonist	Dry mouth, cough, sore throat, insomnia, tremor, and agitation	Class I
Diabetes Management					
GLP-1 agonist (liraglutide and semaglutide)	Type 2 Diabetes Mellitus and PAD	Liraglutide 0.6 mg daily for 1 wk (subQ) then increase to 1.2 mg daily (subQ) Semaglutide 0.25 mg once weekly (subQ) for first 4 wk then 0.5 mg once weekly (subQ) for at least 4 wk	Activate GLP-1 receptor (enhance insulin secretion and slow gastric emptying)	Anxiety, constipation, diarrhea, arrhythmias, nausea, skin rash, and vomiting	Class I
SGLT-2 inhibitors (canagliflozin, dapagliflozin, and empagliflozin)	Type 2 diabetes mellitus and PAD	Canagliflozin 100 mg daily (max 300 mg daily) Dapagliflozin 5 mg daily (max 10 mg daily) Empagliflozin 10 mg daily (max 25 mg daily)	SGLT-2 inhibition in the proximal convoluted tubule (prevent reabsorption of glucose and facilitate excretion in urine)	UTI, yeast infection, and nasopharyngitis	Class I

Abbreviations: ACE, angiotensin-converting enzyme; ACEi, angiotensin-converting enzyme inhibitor; ARB, angiotensin receptor blockers; COX-1, cyclooxygenase 1; GLP-1, glucagon-like peptide-1; HMG-CoA, hydroxymethylglutaryl-CoA; LDL, low-density lipoprotein; PAD, peripheral artery disease; PO, per os; SGLT-2, sodium-glucose cotransporter-2; SubQ, subcutaneous; UTI, urinary tract infection.

management. Comprehensive care, including targeted risk factor modification and evidence-based medical therapies, is essential to optimize outcomes and improve patient quality of life.

CLINICS CARE POINTS

- A team-based strategy is essential for optimizing outcomes, emphasizing the integration of lifestyle changes and medical interventions.
- Despite the high prevalence, PAD remains underdiagnosed and undertreated, highlighting the need for increased awareness and equitable health care access.

DISCLOSURE

The authors have nothing to disclose.

REFERENCES

1. Allison MA, Armstrong DG, Goodney PP, et al. Health disparities in peripheral artery disease: a scientific statement from the American heart association. Circulation 2023;148(3):286–96.
2. Fudim M, Jones WS. New curveball for hypertension guidelines? Circulation 2018;138(17):1815–8.
3. Hirsch AT, Criqui MH, Treat-Jacobson D, et al. Peripheral arterial disease detection, awareness, and treatment in primary care. JAMA 2001;286(11):1317–24.
4. Kennedy M, Solomon C, Manolio TA, et al. Risk factors for declining ankle-brachial index in men and women 65 years or older: the Cardiovascular Health Study. Arch Intern Med 2005;165(16):1896–902.
5. Gornik HL, Aronow HD, Goodney PP, et al, Writing Committee Members. 2024 ACC/AHA/AACVPR/APMA/ABC/SCAI/SVM/SVN/SVS/SIR/VESS guideline for the management of lower extremity peripheral artery disease: a report of the American College of Cardiology/American heart association joint committee on clinical practice guidelines. J Am Coll Cardiol 2024;83(24):2497–604.
6. Lu Y, Ballew SH, Tanaka H, et al. 2017 ACC/AHA blood pressure classification and incident peripheral artery disease: the Atherosclerosis Risk in Communities (ARIC) Study. Eur J Prev Cardiol 2020;27(1):51–9.
7. Wright JT Jr, Williamson JD, Whelton PK, et al, SPRINT Research Group. A randomized trial of intensive versus standard blood-pressure control [published correction appears in N Engl J Med. 2017 Dec 21;377(25):2506. doi: 10.1056/NEJMx170008]. N Engl J Med 2015;373(22):2103–16.
8. Frary JMC, Pareek M, Byrne C, et al. Intensive blood pressure control appears to be effective and safe in patients with peripheral artery disease: the Systolic Blood Pressure Intervention Trial. Eur Heart J Cardiovasc Pharmacother 2021;7(3):e38–40.
9. Mehler PS, Coll JR, Estacio R, et al. Intensive blood pressure control reduces the risk of cardiovascular events in patients with peripheral arterial disease and type 2 diabetes. Circulation 2003;107(5):753–6.
10. Yusuf S, Sleight P, Pogue J, et al, Heart Outcomes Prevention Evaluation Study Investigators. Effects of an angiotensin-converting-enzyme inhibitor, ramipril, on cardiovascular events in high-risk patients. N Engl J Med 2000;342(3):145–53 [published correction appears in 2000 May 4;342(18):1376] [published correction appears in N Engl J Med 2000 Mar 9;342(10):748].
11. Yusuf S, Teo KK, Pogue J, et al, ONTARGET Investigators. Telmisartan, ramipril, or both in patients at high risk for vascular events. N Engl J Med 2008;358(15):1547–59.
12. Armstrong EJ, Chen DC, Singh GD, et al. Angiotensin-converting enzyme inhibitor or angiotensin receptor blocker use is associated with reduced major adverse cardiovascular events among patients with critical limb ischemia. Vasc Med 2015;20:237–44.
13. Chen R, Suchard MA, Krumholz HM, et al. Comparative first-line effectiveness and safety of ACE (Angiotensin-Converting enzyme) inhibitors and angiotensin receptor blockers: a multinational cohort study. Hypertension 2021;78(3):591–603.
14. Khan SZ, O'Brien-Irr MS, Rivero M, et al. Improved survival with angiotensin-converting enzyme inhibitors and angiotensin receptor blockers in chronic limb-threatening ischemia. J Vasc Surg 2020;72(6):2130–8.
15. Fudim M, Hopley CW, Huang Z, et al. Association of hypertension and arterial blood pressure on limb and cardiovascular outcomes in symptomatic peripheral artery disease: the EUCLID trial. Circ Cardiovasc Qual Outcomes 2020;13(9):e006512. https://doi.org/10.1161/CIRCOUTCOMES.120.006512.
16. Cooper-DeHoff RM, Handberg EM, Mancia G, et al. INVEST revisited: a review of findings from the International Verapamil SR-Trandolapril Study. Expert Rev Cardiovasc Ther 2009;7(11):1329–40.
17. Lash JP, Go AS, Appel LJ, et al. Chronic Renal Insufficiency Cohort (CRIC) Study: baseline characteristics and associations with kidney function. Clin J Am Soc Nephrol 2009;4:1302–11.
18. Selvin E, Erlinger TP. Prevalence of and risk factors for peripheral arterial disease in the United States: results from the National Health and Nutrition

Examination Survey, 1999-2000. Circulation 2004; 110:738–43.

19. O'Hare AM, Glidden DV, Fox CS, et al. High prevalence of peripheral arterial disease in persons with renal insufficiency: results from the National Health and Nutrition Examination Survey 1999-2000. Circulation 2004;109(3):320–3.

20. Cooper BA, Penne EL, Bartlett LH, et al. Protein malnutrition and hypoalbuminemia as predictors of vascular events and mortality in ESRD. Am J Kidney Dis 2004;43(1):61–6.

21. Bourrier M, Ferguson TW, Embil JM, et al. Peripheral artery disease: its adverse consequences with and without CKD. Am J Kidney Dis 2020;75:705–12.

22. Hopley CW, Kavanagh S, Patel MR, et al. Chronic kidney disease and risk for cardiovascular and limb outcomes in patients with symptomatic peripheral artery disease: the EUCLID trial. Vasc Med 2019;24(5):422–30.

23. Smilowitz NR, Bhandari N, Berger JS. Chronic kidney disease and outcomes of lower extremity revascularization for peripheral artery disease. Atherosclerosis 2020;297:149–56.

24. Kidney Disease: Improving Global Outcomes (KDIGO) CKD Work Group. KDIGO 2024 clinical practice guideline for the evaluation and management of chronic kidney disease. Kidney Int 2024; 105(4S):S117–314.

25. Steinhubl SR, Berger PB, Mann JT 3rd, et al. Early and sustained dual oral antiplatelet therapy following percutaneous coronary intervention: a randomized controlled trial [published correction appears in JAMA. 2003 Feb 26;289(8):987. JAMA 2002;288(19):2411–20.

26. Gregg EW, Sorlie P, Paulose-Ram R, et al, 1999-2000 national health and nutrition examination survey. 1999-2000 national health and nutrition examination survey. Prevalence of lower-extremity disease in the US adult population >=40 years of age with and without diabetes: 1999-2000 national health and nutrition examination survey. Diabetes Care 2004;27:1591–7.

27. Mohammedi K, Woodward M, Hirakawa Y, et al. Presentations of major peripheral arterial disease and risk of major outcomes in patients with type 2 diabetes: results from the ADVANCE-ON study. Cardiovasc Diabetol 2016;15(1):129.

28. Sen P, Demirdal T, Emir B. Meta-analysis of risk factors for amputation in diabetic foot infections. Diabetes Metab Res Rev 2019;35(7):e3165.

29. Jude EB, Oyibo SO, Chalmers N, et al. Peripheral arterial disease in diabetic and nondiabetic patients: a comparison of severity and outcome. Diabetes Care 2001;24(8):1433–7.

30. Achim A, Stanek A, Homorodean C, et al. Approaches to peripheral artery disease in diabetes: are there any differences? Int J Environ Res Public Health 2022;19(16):9801. Published 2022 Aug 9.

31. Marso SP, Daniels GH, Brown-Frandsen K, et al. Liraglutide and cardiovascular outcomes in type 2 diabetes. N Engl J Med 2016;375(4):311–22.

32. Marso SP, Bain SC, Consoli A, et al. Semaglutide and cardiovascular outcomes in patients with type 2 diabetes. N Engl J Med 2016;375(19):1834–44.

33. Fitchett D, Inzucchi SE, Cannon CP, et al. Empagliflozin reduced mortality and hospitalization for heart failure across the spectrum of cardiovascular risk in the EMPA-REG OUTCOME trial. Circulation 2019;139(11):1384–95.

34. Neal B, Perkovic V, Mahaffey KW, et al. Canagliflozin and cardiovascular and renal events in type 2 diabetes. N Engl J Med 2017;377(7):644–57.

35. Creager MA, Hamburg NM. Smoking cessation improves outcomes in patients with peripheral artery disease. JAMA Cardiol 2022;7(1):15–6.

36. Erb W. Klinische Beiträge zur Pathologie des Intermittierenden Hinkens. Munch Med Wochenschr 1911;2:2487.

37. Wang W, Zhao T, Geng K, et al. Smoking and the pathophysiology of peripheral artery disease. Front Cardiovasc Med 2021;8:704106.

38. Armstrong EJ, Wu J, Singh GD, et al. Smoking cessation is associated with decreased mortality and improved amputation-free survival among patients with symptomatic peripheral artery disease. J Vasc Surg 2014;60(6):1565–71.

39. Hennrikus D, Joseph AM, Lando HA, et al. Effectiveness of a smoking cessation program for peripheral artery disease patients: a randomized controlled trial. J Am Coll Cardiol 2010;56(25): 2105–12.

40. Murphy TP, Cutlip DE, Regensteiner JG, et al. Supervised exercise versus primary stenting for claudication resulting from aortoiliac peripheral artery disease: six-month outcomes from the claudication: exercise versus endoluminal revascularization (CLEVER) study. Circulation 2012;125(1):130–9.

41. Treat-Jacobson D, McDermott MM, Bronas UG, et al. Optimal exercise programs for patients with peripheral artery disease: a scientific statement from the American heart association. Circulation 2019;139(4):e10–33.

42. Larsen OA, Lassen NA. Effect of daily muscular exercise in patients with intermittent claudication. Lancet 1966;2(7473):1093–6.

43. Harwood AE, Cayton T, Sarvanandan R, et al. A Review of the potential local mechanisms by which exercise improves functional outcomes in intermittent claudication. Ann Vasc Surg 2016;30: 312–20.

44. Haas TL, Lloyd PG, Yang HT, et al. Exercise training and peripheral arterial disease. Compr Physiol 2012;2(4):2933–3017.

45. Divakaran S, Carroll BJ, Chen S, et al. Supervised exercise therapy for symptomatic peripheral artery

disease among Medicare beneficiaries between 2017 and 2018: participation rates and outcomes. Circ Cardiovasc Qual Outcomes 2021;14(8): e007953.

46. Cetlin MD, Polonsky T, Ho K, et al. Barriers to participation in supervised exercise therapy reported by people with peripheral artery disease. J Vasc Surg 2023;77(2):506–14.

47. Ward NC, Watts GF, Eckel RH. Statin toxicity. Circ Res 2019;124(2):328–50.

48. Silverman MG, Ference BA, Im K, et al. Association between lowering LDL-C and cardiovascular risk reduction among different therapeutic interventions: a systematic review and meta-analysis. JAMA 2016;316:1289–97.

49. Heart Protection Study Collaborative Group. Randomized trial of the effects of cholesterol-lowering with simvastatin on peripheral vascular and other major vascular outcomes in 20 536 people with peripheral arterial disease and other high-risk conditions. J Vasc Surg 2007;45:645–54. ; discussion 653-654.

50. Arya S, Khakharia A, Binney ZO, et al. Association of statin dose with amputation and survival in patients with peripheral artery disease. Circulation 2018;137:1435–46.

51. Kumbhani DJ, Steg PG, Cannon CP, et al. Statin therapy and long-term adverse limb outcomes in patients with peripheral artery disease: insights from the REACH registry. Eur Heart J 2014;35(41): 2864–72.

52. Page MM, Watts GF. PCSK9 inhibitors - mechanisms of action. Aust Prescr 2016;39(5):164–7.

53. Bonaca MP, Nault P, Giugliano RP, et al. Low-density lipoprotein cholesterol lowering with evolocumab and outcomes in patients with peripheral artery disease: insights from the FOURIER trial (Further Cardiovascular Outcomes Research with PCSK9 Inhibition in Subjects with Elevated Risk). Circulation 2018;137:338–50.

54. Schwartz GG, Steg PG, Szarek M, et al. Peripheral artery disease and venous thromboembolic events after acute coronary syndrome: role of lipoprotein(a) and modification by alirocumab: prespecified analysis of the ODYSSEY OUTCOMES randomized clinical trial. Circulation 2020;141: 1608–17.

55. Phan BA, Dayspring TD, Toth PP. Ezetimibe therapy: mechanism of action and clinical update. Vasc Health Risk Manag 2012;8:415–27.

56. Bonaca MP, Gutierrez JA, Cannon C, et al. Polyvascular disease, type 2 diabetes, and long-term vascular risk: a secondary analysis of the IMPROVE-IT trial. Lancet Diabetes Endocrinol 2018;6:934–43.

57. Berger JS, Krantz MJ, Kittelson JM, et al. Aspirin for the prevention of cardiovascular events in patients with peripheral artery disease: a meta-analysis of randomized trials. JAMA 2009;301:1909–19.

58. CAPRIE Steering Committee. A randomised, blinded, trial of clopidogrel versus aspirin in patients at risk of ischaemic events (CAPRIE). Lancet 1996;348:1329–39.

59. Bonaca MP, Bhatt DL, Simon T, et al. Limb outcomes with ticagrelor plus aspirin in patients with diabetes mellitus and atherosclerosis. J Am Coll Cardiol 2024;83(17):1627–36.

60. Hiatt WR, Fowkes FG, Heizer G, et al. Ticagrelor versus clopidogrel in symptomatic peripheral artery disease. N Engl J Med 2017;376:32–40.

61. Bonaca MP, Scirica BM, Creager MA, et al. Vorapaxar in patients with peripheral artery disease: results from TRA2{degrees}P-TIMI 50. Circulation 2013;127(14):1522–9.e15296.

62. Anand SS, Bosch J, Eikelboom JW, et al, COMPASS Investigators. Rivaroxaban with or without aspirin in patients with stable peripheral or carotid artery disease: an international, randomised, double-blind, placebo-controlled trial. Lancet 2018;391(10117):219–29.

63. Anand SS, Eikelboom JW, Dyal L, et al, COMPASS Trial Investigators. Rivaroxaban plus aspirin versus aspirin in relation to vascular risk in the COMPASS trial. J Am Coll Cardiol 2019;73(25): 3271–80.

64. Bonaca MP, Bauersachs RM, Anand SS, et al. Rivaroxaban in peripheral artery disease after revascularization. N Engl J Med 2020;382(21): 1994–2004.

65. Weintraub WS. The vascular effects of cilostazol. Can J Cardiol 2006;22 Suppl B(Suppl B):56B–60B.

66. Thompson PD, Zimet R, Forbes WP, et al. Meta-analysis of results from eight randomized, placebo-controlled trials on the effect of cilostazol on patients with intermittent claudication. Am J Cardiol 2002;90:1314–9.

67. Farkas K, Kolossvary E, Jarai Z. Simple assessment of quality of life and lower limb functional capacity during cilostazol treatment - results of the SHort-tERm cIlostazol eFFicacy and quality of life (SHERIFF) study. Vasa 2020;49:235–42.

68. Bedenis R, Stewart M, Cleanthis M, et al. Cilostazol for intermittent claudication. Cochrane Database Syst Rev 2014;6(6):CD003748.

69. Soga Y, Hamasaki T, Edahiro R, et al. Sustained effectiveness of cilostazol after endovascular treatment of femoropopliteal lesions: midterm follow-up from the Sufficient Treatment of Peripheral Intervention by Cilostazol (STOP-IC) study. J Endovasc Ther 2018;25:306–12.

70. Zen K, Takahara M, Iida O, et al. Drug-eluting stenting for femoropopliteal lesions, followed by cilostazol treatment, reduces stent restenosis in patients with symptomatic peripheral artery disease. J Vasc Surg 2017;65(3):720–5.

71. Megaly M, Abraham B, Saad M, et al. Outcomes with cilostazol after endovascular therapy of peripheral artery disease. Vasc Med 2019;24(4):313–23.

72. Broderick C, Forster R, Abdel-Hadi M, et al. Pentoxifylline for intermittent claudication. Cochrane Database Syst Rev 2020;10(10):CD005262.

73. Dawson DL, Cutler BS, Hiatt WR, et al. A comparison of cilostazol and pentoxifylline for treating intermittent claudication. Am J Med 2000;109:523–30.

74. Berger JS, Hiatt WR. Medical therapy in peripheral artery disease. Circulation 2012;126(4):491–500.

Vascular Access and Management of Complications

Aman Kansal, MD[a], William Schuyler Jones, MD[a],
Sanjum S. Sethi, MD, MPH[b,c],
Jennifer A. Rymer, MD, MBA, MHS[a,*]

KEYWORDS

- Peripheral artery disease • Vascular access • Femoral access
- Retrograde pedal revascularization • Chronic limb-threatening ischemia • Transradial access

---

KEY POINTS

- The ideal femoral access point is below the inguinal ligament but above the bifurcation into the profunda and superficial femoral arteries. Precision in puncture location is critical to avoid complications such as retroperitoneal bleeding or pseudoaneurysms.
- Ultrasound significantly reduces procedural complications, such as hematomas and accidental venipunctures, and improves first-pass success rates, particularly in patients with high common femoral artery bifurcations or difficult access sites.
- The retrograde pedal/tibial approach offers an alternative to antegrade access in cases of chronic limb-threatening ischemia when the antegrade approach fails. This technique provides better control, especially in crossing long lesions, due to its proximity to the occlusion and the favorable anatomy of the distal cap.
- Transradial access for peripheral vascular interventions (PVI) offers several advantages, including lower risk of severe vascular complications, shorter hospital stays, and improved patient satisfaction, while also avoiding cannulation of runoff vessels. However, challenges like radial spasm, subclavian tortuosity, and limited equipment availability have hindered its widespread adoption for PVI.
- Treatment for complications like retroperitoneal hemorrhage, pseudoaneurysms, and arteriovenous fistulas includes conservative management, compression, or more invasive interventions like embolization or surgical repair, depending on severity.

INTRODUCTION

Peripheral artery disease (PAD), defined as a partial or complete obstruction of at least 1 peripheral artery due to atherosclerotic occlusive disease,[1] is a major health concern affecting more than 200 million people worldwide.[2] Symptoms have varying degrees of severity ranging from asymptomatic, to intermittent claudication, to chronic limb-threatening ischemia (CLTI). Patients with either symptoms refractory to medical therapy and lifestyle modifications or who are at risk of limb loss often undergo revascularization, either surgical or endovascular, to improve quality of life and prevent major adverse limb events.[3]

---

[a] Division of Cardiology, Duke University Medical Center, Durham, NC, USA; [b] Division of Cardiology, Columbia University, New York, NY, USA; [c] Pulmonary Embolism Response Team, Columbia Interventional Cardiovascular Care
* Corresponding author.
E-mail address: jennifer.rymer@duke.edu

Intervent Cardiol Clin 14 (2025) 149–159
https://doi.org/10.1016/j.iccl.2024.11.003

Obtaining appropriate vascular access in the catheterization laboratory is essential to outcomes, safety, and patient satisfaction. Over 97% of peripheral vascular interventions (PVI) are done via transfemoral access (TFA).[4] Alternative access sites, including pedal and radial access, are gaining popularity. The advantages and disadvantages of these methods will be discussed in this article and are represented in Fig. 1. Additionally, TFA is often used for complex coronary interventions,[5] endovascular aneurysm repair, structural cases such as transcatheter aortic valve replacement,[6] and mechanical circulatory support such as intraaortic balloon pump, mechanical circulatory support devices (eg, Impella), and venoarterial extracorporeal membrane oxygenation.[7] This article reviews techniques to optimize peripheral vascular access and manage vascular complications.

CONTRALATERAL RETROGRADE TRANSFEMORAL ACCESS

Optimal femoral access requires understanding anatomic, fluoroscopic, and ultrasound- guided principles. Combining these modalities allows for efficient, reproducible, and safe results. In this section, we will discuss each of these strategies.

Anatomic
The primary anatomic principle for ideal femoral access is to enter the common femoral artery (CFA) below the inguinal ligament and above the bifurcation into the profunda artery and superficial femoral artery (SFA) over the femoral head. This is important to facilitate vessel access and closure as well as avoid complications. Puncture above the inguinal ligament is associated with a higher risk of retroperitoneal bleeding and puncture of either the SFA or profunda below the bifurcation of the CFA is associated with higher risk of pseudoaneurysms.[8] The common approach is to mark 2 to 3 cm below the mid-point between the pubic symphysis and anterior superior iliac crest. Additional anatomic landmarks include femoral artery palpation, inguinal skin crease, and bony structures. Although basic anatomic principles can be helpful, each can be unreliable. The femoral artery should be palpated; however, the greatest point of pulsation does not necessarily correspond to the point of optimal entry. The inguinal skin crease is also unreliable as over 70% of patients have the crease below the bifurcation leading to low stick access.[9] Bony landmarks can be variable with height and body mass index.

The importance of access precision was highlighted in a 2005 study by Sherev and colleagues which looked at a prospective cohort of 33 patients with femoral access site complications.[10] Patients were divided into 4 groups based on the location of vascular entry. Group 1 was the low arteriotomy group accessed below the CFA bifurcation. Group 2 was the middle above the femoral bifurcation and below the most inferior border of the inferior epigastric artery (IEA) seen on angiogram post access. Group 3 was the high middle group above the most inferior border of the IEA and below the origin of the IEA. Group 4 was the high group above the origin of the IEA. This study found that all life-threatening complications of retroperitoneal hemorrhage occurred in groups 3 and 4, and all pseudoaneurysms occurred in group 1. Group 2 was associated with the least number of complications and no serious life-threatening adverse events.[10] While this study highlighted the importance of basic anatomic understanding, it also suggested that a sole anatomic strategy may lead to unnecessary complications.

Fluoroscopic
A subsequent study by Garrett and colleagues discussed how fluoroscopic landmarks can improve the accuracy of CFA access.[11] The purpose of the study was to define the relationship of the CFA to the inguinal ligament, femoral head, and inguinal skin crease. This was performed as a descriptive study in a prospective design of 158 patients undergoing catheterization through the

Retrograde Femoral	Retrograde Pedal	Radial to Peripheral
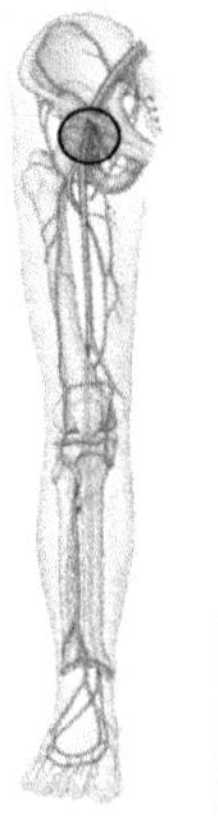 **Advantages** • Large vessel size to accommodate large bore devices • Operator experience • Flexibility especially for complex procedure • Immediate access • Minimal tortuosity and risk for spasm	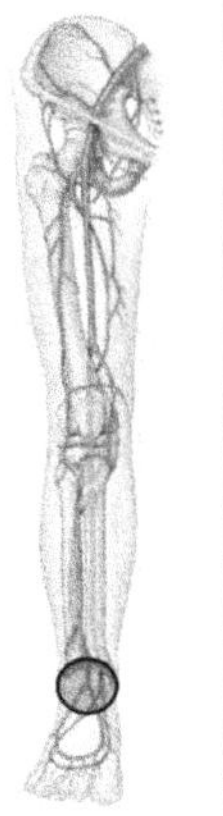 **Advantages** • Usually closer to occlusion allowing for greater control • Less likely to divert into branch or collateral vessel	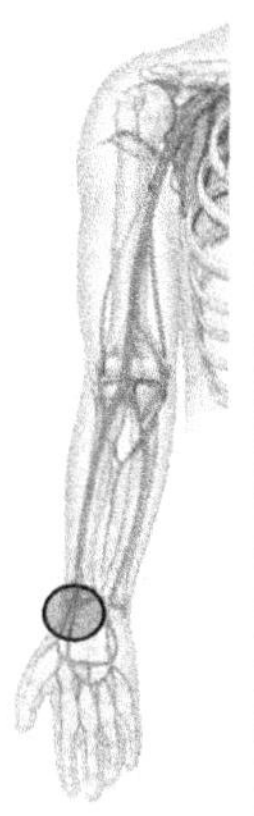 **Advantages** • Lower risk of vascular complications • Ability to intervene on both legs in one procedure • Shorter hospital stay • Improved patient satisfaction
Challenges • Retroperitoneal hemorrhage • Small vessel perforation • Pseudoaneurysms • Groin site hematoma • Arteriovenous fistula • Ischemic complications	**Challenges** • Cannulation of outflow vessel • Limited operator experience • Limited visualization	**Challenges** • Radial spasm • Subclavian tortuosity • Possible risk of stroke

Fig. 1. Advantages and disadvantages of retrograde femoral, pedal, and radial to peripheral access.

femoral approach. The study found the CFA bifurcation was below the inguinal ligament and middle of the femoral head in 99%, below the inferior femoral head in 80%, and above the inguinal crease in 78% of the patients. These results suggested a safe access of the CFA is reliably located between the inferior and middle femoral head and that fluoroscopy can be used to improve CFA access.[11]

Although fluoroscopic guidance had compelling nonrandomized data, Abu-Fadel et al conducted the first prospective, randomized clinical trial in 2009 comparing fluoroscopic guidance to traditional anatomic landmark guidance.[8] Nearly 1000 patients were randomized in a 1:1 fashion. The primary endpoint was the suitability for vascular closure devices (VCD) which was deemed unsuitable if the arteriotomy was above the IEA, distal to the CFA bifurcation, in a side branch, dissection, or other angiographic abnormalities. The study found that although fluoroscopy did decrease the incident of low arteriotomies, it was overall not superior to a traditional anatomic-only approach when determining suitability for VCD or CFA access.[8]

Ultrasound

Ultrasound (US) guidance was the next strategy investigated to improve femoral access safety. The Femoral Arterial Access with Ultrasound (FAUST) trial was a 2010 prospective, randomized, single-blinded trial conducted at 4 US medical centers.[12] Approximately 1000 patients were randomized in a 1:1 fashion to either US or fluoroscopic guidance. All patients underwent manual palpation of anatomic landmarks. The study demonstrated that US guidance did not improve rate of CFA cannulation, except in patients with high CFA bifurcations. However, US guidance did result in a statistically significant improvement in secondary procedural outcomes including number of attempts, first pass success, accidental venipuncture, and time to insertion. US guidance was associated with a statistically significant decrease in rates of hematoma (2.2% vs 0.6%, P =.034) and any vascular complication (3.4% vs 1.4%, P =.041). Furthermore, increasing experience with ultrasound demonstrated a trend toward improved CFA cannulation (87.6% vs 83.3% success rate, P=.076). Overall, this trial suggested US guidance can facilitate arterial access, especially in difficult cases such as high CFA bifurcations, and reduce complications.[12]

The case for ultrasound-guided access has continued to grow. A 2013 randomized trial of approximately 200 patients compared US to traditional palpation and fluoroscopy techniques for CFA access. The study showed that US-guided access trended toward increased technical success and decreased access-related complications, but the difference did not reach statistical significance. However, technical success would have been higher if patients without a palpable pulse were included. Additionally, US guidance was superior for secondary procedural outcomes including first pass success, total number of attempts, and time to sheath insertion.[13] A 2015 retrospective, observational study analyzed post procedural groin hematoma rates after ~7400 PVI. Routine US guidance was significantly protective against hematoma (RR 0.62; 95% CI, 0.46–0.84; P<.01).[14] A 2015 meta-analysis of randomized controlled trials found US guidance was associated with reduction in overall complications, including hematoma and accidental venipuncture (relative risk, 0.51; 95% CI, 0.28–0.91) and improvement in first-attempt success (relative risk, 1.42; 95% CI 1.01–2.00).[15] More recently, the 2022 UNIVERSAL (Routine Ultrasound Guidance for Vascular Access for Cardiac Procedures) trial was an approximately 600-patient, 1:1 randomized, multicenter, prospective trial of US-guided versus palpation and fluoroscopy for femoral access. There was not a significant difference in the primary outcome of major bleeding or vascular complication (12.9% vs 16.1%, $P = .25$). However, US guidance again improved first pass success, reduced puncture attempts, and reduced venipuncture.[16]

US guidance has also been studied in structural cases. A 2020 single-center 3-armed cohort study compared US to fluoroscopic-guided TFA in transcatheter aortic valve replacement (TAVR) cases.[17] The 2 arms included US-guided second generation TAVR, fluoroscopic-guided second generation TAVR, and US-guided third generation TAVR. All vascular and bleeding complications were reduced in the US-guided second generation group compared with fluoroscopic-guided second generation group (6.3% vs 16.8%; $P = .023$). These were further decreased in the US-guided third generation group.[17]

Micropuncture

Along with access guidance, access equipment has also gone through changes to try and improve access site accuracy and decrease complications. The micropuncture 21-gauge (G) needle set is a commonly used kit.[18] The needle set is composed of the 21G needle, 0.018-inch guidewire, and micro puncture dilator. A 2012 study analyzed a cohort of ~3200 consecutive patients. Micropuncture access was used in ~550 and standard 18G in ~2700 patients. Overall, there was no significant difference in access site complications. However, the micropuncture group did have significantly higher retroperitoneal bleeding (0.7% vs 0.18%, $P = .04$) though this was based on very small numbers. This may be explained by the micropuncture guide wire having an angled tip unlike the standard J-tip and also being thinner than the standard 0.035-inch wire. These features allow the micropuncture guide wire to be diverted from the main vessel into small side branches more susceptible to perforation.[18] This can then be exacerbated by following with a dilator, resulting in an even larger perforation with hemodynamic consequences.

A subsequent 2014 study randomized ~400 patients in a 1:1 fashion to micropuncture versus an 18G needle for TFA. The primary endpoint was a composite of access site bleeding. Although this endpoint was not statistically significant between the 2 groups, there was a trend toward improvement with micropuncture (event rate 9.4% vs 15.5%, P=.10). Additionally, micropuncture was superior in certain subgroups with low bleeding risk profile including procedures without percutaneous coronary intervention (PCI), without thrombin inhibitor, elective, and final sheath size $\leq$ 6 Fr. This study suggests potential benefits of micropuncture in TFA.[19]

While contralateral retrograde TFA is the most common approach for PAD interventions and the most well studied, antegrade femoral access has been used especially when approaching distal vessels in the lower leg and foot. The principles regarding anatomy, fluoroscopy, and cannulation still apply with ideal access occurring in the CFA as previously discussed. Antegrade ipsilateral transfemoral access appears to be associated with a higher rate of bleeding complications and thus should be used judiciously as needed.

Overall, there is significant value in understanding the anatomic, fluoroscopic, and ultrasound principles of TFA. Ultrasound guidance has strong data supporting reduced vascular and bleeding complications along with improved procedural outcomes. Ultrasound guidance should be routinely used to obtain TFA. However, integrating information across all 3 domains and using them in combination allows the operator the best opportunity to achieve procedural success while minimizing complications.

RETROGRADE PEDAL REVASCULARIZATION

CLTI is a severe form of PAD associated with a high degree of morbidity and mortality. CLTI usually requires prompt surgical or endovascular intervention to avoid limb loss. While intervention is effective, it is often challenging, given comorbidities, multilevel disease, long occlusive lesions, and involvement of smaller caliber vessels. The failure rate of antegrade approach can reach up to 20%.[20] The main reason for an unsuccessful antegrade approach can include both the inability of the guidewire to cross the lesion and the inability to access the true lumen distal to the occlusion.[20]

In 1990, Iyer and colleagues first described the retrograde pedal/tibial approach as an alternative in cases where the typical antegrade approach had failed. Access was initially obtained via cut down and but has now become percutaneous.[21] A 2008 study analyzed an observational registry of ~50 retrograde revascularizations done in limbs and patients who had antegrade failures. The overall success rate was 86.3% (44/51) with adjunctive stenting needed in 21 (41.4%) to optimize results. This study suggested that in complex popliteal to infrapopliteal occlusions, the additional use of the retrograde pedal approach can improve outcomes.[20] This was further supported by Bazan and colleagues in 2014 showing retrograde pedal access is a relatively feasible and safe choice for high-risk patients who have failed antegrade intervention and are poor candidates for bypass.[22] The reasons for retrograde access facilitating successful intervention are likely multifactorial. The access point is usually closer to the occlusive segment which allows for more control in crossing the lesion. The distal cap may have a more favorable anatomy for a retrograde approach. Lastly, there is also less likelihood of diverting from the main into a branch or collateral vessel as these all point downwards against the retrograde wire.[23]

The retrograde access technique has 2 steps. The first step focuses on gaining access into a pedal vessel. The second step focuses on retrograde crossing of the occlusion. All pedal vessels, namely the anterior tibial, posterior tibial, and peroneal arteries, can be successfully accessed in a retrograde fashion. More advanced techniques allow for successful cannulation of the dorsalis pedis and other plantar branches as well. The choice of pedal artery access site depends on the intended target vessel, any tortuosity, and the overall number and amount of disease in the runoff vessels. It is important to remember the peroneal is deep and posterior to the tibia. For these reasons, it should be used only when the target is inaccessible by other entry sites and there is a plan for bleeding management which typically involves surgical planning and backup.[23]

Pedal vessel access is most commonly and reliably achieved via ultrasound guidance. The vessel is identified on ultrasound in the longitudinal or transverse position. Color flow can be used to identify flow in the target vessel. Then, gray scale is used to access the vessel. The hockey stick probe can improve the resolution to facilitate access. Ultrasound can be suboptimal in heavily calcified vessel due to significant acoustic shadowing. In these situations, fluoroscopy will easily highlight calcified vessels.

Alternatively, the road mapping technique can be used via antegrade vessel runoff from the femoral access site.[23] Access is typically achieved with 21G needles and either 0.014-inch or 0.018-inch guide wires. The operator may then choose whether to place a sheath or proceed sheathless based on the overall procedural strategy. One common technique is to obtain concomitant retrograde contralateral transfemoral access or antegrade transfemoral access antegrade access. Once the retrograde wire crosses the lesion, the wire can be snared from the antegrade approach and externalized, creating through-and-through guide wire access for the remainder of the procedure. For this reason, it is important to make sure the retrograde wire is exchange-length.[24] Alternatively, a pedal-only approach has been successfully using devices that are compatible with smaller sheath sizes.[25]

RADIAL TO PERIPHERAL

Transradial access (TRA) for PCI has shown to reduce mortality, reduce MACE, and improve safety when compared to TFA across the spectrum of patients with coronary disease. TRA is now the preferred approach for coronary intervention.[26] TRA for PVI has been increasingly explored. The numerous potential benefits include lower risk of severe vascular access complications, ability to intervene on both legs during one procedure, shorter hospital stay, improved patient satisfaction, and avoiding cannulation of runoff vessels. While coronary data suggest lower mortality and hospital costs, this has not yet been demonstrated in the PAD population. Potential challenges include radial spasm and subclavian tortuosity, unknown risk of stroke given interaction with the aortic arch especially from right radial access, ergonomic challenges for the operator, insufficient shaft lengths on commonly used equipment, and the possibility of higher procedural complexity leading to increased radiation exposure.[27]

An additional important reason radial access has not been used in PVI is because of the lack of equipment to support these procedures via TRA. However, newly developed and evolving radial to peripheral (R2P) devices are able to support PVI, warranting reevaluation of benefits and challenges.

A recent 2023 prospective, multicenter, and observational study evaluated the safety and feasibility of radial access for peripheral intervention.[28] In this study, 120 patients from 8 US centers were enrolled. The 224 lesions treated comprised iliac (12.9%), femoropopliteal (55.3%), isolated popliteal (11.9%), and tibial (19.5%). The primary efficacy end point was procedural success defined as completion without conversion to femoral access and without radial access complications. The primary safety endpoint was any radial access complication at 30 days. The primary efficacy and safety end points were achieved in 93.3% and 92.7% of the patients, respectively. Additionally, 93.3% of the patients had same-day discharge.[28] These results suggest radial access as a promising additional approach to peripheral intervention. As more devices are developed, clinical trials directly comparing TRA to TFA in PVI will be necessary.

Other alternative access sites have been used for peripheral interventions including the brachial artery, axillary artery, popliteal artery, and superficial femoral artery. These access sites are used relatively sparingly and tend to have a higher rate of bleeding complications. Access should be reserved for operators with expertise in the management of access sites.

VASCULAR ACCESS COMPLICATIONS

Intervention for lower extremity PAD carries the risk of vascular access complications. The Society for Vascular Surgery's Vascular Quality Initiative (VQI) analyzed 22,226 patients who underwent 27,048 PVI from August 2007 to May 2013. The VQI found access site complications in 936 procedures (3.5%). Although the majority was minor not requiring treatment, 240 procedures (0.9%) required treatment (thrombin injection, transfusion, surgery).[4] Other series have found this number to be as high as 11%.[29] Additionally, access site complications increased mean hospitalization (1.6 vs 1.2 days), are less likely to be discharged home (62.1% vs 89.1%), and have higher 30-day mortality (6.1% vs 1.4%).[4] Understanding, preventing, and managing access site complications is critical.

Retroperitoneal hemorrhage (RPH) is the most life-threatening complication of TFA. Although the incidence is relatively low (up to 0.7% in larger series),[30] the associated frequency of postprocedural myocardial infarction (5.8% vs 1.7%), infection (17.4% vs 3.0%), heart failure (8.0% vs 1.6%), and in-hospital mortality (6.6% vs 1.1%) is among the highest of access complications.[31] This is because the retroperitoneal (RP) cavity can hold a large amount of rapidly accumulating blood and often shows few symptoms until hemodynamic collapse. This can lead to delayed recognition, rapid deterioration, and a resultant poor outcome. The mechanism

of RPH is associated with higher femoral arterial puncture, defined as above the middle third of the femoral head on fluoroscopy.[32] Arteriotomy in this area is at higher risk of being above the inguinal ligament and above the inferior-most segment of the inferior epigastric artery, allowing access to the RP space. Additional predictors include low body weight, female gender, and larger sheath size. RPH can present with hemodynamic instability, decreasing blood counts, suprainguinal tenderness and fullness, severe back and lower quadrant pain, and femoral neuropathy in up to one-third of patients.[33] Strategies for prevention include deliberate imaging-guided access to ensure arteriotomy below the inguinal ligament and inferior epigastric artery, routine femoral angiography to evaluate sheath placement prior to intervention, and effective hemostasis whether through compression or closure device. The majority of RPH will respond to conservative management; however, more severe cases require intervention through endovascular stent, coiling, embolization, or surgical repair.[33]

It is also important to be vigilant for small vessel perforation. These are more common with the micropuncture 0.018-inch wire entering small side branches. These are usually asymptomatic though can certainly still lead to RPH. To prevent these smaller perforations, watch wire advancement under fluoroscopy. If deviation detected, pull wire back from side branch, hold pressure, and recheck that extravasation has resolved before readvancing the wire.

Access site pseudoaneurysms (PA) are one of the most common complications, occurring in up to 8% of PVI,[34] and in some studies up to nearly 70% of access site complications.[35] The mechanism is local hemorrhage of an injured vessel into adjacent soft tissue sac.[12] Puncture below the CFA bifurcation increases the risk of pseudoaneurysm. The symptoms of PA are pain, swelling, severe bruising, pulsatile mass, and palpable thrill or bruit at the puncture site. Ultrasound is used to confirm PA by looking for an echo-lucent mass communicating with the access artery.[30] To prevent PA, use ultrasound to precisely locate the CFA bifurcation. Appropriate vessel closure is also important to prevent pseudoaneurysm formation. Treatment should be considered in PA $\geq$ 3 cm, patients on anticoagulation, or patients unable to have serial duplex examinations. Complications from untreated PA include rupture, local pain secondary to compression syndrome, and late distal embolization. Most common treatment involves compression of the communicating tract, most often performed with ultrasound guidance, and ultrasound-guided thrombin injection.[33] Further treatment such as endovascular stent repair or open surgical repair can be considered when other options are not successful.

Access site hematomas are another common complication of PVI.[34] The mechanism is by local hemorrhage of an injured vessel into the adjacent soft tissue. Access site hematomas complicating PVI are associated with increased hospital length of stay, 30-day, and 1-year mortality.[4] Hematomas present as nonpulsatile mass unlike PA, often with ecchymosis at the puncture site.

Arteriovenous fistulas (AVF) are more likely when undergoing a distal puncture during retrograde transfemoral access.[34] The mechanism is through a vascular channel connecting artery and adjacent vein created by simultaneous arterial and venous injury from needle tract. AVF present with a palpable thrill over the arterial site, often with audible bruit. To prevent AVF formation, limit puncture attempts, avoid posterior arterial wall, and be careful with larger gauge needles which have increased risk of AVF. AVF do not need treatment in the immediate period as there are usually no clinical signs or hemodynamic significance and small AVF will spontaneously occlude. However, longstanding AVF can lead to high-output heart failure, aneurysmal degeneration of the artery, and limb edema. Treatment for symptomatic AVF includes ultrasound-guided compression, endovascular embolization, stent-graft (both balloon-expanding and self-expanding), and surgical ligation.[34]

Ischemic complications following PVI are less common but need to be quickly identified and addressed to prevent limb loss. Common mechanisms are cholesterol embolism, thromboembolism, arterial dissection, and thrombosis. The presentation of cholesterol embolization syndrome (CES) includes leg and foot pain and livedo reticularis. Ischemic complications are best prevented by adhering to meticulous access technique, using soft guidewires, and smallest sheath possible. Treatment for acute limb ischemia is endovascular treatment via contralateral femoral approach or surgical repair (thrombectomy, endarterectomy, bypass). Treatment for CES is usually supportive care.[36] Arterial dissection is primarily caused by a wire or catheter entering the subintimal space creating a false lumen. This allows for early recognition which usually guides the operator to either try another arterial access or postpone the procedure due to safety. Dissection can be prevented by watching the needle under ultrasound and

wire under fluoroscopy to ensure true lumen entry. The wire should not be advanced against resistance. The majority of dissections are nonflow limiting and can be observed as they will heal and remain asymptomatic. Some dissection will remain persistent and need endovascular and surgical treatment due to persistent symptoms of claudication or limb ischemia.

LARGE-BORE ACCESS

In addition to PVI, complex coronary interventions, mechanical circulatory support, and structural heart cases often require large-bore femoral arterial access. Vascular and bleeding complications are reported as high as 20%.[37] This section focuses on strategies to optimize large-bore femoral access.

Initial access puncture uses the same anatomic, fluoroscopic, and ultrasound-guided techniques discussed earlier. Access can be obtained with either the 18F or 21F systems. A 6 F sheath is placed over the wire. A stiff 0.035-inch wire is then advanced through the 6 Fr sheath. Often, 2 Perclose ProGlide suture-mediated closure systems are deployed at 10' and 2' o'clock positions. This technique allows for future successful closure of the large-bore access site.[38] This is known as the "preclose" technique, and is required before using sheath sizes greater than 14 Fr. Once sutures are secure, the large bore sheath is placed through a series of upsizing dilators over the 0.035-inch stiff wire.

Once access is obtained and prior to upsizing the sheath, angiography is performed in an ipsilateral oblique projection to confirm optimal CFA access without vascular complication and to also define vessel size, tortuosity, degree of atherosclerosis/calcification, and distal perfusion. This should be routinely done in all cases to assess the likelihood of potential complication. After the large bore sheath is in place, an aorto-iliac angiogram is most commonly performed via contrast injection into the large bore sheath's side arm.[38] It is crucial to carefully assess the iliofemoral artery and distal perfusion, given the relatively higher risk of vessel occlusion and consequent acute limb ischemia with large-bore access. In situations when occlusion is expected (ie, extracorporeal membrane oxygenation [ECMO]), antegrade SFA access with a 5 Fr or 6 Fr sheath can be placed preemptively prior to large-bore sheath insertion.[38] In unexpected occlusion, there are strategies to restore distal perfusion. These include external contralateral, external ipsilateral, and internal contralateral bypass circuits.[38]

VASCULAR CLOSURE DEVICES

Adequate hemostasis after sheath removal is critical to avoid vascular and bleeding complications including pseudoaneurysm formation. Manual compression is often used to achieve hemostasis for smaller arterial sheaths (5–8 Fr); however, this is inadequate for large-bore access due to lack of direct visualization and control over the puncture site. This has led to the increasing usage of VCDs.[38]

Suture-Based

The Perclose Proglide is a commonly used suture-mediated VCD. The mechanism involves a combination of a suture-based closure system and delivery mechanism. After the arterial sheath is removed from the puncture site, the Perclose Proglide is then introduced through a delivery catheter. The device is designed with a preloaded monofilament polypropylene suture that is then deployed across the arterial puncture. The device includes a needle that is inserted through the vessel wall, which creates a path for the suture to be placed. After the suture is placed, a slipknot is deployed inside the artery to securely close the puncture. Once the knot is secure, the device is withdrawn from the puncture site. The suture remains to maintain hemostasis, and, over time, the suture is absorbed by the body as the artery also heals.

There are several advantages to suture-mediated VCDs. The arteriotomy is physically closed and vessel integrity is maintained which is crucial for maintaining future access and preventing injury. Deployment can be done quickly improving patient satisfaction and clinical workflow. The "preclose" technique can be used for large-bore access, allowing these devices to safely accommodate up to 21F devices as shown in the PEVAR trial.[39] The main disadvantage is technical complexity requiring adequate operator experience and potential for vascular injury leading to bleeding or limb ischemia.

Collagen Plug

The collagen plug VCDs use a combination of a biocompatible collagen-based plug and supporting anchor to achieve hemostasis. After the arterial sheath is removed, the Angioseal device is introduced into the puncture site. The device features a small, expandable anchor that is deployed on the inner side of the artery. The anchor is designed to press against the arterial wall, providing support and stability. Once the anchor is in place, a collagen-based plug is placed on the outside of the arterial wall. The anchor and plug are then brought together sealing the puncture site. The collagen plug acts as a scaffold for natural healing and tissue repair. After the anchor and plug have been properly positioned and the puncture site sealed, the device is withdrawn from the vessel. Over time, the collagen plug is absorbed by the body.

Collagen plug VCDs have some similar advantages to suture-mediated VCDs including effective hemostasis, minimally invasive, biocompatibility, and faster recovery. The process is also relatively straightforward, which, in theory, requires less technical expertise to use effectively. Although the intraluminal anchor promotes effective hemostasis, the disadvantage is it also allows the potential of distal embolization or infection. This is particularly relevant if reaccess is required.[40] Additionally, it is not as versatile as suture-mediated VCDs as there is no equivalent "preclose" technique for large-bore access.

Clip-Based

Clip-based VCDs use a mechanical "clamp" mechanism to achieve hemostasis. After the arterial sheath is removed, the device is introduced and contains a biocompatible clip to be placed around the puncture site. The mechanism involves opening and closing the clip to clamp the vessel walls together. The clip is then secured in place using a locking mechanism. The delivery system is then withdrawn from the vessel.

Unique advantages of this system include mechanical closure of the puncture site and rapid deployment. Disadvantages include puncture size range limited by clip size.

Sealant-Based

Sealant-based VCDs use specialized synthetic or biologically derived materials to achieve hemostasis. After the arterial sheath is removed, the device is introduced, and the sealant material is applied to the inner side of the artery. Once applied, the sealant interacts with blood and the arterial wall to promote clotting, form a solid or semi-solid plug, and create a stable seal. The sealant material further integrates with the surrounding tissue as it hardens or sets creating a stronger seal.

The sealant delivery system similarly allows for rapid deployment. Additionally, because the sealant does not have a predetermined body, it conforms to the arteriotomy and can theoretically be used for a large range of puncture sizes. Disadvantages include risk of sealant failure and material incompatibility which may not be suitable for all patients.[40]

Importantly, VCDs have not been shown to be definitively superior to manual compression with respect to vascular complications. A recent meta-analysis showed that while VCDs might be associated with a lower risk of vascular complications, when the analysis was limited to randomized controlled trials, there was no significant difference.[41] A separate, recent gender-based analysis similarly showed that VCD and manual compression provided comparable safety.[42]

SUMMARY

Vascular access requires a deliberate and thoughtful approach. Management starts pre procedurally by practicing anatomic, fluoroscopic, and ultrasound-guided techniques, becoming comfortable with various access sites, and planning for potential large-bore access. It continues post procedurally by optimizing hemostasis, now through a diverse group of vascular closure devices. Awareness of potential complications allows for proactive measures. Early recognition and intervention of complications can significantly improve patient outcomes and reduce the risk of life-threatening injury. A comprehensive understanding of vascular access and complications is essential for performing safe, effective, and efficient peripheral vascular interventions. It enhances patient safety, improves procedural outcomes, and ensures optimal care throughout the intervention and recovery process.

CLINICS CARE POINTS

- Integrating anatomic, fluoroscopic, and ultrasound principles allows operators the best opportunity to achieve safe procedural success.
- Retrograde pedal/tibial and transradial access offer alternative access approaches when planning peripheral intervention.
- Interventional cardiologists have several strategies to reduce the risk of vascular complications in patients undergoing peripheral vascular intervention.

DISCLOSURE

No disclosures.

REFERENCES

1. Hiatt WR, Goldstone J, Smith SC Jr, et al. Atherosclerotic peripheral vascular disease symposium II: nomenclature for vascular diseases. Circulation 2008;118(25):2826–9.
2. Criqui MH, Aboyans V. Epidemiology of peripheral artery disease. Circ Res 2015;116(9):1509–26.
3. Diamantopoulos A, Katsanos K. Treating femoropopliteal disease: established and emerging technologies. Semin Intervent Radiol 2014;31(4). https://doi.org/10.1055/s-0034-1393971.
4. Ortiz D, Jahangir A, Singh M, et al. Access site complications after peripheral vascular interventions: incidence, predictors, and outcomes. Circ Cardiovasc Interv 2014;7(6):821–8.
5. Tanaka Y, Moriyama N, Ochiai T, et al. Transradial coronary interventions for complex chronic total occlusions. JACC Cardiovasc Interv 2017;10(3). https://doi.org/10.1016/j.jcin.2016.11.003.
6. Webb JG, Wood DA. Current status of transcatheter aortic valve replacement. J Am Coll Cardiol 2012;60(6). https://doi.org/10.1016/j.jacc.2012.01.071.
7. Sandoval Y, Basir MB, Lemor A, et al. Optimal large-bore femoral access, indwelling device management, and vascular closure for percutaneous mechanical circulatory support. Am J Cardiol 2023;206. https://doi.org/10.1016/j.amjcard.2023.08.024.
8. Abu-Fadel MS, Sparling JM, Zacharias SJ, et al. Fluoroscopy vs. traditional guided femoral arterial access and the use of closure devices: a randomized controlled trial. Cathet Cardiovasc Interv 2009;74(4). https://doi.org/10.1002/ccd.22174.
9. Cox N. Managing the femoral artery in coronary angiography. Heart Lung Circ 2008;17(SUPPL. 4). https://doi.org/10.1016/j.hlc.2008.08.007.
10. Sherev DA, Shaw RE, Brent BN. Angiographic predictors of femoral access site complications: implication for planned percutaneous coronary intervention. Cathet Cardiovasc Interv 2005;65(2). https://doi.org/10.1002/ccd.20354.
11. Garrett PD, Eckart RE, Bauch TD, et al. Fluoroscopic localization of the femoral head as a landmark for common femoral artery cannulation. Cathet Cardiovasc Interv 2005;65(2). https://doi.org/10.1002/ccd.20373.
12. Seto AH, Abu-Fadel MS, Sparling JM, et al. Real-time ultrasound guidance facilitates femoral arterial access and reduces vascular complications: FAUST (Femoral Arterial Access with Ultrasound Trial). JACC Cardiovasc Interv 2010;3(7). https://doi.org/10.1016/j.jcin.2010.04.015.
13. Gedikoglu M, Oguzkurt L, Gur S, et al. Comparison of ultrasound guidance with the traditional palpation and fluoroscopy method for the common femoral artery puncture. Cathet Cardiovasc Interv 2013;82(7). https://doi.org/10.1002/ccd.24955.
14. Kalish J, Eslami M, Gillespie D, et al. Routine use of ultrasound guidance in femoral arterial access for

peripheral vascular intervention decreases groin hematoma rates. J Vasc Surg 2015;61(5). https://doi.org/10.1016/j.jvs.2014.12.003.

15. Sobolev M, Slovut DP, Chang AL, et al. Ultrasound-guided catheterization of the femoral artery: a systematic review and meta-analysis of randomized controlled trials. J Invasive Cardiol 2015;27(7). https://doi.org/10.1378/chest.9861.

16. Jolly SS, AlRashidi S, d'Entremont MA, et al. Routine ultrasonography guidance for femoral vascular access for cardiac procedures. JAMA Cardiol 2022;7(11). https://doi.org/10.1001/jamacardio.2022.3399.

17. Vincent F, Spillemaeker H, Kyheng M, et al. Ultrasound guidance to reduce vascular and bleeding complications of percutaneous transfemoral transcatheter aortic valve replacement: a propensity score–matched comparison. J Am Heart Assoc 2020;9(6). https://doi.org/10.1161/JAHA.119.014916.

18. Ben-Dor I, Maluenda G, Mahmoudi M, et al. A novel, minimally invasive access technique versus standard 18-gauge needle set for femoral access. Cathet Cardiovasc Interv 2012;79(7). https://doi.org/10.1002/ccd.23330.

19. Ambrose JA, Lardizabal J, Mouanoutoua M, et al. Femoral micropuncture or routine introducer study (FEMORIS). Cardiology (Switzerland) 2014;129(1). https://doi.org/10.1159/000362536.

20. Montero-Baker M, Schmidt A, Bräunlich S, et al. Retrograde approach for complex popliteal and tibioperoneal occlusions. J Endovasc Ther 2008;15(5). https://doi.org/10.1583/08-2440.1.

21. Iyer SS, Dorros G, Zaitoun R, et al. Retrograde Recanalization of an occluded posterior tibial artery by using a posterior tibial cutdown: two case reports. Cathet Cardiovasc Diagn 1990;20(4). https://doi.org/10.1002/ccd.1810200408.

22. Bazan HA, Le L, Donovan M, et al. Retrograde pedal access for patients with critical limb ischemia. J Vasc Surg 2014;60(2). https://doi.org/10.1016/j.jvs.2014.02.038.

23. El-Sayed HF. Retrograde pedal/tibial artery access for treatment of infragenicular arterial occlusive disease. Methodist Debakey Cardiovasc J 2013;9(2). https://doi.org/10.14797/mdcj-9-2-73.

24. Vance AZ, Leung DA, Clark TW. Tips for pedal access: technical evolution and review. J Cardiovasc Surg 2018;59(5). https://doi.org/10.23736/S0021-9509.18.10627-6.

25. Adams GL, Khanna PK, Staniloae CS, et al. Optimal techniques with the diamondback 360° system achieve effective results for the treatment of peripheral arterial disease. J Cardiovasc Transl Res 2011;4(2). https://doi.org/10.1007/s12265-010-9255-x.

26. Ferrante G, Rao SV, Jüni P, et al. Radial versus femoral access for coronary interventions across the entire spectrum of patients with coronary artery disease: a meta-analysis of randomized trials. JACC Cardiovasc Interv 2016;9(14). https://doi.org/10.1016/j.jcin.2016.04.014.

27. Fanaroff AC, Rao SV, Swaminathan RV. Radial access for peripheral interventions. Interv Cardiol Clin 2020;9(1):53–61.

28. Castro-Dominguez Y, Li J, Lodha A, et al. Prospective, multicenter registry to assess safety and efficacy of radial access for peripheral artery interventions. J Soc Cardiovasc Angiogr Interv 2023;2(6). https://doi.org/10.1016/j.jscai.2023.101107.

29. Sheikh IR, Ahmed SH, Mori N, et al. Comparison of safety and efficacy of bivalirudin versus unfractionated heparin in percutaneous peripheral intervention. A single-center experience. JACC Cardiovasc Interv 2009;2(9). https://doi.org/10.1016/j.jcin.2009.06.015.

30. Dangas G, Mehran R, Kokolis S, et al. Vascular complications after percutaneous coronary interventions following hemostasis with manual compression versus arteriotomy closure devices. J Am Coll Cardiol 2001;38(3). https://doi.org/10.1016/S0735-1097(01)01449-8.

31. Trimarchi S, Smith DE, Share D, et al. Retroperitoneal hematoma after percutaneous coronary intervention: prevalence, risk factors, management, outcomes, and predictors of mortality: a report from the BMC2 (Blue Cross Blue Shield of Michigan Cardiovascular Consortium) registry. JACC Cardiovasc Interv 2010;3(8). https://doi.org/10.1016/j.jcin.2010.05.013.

32. Farouque HMO, Tremmel JA, Shabari FR, et al. Risk factors for the development of retroperitoneal hematoma after percutaneous coronary intervention in the era of glycoprotein IIb/IIIa inhibitors and vascular closure devices. J Am Coll Cardiol 2005;45(3). https://doi.org/10.1016/j.jacc.2004.10.042.

33. Stone PA, Campbell JE. Complications related to femoral artery access for transcatheter procedures. Vasc Endovascular Surg 2012;46(8). https://doi.org/10.1177/1538574412457475.

34. Tsetis D. Endovascular treatment of complications of femoral arterial access. Cardiovasc Intervent Radiol 2010;33(3). https://doi.org/10.1007/s00270-010-9820-3.

35. Hetrodt J, Engelbertz C, Reinecke H, et al. Access site related vascular complications following percutaneous cardiovascular procedures. J Cardiovasc Dev Dis 2021;8(11). https://doi.org/10.3390/jcdd8110136.

36. Schumacher PM, Ross CB, Wu YC, et al. Ischemic complications of percutaneous femoral artery catheterization. Ann Vasc Surg 2007;21(6). https://doi.org/10.1016/j.avsg.2007.05.001.

37. Van Wiechen MP, Ligthart JM, Van Mieghem NM. Large-bore vascular closure: new devices and techniques. Intervent Cardiol: Reviews, Research,

Resources 2019;14(1). https://doi.org/10.15420/icr.2018.36.1.

38. Kaki A, Blank N, Alraies MC, et al. Access and closure management of large bore femoral arterial access. J Interv Cardiol 2018;31(6). https://doi.org/10.1111/joic.12571.

39. Nelson PR, Kracjer Z, Kansal N, et al. A multicenter, randomized, controlled trial of totally percutaneous access versus open femoral exposure for endovascular aortic aneurysm repair (the PEVAR trial). J Vasc Surg 2014;59(5). https://doi.org/10.1016/j.jvs.2013.10.101.

40.. Hon LQ, Ganeshan A, Thomas SM, et al. An overview of vascular closure devices: what every radiologist should know. Eur J Radiol 2010;73(1):181–90.

41. Pang N, Gao J, Zhang B, et al. Vascular closure devices versus manual compression in cardiac interventional procedures: systematic review and meta-analysis. Cardiovasc Ther 2022;2022. https://doi.org/10.1155/2022/8569188.

42. Gewalt SM, Helde SM, Ibrahim T, et al. Comparison of vascular closure devices versus manual compression after femoral artery puncture in women. Circ Cardiovasc Interv 2018;11(8):e006074.

Intravascular Imaging in Peripheral Endovascular Intervention: A Contemporary Review

Daniel J. Snyder, MD[a,b], Robert S. Zilinyi, MD[a,b],
Takehiko Kido, MD[a,b], Sahil A. Parikh, MD, FSCAI[a,b,*]

KEYWORDS

- Peripheral artery disease • Endovascular intervention • Intravascular imaging
- Intravascular ultrasound • Optical coherence tomography

KEY POINTS

- The use of intravascular imaging modalities including intravascular ultrasound (IVUS) and optical coherence tomography (OCT) is increasing in peripheral endovascular intervention (PVI).
- Adjunctive use of intravascular imaging confers many advantages, ranging from assessment of vessel size and plaque morphology pre-intervention to identification of complications and opportunities for optimization post-intervention.
- Large observational studies and RCTs have demonstrated IVUS use improves long-term patency and amputation rates, leading to recent consensus statements and expert opinions recommending IVUS use in PVI.

BACKGROUND

Peripheral artery disease (PAD) affects greater than 10 million individuals in the United States and greater than 200 million people worldwide.[1] While open bypass surgery was traditionally the main treatment option for patients with symptomatic PAD and chronic limb-threatening ischemia (CLTI), recent trials have suggested that percutaneous endovascular treatment may provide similar outcomes in terms of amputation-free survival, particularly for patients lacking a suitable great saphenous vein graft.[2–4] In light of this data and the fact that patients with PAD often carry comorbidities that make them poor surgical candidates, an increasing number of patients are being treated with peripheral endovascular intervention (PVI).

Within PVI, angiography has long been the primary imaging modality used during intervention. While it has many benefits including ease of use and accurate estimation of flow, its limitations as a contrast-based 2-dimensional imaging modality have been well-described.[5–7] In light of these limitations, the use of intravascular imaging modalities including intravascular ultrasound (IVUS) and optical coherence tomography (OCT) has been increasing. While the use of these modalities has become commonplace in the coronary circulation given high-quality randomized controlled trial (RCT) data demonstrating improvements in mortality, stent thrombosis, and target-lesion revascularization, the use of IVUS and OCT in PVI has been relatively low.[8] This trend is changing, however, with the foundation of research supporting the use of intravascular imaging in PVI becoming more robust in recent years.

This article will review the use of intravascular imaging in peripheral arterial intervention; the role of intravascular imaging in lower extremity (LE) venous intervention has been detailed

---

[a] Department of Medicine, Division of Cardiology, Columbia University Irving Medical Center and Columbia University Vagelos College, 161 Fort Washington Avenue, 6th Floor, New York, NY 10032, USA; [b] Clinical Trials Center, Cardiovascular Research Foundation, 1700 Broadway, New York, NY 10019, USA
* Corresponding author. Department of Medicine, Division of Cardiology, Columbia University Irving Medical Center and Columbia University Vagelos College, 161 Fort Washington Avenue, 6th Floor, New York, NY, 10032.
E-mail address: sap2196@cumc.columbia.edu

Intervent Cardiol Clin 14 (2025) 161–171
https://doi.org/10.1016/j.iccl.2024.11.004

Abbreviations	
AVF	American Venous Forum
AVLS	American Vein & Lymphatic Society
BTK	below-the-knee
CLTI	chronic limb-threatening ischemia
CMS	Centers for Medicare and Medicaid Services
CSA	cross-sectional area
DCB	drug-coated balloons
IVUS	intravascular ultrasound
LE	lower extremity
OCT	optical coherence tomography
PAD	peripheral artery disease
PVI	peripheral endovascular intervention
RCT	randomized controlled trial
RVD	reference vessel diameter
SCAI	Society for Cardiovascular Angiography & Interventions
SIR	Society of Interventional Radiology
SVM	Society for Vascular Medicine
SVS	Society for Vascular Surgery

elsewhere.[9] First, the fundamentals of intravascular imaging will be reviewed, followed by a description of the literature supporting the use of intravascular imaging in peripheral arterial intervention. These data will be used to explain the current expert opinions and consensus statements put forth by the Society for Cardiovascular Angiography & Interventions (SCAI), Society of Interventional Radiology (SIR), Society for Vascular Medicine (SVM), Society for Vascular Surgery (SVS), American Venous Forum (AVF), and American Vein & Lymphatic Society (AVLS), as well as the trends in usage across the United States. Finally, current limitations and future directions will be discussed.

THE FUNDAMENTALS OF INTRAVASCULAR IMAGING

IVUS obtains images using a piezoelectric ultrasound transducer which is mounted on the tip of a catheter. This transducer, when delivered intravascularly, produces sound waves that differentially reflect off components of the vessel and vessel wall and are captured back by the transducer, generating a 360-degree grayscale ultrasound image. The IVUS catheters available

on the market rely on either a single mechanically rotating piezoelectric transducer or a phased array of multiple stationary transducers. The resolution and penetration of the image are highly dependent on the frequency of the ultrasound transducer, with higher frequency transducers (eg, 20–45 mHz) producing spatial resolutions of 200 to 500 μm and penetration depths of up to 10 mm and lower frequency transducers (eg, 8–12 mHz) producing resolutions of 150 μm at the cost of decreased penetration depth.[10]

OCT, on the other hand, obtains images by using a light source mounted on the tip of a catheter. This light source emits light waves that are initially split and then scatter differentially based on the composition of tissue. These light waves are then captured by an interferometer which uses the interference pattern to create a high-resolution cross-sectional image of the vessel.[11] Because these interference patterns are highly sensitive, resolutions of up to 25 μm can be achieved. The penetration depth, however, is limited to a maximum of 3 mm because light waves are absorbed by biological tissues.[10] Given that blood scatters light, a flush medium has to be used to clear blood from the vessel prior to OCT imaging. While some success has been demonstrated with the use of heparinized saline and dextran, iodinated contrast remains the most commonly utilized flush medium.[12,13]

UTILITY OF INTRAVASCULAR IMAGING PREINTERVENTION

One of the main benefits of intravascular imaging is the ability to generate precise measurements of the target vessel lumen. On IVUS imaging, the borders of the vessel lumen and vessel wall are clearly demarcated by the bright, echogenic intima and adventitia. This enables operators to make precise measurements of the lumen diameter, cross-sectional area (CSA), and reference vessel diameter (RVD) (Fig. 1). These measurements are often significantly larger than those guided by angiography. In the femoropopliteal circulation, Iida and colleagues demonstrated using a population of 1725 patients that IVUS generated RVD estimates that were 1 mm larger than angiographically derived estimates (6 mm vs 5 mm, <0.001), with almost half of the study population having measurements discrepancies of greater than 1 mm.[14] Pliagas and colleagues demonstrated similar results in a smaller population of patients with infra-inguinal PAD, revealing IVUS-derived

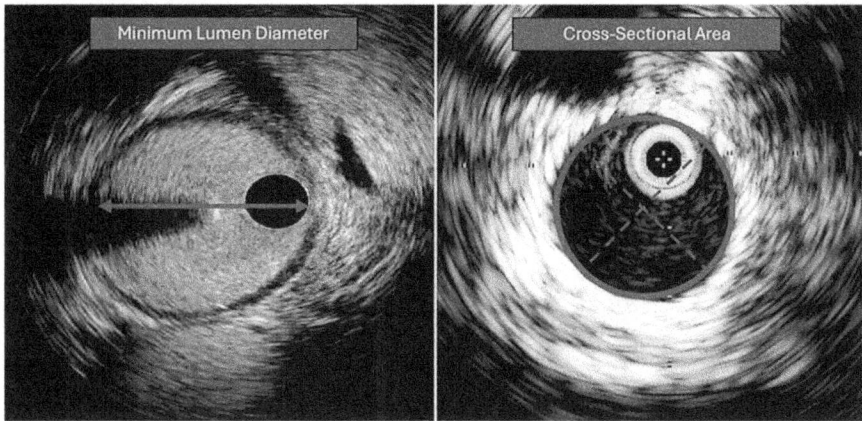

Fig. 1. Measurement of minimum lumen diameter and CSA using IVUS.

RVD estimates were between 0.6 and 1.3 mm larger than angiographically derived estimates.[15] This pattern holds true in the smaller caliber vessels in the infrapopliteal circulation as well; in the population of 20 patients with below-the-knee (BTK) PAD enrolled in the BTK Calibration study, IVUS produced RVD estimates that were 0.5 mm larger than angiographically derived measurements.[16] These measurements have been shown to hold predictive value for patency rates after drug-coated balloons (DCB) and stenting as well.[17,18] Because of its higher spatial resolution, OCT is also able to generate precise measurements of the vessel and its lumen (Fig. 2). In a study comparing 112 IVUS and OCT images of the same popliteal and infrapopliteal segments, Eberhardt and colleagues demonstrated that OCT provided better vessel wall discriminability than IVUS, although this did not translate into any appreciable difference in vessel measurements between the 2 imaging modalities.[19]

Intravascular imaging also provides operators the opportunity to gain a better understanding of plaque composition and morphology. On IVUS, plaque can be identified as fibrous, fibro-fatty, fatty, or calcific based on echogenicity and the presence or absence of posterior acoustic shadowing.[20] IVUS has substantial benefits when it comes to identifying calcified plaques in particular (Fig. 3). In an independent core-lab analysis of 47 patients with femoropopliteal PAD and severe calcification performed by Yin and colleagues, IVUS detected calcium in almost 40% more lesions than angiography.[21] When compared with IVUS, this gave angiography a sensitivity of 59% for identifying calcium, explaining why IVUS has been used to validate many of the existing angiographic calcium scoring systems. Given that IVUS provides a 360-degree view of the vessel, it can also delineate plaque morphology (eg, eccentric vs concentric) and quantify the degree of circumferential calcium involvement (eg, the calcium

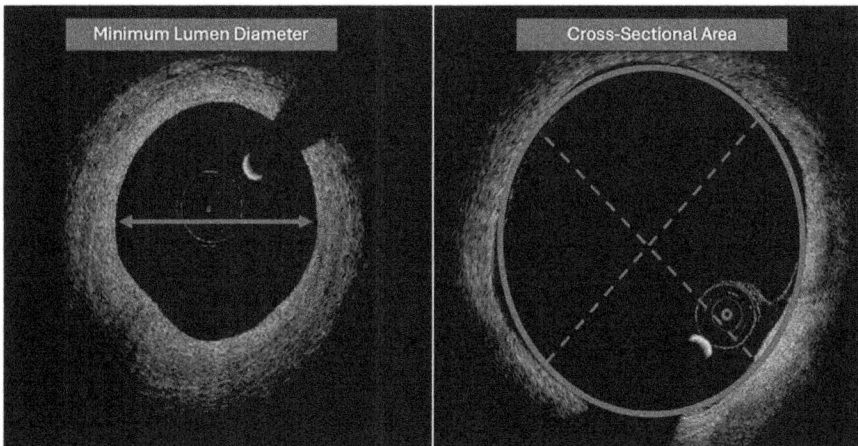

Fig. 2. Measurement of minimum lumen diameter and CSA using OCT.

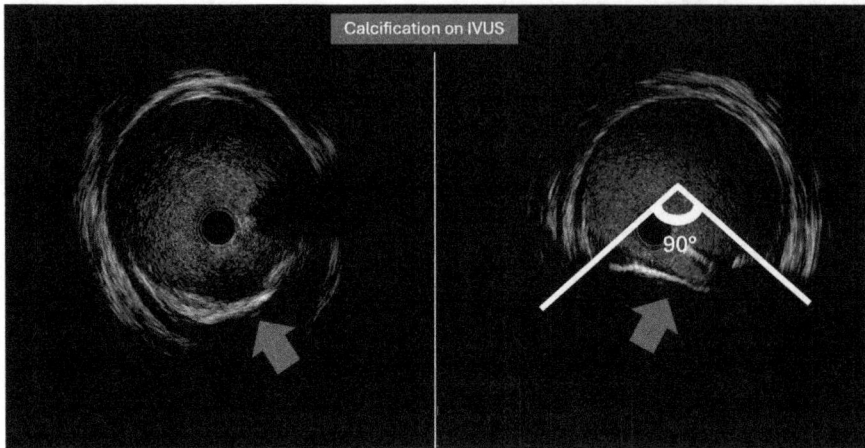

Fig. 3. Identification of calcification and measurement of the calcium arc using IVUS.

arc) if calcification is present.[22] This morphologic assessment has been shown to predict response to treatment along with the risk of complications such as stent malapposition and restenosis.[23] OCT also provides a detailed characterization of plaque composition based on the level of brightness and signal attenuation.[24] Two small studies suggest that the higher spatial resolution of OCT translates into better plaque characterization than IVUS, although these assessments have been limited to qualitative evaluations by operators.[19,25]

In addition to characterizing plaque, intravascular imaging has also been demonstrated to be effective at identifying thrombus (Fig. 4A, B). In a study of 17 patients with infra-inguinal PAD and associated thrombus performed by Shammas and colleagues, IVUS was able to identify definite thrombus in 16 of the 17 patients.[26] Angiography, on the other hand, was only able to identify definite thrombus in 2 of the 17 cases, underscoring the added value of intravascular imaging evaluation. OCT also provides information regarding the presence of thrombus. On OCT, thrombi appear bright, with white and red thrombi being differentiable by the level of backscattering present.[27] In a cohort of 27 femoropopliteal lesions, Karnabatidis demonstrated the utility of OCT in identifying thrombus, and subsequent articles have been published showing the utility of OCT in guiding thrombectomy in acute limb ischemia and evaluating for postprocedural stent thrombosis.[12,28,29]

INTRAPROCEDURAL BENEFITS OF INTRAVASCULAR IMAGING

Intraprocedurally, the precise vessel measurements and added characterization of plaque composition and morphology yielded from intravascular imaging can be used to guide clinical decision-making regarding device sizing and the need for vessel preparation or stenting. In femoropopliteal and infrapopliteal interventions, adjunctive IVUS usage has consistently been associated with the use of larger-diameter balloons when compared with angiography. In a RCT of 150 patients with femoropopliteal PAD assigned to either angiography alone or IVUS plus angiography, Allan and colleagues demonstrated that the DCB used in IVUS-guided procedures were 0.4 mm larger in diameter on average than those used in angiography-guided procedures.[30] A similar finding was demonstrated in the study of 155 patients with infrapopliteal CLTI performed by Soga and colleagues, where IVUS use was associated with a +0.5 mm difference in average balloon diameter when compared with angiography.[31] This change in device sizing becomes especially important when using DCB, as more accurate balloon sizing helps optimize the amount of drug delivered into the vessel walls, which may in turn help to improve patency over time.

Prior to angioplasty or stenting, intravascular imaging also helps operators determine if vessel preparation techniques are required. In the JETSTREAM trial, IVUS was utilized by Maehara and colleagues to evaluate severely calcified femoropopliteal artery lesions prior to the use of the JETSTREAM Atherectomy System (Boston Scientific, Marlborough, MA, USA).[32] Bastante and colleagues used a case of in-stent restenosis to demonstrate how OCT could also be useful in helping operators determine if atherectomy was necessary.[33] Once the decision to perform vessel preparation has been made, intravascular imaging can also provide data regarding how vessel preparation is

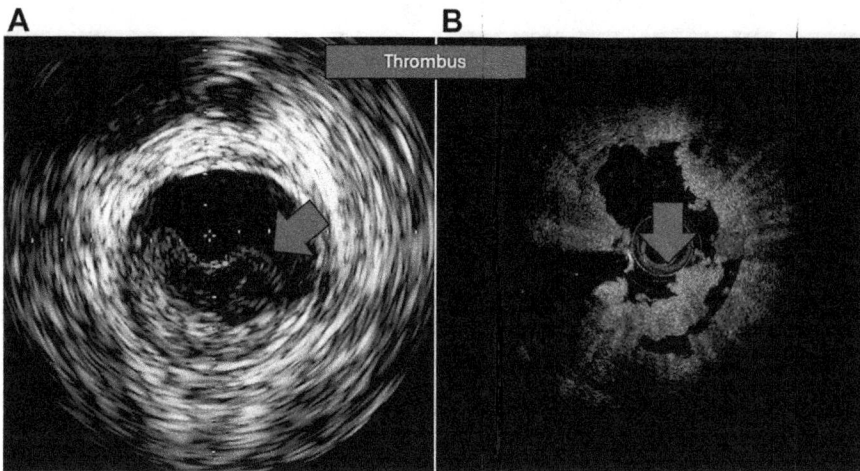

Fig. 4. Appearance of thrombus on IVUS (A) and OCT (B).

progressing. In a cohort of 40 patients with femoro-popliteal PAD undergoing atherectomy, Tielbeek and colleagues found that IVUS use prompted additional passes of the atherectomy device in 83% of the cases where it was utilized.[34] OCT has been incorporated into an atherectomy device (Pantheris Atherectomy System, Avinger Inc, Redwood City, CA, USA) to provide real-time intravascular imaging guidance during plaque debulking. In the VISION trial, the use of OCT during atherectomy was associated with sparing of the adventitia in greater than 80% of samples, highlighting the precision that can be provided using intravascular imaging guidance during interventions.[35]

Intravascular imaging also has well-demonstrated utility in LE chronic total occlusion (CTO) intervention. Technical success rates of ≥90% have been described when using IVUS-guided reentry devices to recanalize LE CTOs.[36] Novel techniques using IVUS in a parallel vein to facilitate guidewire crossing have also been described, with Takahashi and colleagues reporting a 96% success rate using this technique to cross 50 femoropopliteal and tibioperoneal CTOs.[37] OCT, on the other hand, has been incorporated directly into catheters (Ocelot, Avinger Inc, Redwood City, CA, USA) which provide real-time imaging from the catheter tip during CTO recanalization.[38] The Ocelot system has been demonstrated to be effective in several different studies performed in the United States and Europe, with technical success rates being reported as high as 94%.[39–41]

POSTINTERVENTION BENEFITS OF INTRAVASCULAR IMAGING

Some of the main benefits of intravascular imaging in LE PVI stem from the ability to identify

opportunities for device optimization (eg, stent malapposition or underexpansion) prior to the end of the case. With the high-resolution cross-sectional imaging of IVUS and OCT, stent malapposition can be readily identified after stent deployment when the stent strut fails to abut the vessel wall and blood is visible between the 2 structures (Fig. 5A, B).[10] Stent underexpansion, one of the main predictors of thrombosis and need for revascularization in the coronary circulation, can also be identified by measuring the minimum stent diameter and comparing this to the reference lumen diameter.[42] Separate studies of 32 and 36 patients undergoing aortoiliac PVI with angioplasty and stenting found evidence of stent under-deployment after IVUS use in 40% of cases, all of which appeared to have adequate expansion on angiography.[43,44] This identification of under-deployment led to substantial changes in management prior to the end of the case. Similar results have been demonstrated in case series of patients undergoing femoropopliteal PVI with OCT use.[45]

Intravascular imaging also provides the opportunity to identify procedural complications that may not be immediately apparent on angiography. Because IVUS and OCT provide a 360-degree view of all of the components of the vessel wall, dissections can be readily identified by evaluating for breaks in the continuity of the wall and the presence of blood outside of the vessel lumen (Fig. 6A, B). The depth of the dissection (eg, intimal, medial, extra-medial) and length can also be used to gain an idea of the dissection severity. The increased sensitivity of both IVUS and OCT in identifying dissections as compared with angiography has been well-demonstrated in cohort studies of patients undergoing

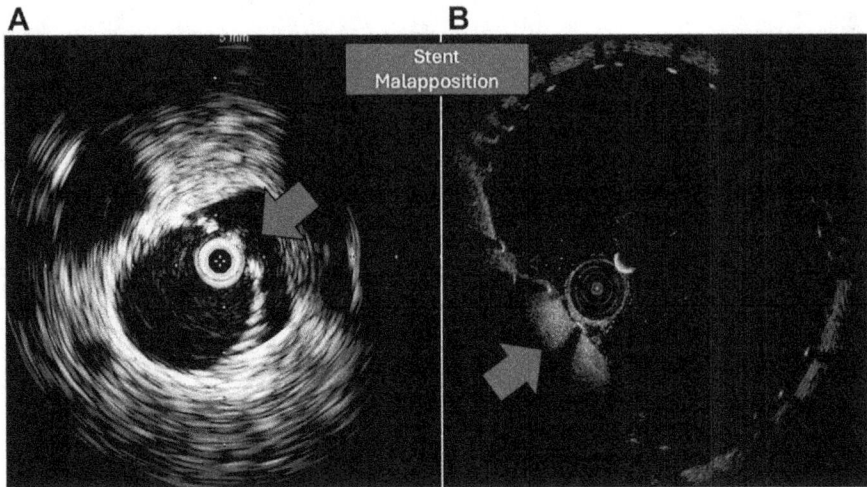

Fig. 5. Identification of stent malapposition on IVUS (A) and OCT (B).

aortoiliac, femoropopliteal, and infrapopliteal interventions, with intravascular imaging identifying between 2.5 and 5.8 times as many dissections as angiography.[12,46–48] Identification of these dissections is critical, as it allows them to be addressed with either postdilation of a noncompliant balloon or further stenting prior to the end of the case. This was well-demonstrated in a case of superficial femoral artery intervention published by Stefano and colleagues, where OCT use prompted stenting after the identification of a spiral dissection following an initial angioplasty.[49]

With intravascular imaging, operators also have the opportunity to assess the response to their initial intervention, which may dictate the need for further treatment prior to closing. With IVUS use, investigators have described the ability to quantify the degree of calcium removal by comparing the calcium arc preatherectomy and postatherectomy.[32,50,51] With both IVUS and OCT, investigators can also measure the change in minimum lumen area predevice and postdevice deployment to gain an idea of the luminal gain from an intervention.[32,50–52]

THE IMPACT OF INTRAVASCULAR IMAGING USE ON CLINICAL OUTCOMES

In the coronary circulation, adjunctive intravascular imaging usage has been well-demonstrated to improve rates of major adverse cardiovascular events, the need for repeat revascularization, and stent thrombosis in both RCTs

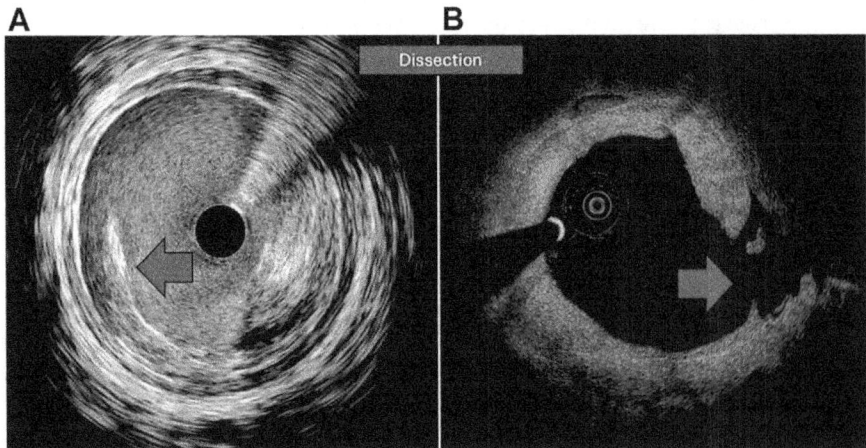

Fig. 6. Identification of dissection on IVUS (A) and OCT (B).

and large-scale observational analyses.[8,53] While the data in LE PVI has been limited to mostly observational studies, existing data suggest that these findings extend to the LE circulation as well. The largest observational study of IVUS use in LE PVI in the United States was performed by Divakaran and colleagues using the Centers for Medicare and Medicaid Services (CMS) data set. In this study of greater than 500,000 patients, authors demonstrated a 27% reduction in the risk of major adverse limb events at a median follow-up of 1.5 years when IVUS was utilized along with significantly lower rates of minor and major amputation.[54] In Japan, similar findings were identified when evaluating a population of 85,649 patients undergoing LE PVI. In this propensity-scored analysis, IVUS use was associated with a significantly lower incidence of amputation at 1 year when compared with procedures guided by angiography alone.[55] As of 2022, these findings are now further supported by randomized data. Allan and colleagues randomized 150 patients undergoing femoropopliteal PVI to either IVUS plus angiography or angiography alone and demonstrated a significantly higher rate of freedom from binary restenosis at 1 year with IVUS use (72% vs 55%).[30] Importantly, the usage of IVUS led to changes in management in the majority of cases where it was used. This was recently followed by the IVUS-DCB RCT which demonstrated improvements in primary patency and freedom from clinically driven target lesion revascularization at 1 year with IVUS-guided as opposed to angiography-guided femoropopliteal PVI.[56] While additional prospective data are needed, these findings support an association of improved outcomes with adjunctive IVUS usage. To the authors' knowledge, minimal research exists investigating the association between OCT usage and outcomes following LE PVI.

CONSENSUS DOCUMENTS AND EXPERT OPINIONS

In recent years, the body of evidence supporting the use of intravascular imaging has grown strong enough to support recent consensus statements and expert opinions that recommend the use of IVUS in LE PVI. In 2022, the first consensus document regarding the appropriate use of IVUS in LE arterial and venous intervention was published.[57] In this document, a series of clinical vignettes designed by a writing committee of interventional cardiologists, interventional radiologists, vascular medicine specialists, and vascular surgeons were distributed to 30 different experts in PVI. These vignettes included different scenarios operators commonly encountered in iliac, femoropopliteal, and tibial cases both preintervention (eg, sizing the vessel, evaluating plaque morphology), intraprocedurally (eg, sizing the device, deciding the next therapeutic step), and postintervention (eg, identifying dissections, optimizing stents) and asked experts to grade the appropriateness of IVUS use in each scenario. Experts determined IVUS was appropriate (eg, would be a reasonable approach for the indication that was likely to improve patient outcomes) in all phases and scenarios of tibial PVI, most scenarios preintervention in iliac and femoropopliteal PVI, and almost all scenarios intraintervention and postintervention in iliac and femoropopliteal PVI. This consensus document was followed more recently by a multidisciplinary expert opinion put forth by members of SCAI, AQVF, AVLS, SIR, SVM, and SVS which supported the role of IVUS in LE PVI, reviewed key barriers to IVUS adoption, and set out next steps to address these barriers.[58]

TRENDS IN CURRENT USAGE

While limited data exist evaluating rates of OCT usage in LE PVI, the use of IVUS has been demonstrated to be increasing across the United States. In an analysis of all Medicare beneficiaries undergoing LE PVI between 2016 and 2019, Secemsky and colleagues identified IVUS utilization in ~12% of cases performed during the study period.[54] This usage rate was more than 8x higher than the frequency of IVUS use noted in a similar analysis of the National Inpatient Sample from 2006 to 2011.[59] Notably, IVUS utilization was mainly localized to ambulatory surgical centers and office-based laboratories (27% of total cases), while use in the inpatient setting was limited to 4% of total cases. Usage was also highly variable between physician subspecialties, with interventional radiologists having the highest utilization of IVUS (17.4% of cases) and interventional cardiologists having the lowest utilization of all subspecialty groups (10.3% of cases). While trends toward increasing usage are encouraging, these data highlight how much opportunity there is to continue integrating IVUS usage into practice, especially in the inpatient setting. Other countries' experiences incorporating IVUS into LE PVI are encouraging; in a recent analysis using the Japanese Diagnosis Procedure Combination database which includes the majority of inpatients in Japan, IVUS was found to be utilized in almost 60% of endovascular cases.[55]

LIMITATIONS OF INTRAVASCULAR IMAGING IN THE PERIPHERAL CIRCULATION

While intravascular imaging has many substantial benefits, it also has its limitations. One of the major drawbacks is the additional time that it adds to the procedure. To obtain IVUS images, the catheter needs to be guided to the vessel of interest and advanced past the target lesion. In the long vessels of the LE, this can take a substantial amount of time, especially if vessel preparation techniques need to be employed for the IVUS catheter to be able to cross the target lesion. Once the lesion has been crossed, the images can then be obtained through either manual or mechanical pullback. To ensure high-quality images, pullback has to be slow and speeds are typically limited to ≤1 mm per second. After a device is deployed, this process must be repeated to recognize the benefits of device optimization and complication identification. IVUS use is also associated with substantial costs. For hospitals, an upfront capital expenditure is required to purchase the IVUS technology and make it accessible to physicians in the catheterization laboratory or operating room. For the payer, IVUS use has been associated with an added cost of ~$1200 per index procedure.[59] IVUS is also only useful if operators are adequately trained in how to interpret the images and apply them to the case. Unfortunately, IVUS use is also the most limited in the inpatient setting where most operators gain their training, and as a result a substantial number of operators around the United States are not familiar with its use.

OCT is limited by many of the same drawbacks of IVUS. A notable differentiating limitation is the requirement for a flush medium to clear the blood from the target vessel prior to imaging. While other solutions have shown some promise in small studies, iodinated contrast remains the most commonly used medium.[12,13] This poses a problem in a population of PAD patients who have a high rate of comorbid chronic kidney disease and increases their risk of contrast-induced nephropathy.[5] When compared with IVUS, although the depth of OCT is fairly limited, the speed of image acquisition is substantially faster. With current-generation Fourier-domain OCT devices, pullback speeds can now reach up to 20 mm per second, and frame rates are also much higher (100 fps as opposed to 30 fps with IVUS).[10]

TAKEAWAYS AND FUTURE DIRECTIONS

This review demonstrates many of the applications and benefits of intravascular imaging in LE PVI, from assessment of vessel size and plaque morphology preintervention to identification of complications and opportunities for device optimization postintervention. With IVUS in particular, these applications have been demonstrated to translate into better patency rates and lower rates of amputation at follow-up, leading to the release of recent consensus statements and expert opinions that recommend the use of IVUS in LE PVI. With OCT, although the safety and feasibility of use in the LE have been demonstrated, additional data are needed to establish a connection between OCT usage and improvements in outcomes after PVI.

Given the strength of literature supporting IVUS use, uptake has been increasing around the country. Usage rates remain limited, however, and substantial opportunity exists to address the limitations mentioned earlier and spur further uptake. The first step toward making this happen involves addressing gaps in the existing data. Additional prospective research is needed to substantiate the impact of IVUS usage on outcomes postintervention, with a particular focus on clinical outcomes (eg, amputation, clinically driven target lesion revascularization). If level 1 evidence can be produced demonstrating improvements in amputation and revascularization rates, additional physicians are likely to be convinced to start using IVUS, hospital administration can be better convinced that the technology is worth the capital expenditure, and arguments for cost-effectiveness and reimbursement can start to be made.

CLINICS CARE POINTS

- Pre-intervention, the use of intravascular imaging provides operators with additional information regarding vessel sizing and plaque morphology and can help guide clinical decision-making regarding device sizing and the need for vessel preparation or stenting.

- Post-intervention, the use of intravascular imaging can help operators identify complications (ex. dissection) and discern whether additional steps are needed to optimize the device prior to ending the case.

- These benefits have been shown to translate into improved patency and amputation rates in large observational studies and two RCTs.

DISCLOSURE

Sahil Parikh receives institutional grants/research support from Abbott Vascular, United States, Shockwave Medical, United States, TriReme Medical, United States, Surmodics, Silk Road Medical, and the National Institutes of Health, United States. He has received consulting fees from Terumo and Abiomed and served on the advisory boards of Abbott, Medtronic, Boston Scientific, CSI, Janssen, and Philips. Sanjum Sethi reports honoraria from Janssen and Chiesi Inc. All other authors have no conflicts of interest to report.

REFERENCES

1. Allison MA, Armstrong DG, Goodney PP, et al. Health disparities in peripheral artery disease: a scientific statement from the American Heart Association. Circulation 2023;148(3):286–96.
2. Bradbury AW, Moakes CA, Popplewell M, et al. A vein bypass first versus a best endovascular treatment first revascularisation strategy for patients with chronic limb threatening ischaemia who required an infra-popliteal, with or without an additional more proximal infra-inguinal revascularisation procedure to restore limb perfusion (BASIL-2): an open-label, randomised, multicentre, phase 3 trial. Lancet 2023;401(10390):1798–809.
3. Bradbury AW, Adam DJ, Bell J, et al. Bypass versus angioplasty in severe ischaemia of the leg (BASIL) trial: an intention-to-treat analysis of amputation-free and overall survival in patients randomized to a bypass surgery-first or a balloon angioplasty-first revascularization strategy. J Vasc Surg 2010;51(5 Suppl):5S–17S.
4. Farber A, Menard MT, Conte MS, et al. Surgery or endovascular therapy for chronic limb-threatening ischemia. N Engl J Med 2022;387(25):2305–16.
5. Safley DM, Salisbury AC, Tsai TT, et al. Acute kidney injury following in-patient lower extremity vascular intervention: from the national cardiovascular data registry. JACC Cardiovasc Interv 2021;14(3):333–41.
6. Zilinyi RS, Alsaloum M, Snyder DJ, et al. Surgical and endovascular therapies for below-the-knee peripheral arterial disease: a contemporary review. J Soc Cardiovasc Angiogr Interv 2024;3(3):101268.
7. Loffroy R, Falvo N, Galland C, et al. Intravascular ultrasound in the endovascular treatment of patients with peripheral arterial disease: current role and future perspectives. Front Cardiovasc Med 2020;7.
8. Darmoch F, Alraies MC, Al-Khadra Y, et al. Intravascular ultrasound imaging–guided versus coronary angiography–guided percutaneous coronary intervention: a systematic review and meta-analysis. J Am Heart Assoc 2020;9(5).
9. Secemsky EA, Parikh SA, Kohi M, et al. Intravascular ultrasound guidance for lower extremity arterial and venous interventions. EuroIntervention 2022;18(7):598.
10. Snyder D, Zilinyi R, Pruthi S, et al. Intravascular imaging for infra-inguinal peripheral artery disease intervention: a review of current methods and existing data. Vascular Disease Management 2023;20(7):E130–9.
11. Marschall S, Sander B, Mogensen M, et al. Optical coherence tomography-current technology and applications in clinical and biomedical research. Anal Bioanal Chem 2011;400(9):2699–720.
12. Karnabatidis D, Katsanos K, Paraskevopoulos I, et al. Frequency-domain intravascular optical coherence tomography of the femoropopliteal artery. Cardiovasc Intervent Radiol 2011;34(6):1172–81.
13. Kendrick DE, Allemang MT, Gosling AF, et al. Dextran or saline can replace contrast for intravascular optical coherence tomography in lower extremity arteries. J Endovasc Ther 2016;23(5):723–30.
14. Iida O, Takahara M, Soga Y, et al. Vessel diameter evaluated by intravascular ultrasound versus angiography. J Endovasc Ther 2022;29(3):343–9.
15. George Pliagas. Intravascular ultrasound imaging versus digital subtraction angiography in patients with peripheral vascular disease. J Invasive Cardiol 2020;32(3). Available at: https://www.hmpglobaleearningnetwork.com/site/jic/articles/intravascular-ultrasound-imaging-versus-digital-subtraction-angiography-patients-peripheral-vascular-disease. Accessed April 9, 2023.
16. Kuku KO, Garcia-Garcia HM, Finizio M, et al. Comparison of angiographic and intravascular ultrasound vessel measurements in infra-popliteal endovascular interventions: the below-the-knee calibration study. Cardiovasc Revascularization Med 2022;35:35–41.
17. Soga Y, Takahara M, Iida O, et al. Vessel patency and associated factors of drug-coated balloon for femoropopliteal lesion. J Am Heart Assoc 2022;12(1):e025677.
18. Miki K, Fujii K, Tanaka T, et al. Impact of IVUS-derived vessel size on midterm outcomes after stent implantation in femoropopliteal lesions. J Endovasc Ther 2020;27(1):77–85.
19. Eberhardt KM, Treitl M, Boesenecker K, et al. Prospective evaluation of optical coherence tomography in lower limb arteries compared with intravascular ultrasound. J Vasc Intervent Radiol 2013;24(10):1499–508.
20. Nissen SE, Yock P. Intravascular ultrasound novel pathophysiological insights and current clinical applications. 2001. Available at: http://www.circulatio-naha.org. Accessed April 9, 2023.
21. Yin D, Maehara A, Shimshak TM, et al. Intravascular ultrasound validation of contemporary angiographic scores evaluating the severity of

calcification in peripheral arteries. J Endovasc Ther 2017;24(4):478–87.

22. Arthurs ZM, Bishop PD, Feiten LE, et al. Evaluation of peripheral atherosclerosis: a comparative analysis of angiography and intravascular ultrasound imaging. J Vasc Surg 2010;51(4):933–9.

23. Fujihara M, Yazu Y, Takahara M. Intravascular ultrasound-guided interventions for below-the-knee disease in patients with chronic limb-threatening ischemia. J Endovasc Ther 2020;27(4): 565–74.

24. Bezerra HG, Costa MA, Guagliumi G, et al. Intracoronary optical coherence tomography: a comprehensive review clinical and research applications. JACC Cardiovasc Interv 2009;2(11):1035–46.

25. Pavillard E, Sewall L. A post-market, multi-vessel evaluation of the imaging of peripheral arteries for diagnostic purposeS comparing optical Coherence tomogrApy and iNtravascular ultrasound imaging (SCAN). BMC Med Imag 2020;20(1).

26. Shammas NW, Dippel EJ, Shammas G, et al. Dethrombosis of the lower extremity arteries using the power-pulse spray technique in patients with recent onset thrombotic occlusions: results of the DETHROMBOSIS registry. J Endovasc Ther 2008; 15(5):570–9.

27. Kume T, Akasaka T, Kawamoto T, et al. Assessment of coronary arterial thrombus by optical coherence tomography. Am J Cardiol 2006;97(12):1713–7.

28. Yamamoto Y, Kawarada O, Sakamoto S, et al. Progression of intimal hyperplasia and multiple-channel formation after fogarty thrombectomy: insight into vasculopathy from optical coherence tomography and intravascular ultrasound findings. JACC Cardiovasc Interv 2015;8(15):e251–3.

29. Yang X, Leesar MA, Ahmed H, et al. Impact of ticagrelor and aspirin versus clopidogrel and aspirin in symptomatic patients with peripheral arterial disease: thrombus burden assessed by optical coherence tomography. Cardiovasc Revascularization Med 2018;19(7):778–84.

30. Allan RB, Puckridge PJ, Spark JI, et al. The impact of intravascular ultrasound on femoropopliteal artery endovascular interventions: a randomized controlled trial. JACC Cardiovasc Interv 2022; 15(5):536–46.

31. Soga Y, Takahara M, Ito N, et al. Clinical impact of intravascular ultrasound-guided balloon angioplasty in patients with chronic limb threatening ischemia for isolated infrapopliteal lesion. Cathet Cardiovasc Interv 2021;97(3):E376–84.

32. Maehara A, Mintz GS, Shimshak TM, et al. Intravascular ultrasound evaluation of JETSTREAM atherectomy removal of superficial calcium in peripheral arteries. EuroIntervention 2015;11(1):96–103.

33. Bastante T, Rivero F, Cuesta J, et al. Calcified neo-atherosclerosis causing "undilatable" in-stent restenosis: insights of optical coherence tomography and role of rotational atherectomy. JACC Cardiovasc Interv 2015;8(15):2039–40.

34. Tielbeek AV, Vroegindeweij D, Buth J, et al. Comparison of intravascular ultrasonography and intra-arterial digital subtraction angiography after directional atherectomy of short lesions in femoro-popliteal arteries. J Vasc Surg 1996;23(3):436–45.

35. Schwindt AG, Bennett JG, Crowder WH, et al. Lower Extremity Revascularization Using Optical Coherence Tomography-Guided Directional Atherectomy: Final Results of the e v aluat i on of the Pantheri S Opt i cal C O herence Tomography Imagi N g Atherectomy System for Use in the Peripheral Vasculature (VISION) Study. J Endovasc Ther 2017;24(3):355–66.

36. Baker AC, Humphries MD, Noll RE, et al. Technical and early outcomes using ultrasound-guided reentry for chronic total occlusions. Ann Vasc Surg 2015;29(1):55–62.

37. Takahashi Y, Sato T, Okazaki H, et al. Transvenous intravascular ultrasound-guided endovascular treatment for chronic total occlusion of the infrainguinal arteries. J Endovasc Ther 2017;24(5):718–26.

38. Marmagkiolis K, Lendel V, Cawich I, et al. Ocelot catheter for the recanalization of lower extremity arterial chronic total occlusion. Cardiovasc Revascularization Med 2014;15(1):46–9.

39. Schwindt A, Reimers B, Scheinert D, et al. Crossing chronic total occlusions with the Ocelot system: the initial European experience. EuroIntervention 2013; 9(7):854–62.

40. Selmon MR, Schwindt AG, Cawich IM, et al. Final results of the chronic total occlusion crossing with the ocelot system II (CONNECT II) study. J Endovasc Ther 2013;20(6):770–81.

41. Schaefers JF, Schwindt AG, Maritati G, et al. Outcome after crossing femoropopliteal chronic total occlusions based on optical coherence tomography guidance. Vasc Endovasc Surg 2018; 52(1):27–33.

42. Fujii K, Carlier SG, Mintz GS, et al. Stent underexpansion and residual reference segment stenosis are related to stent thrombosis after sirolimus-eluting stent implantation: an intravascular ultrasound study. J Am Coll Cardiol 2005;45(7):995–8.

43. Arko F, McCollough R, Manning L, et al. Use of intravascular ultrasound in the endovascular management of atherosclerotic aortoiliac occlusive disease. Am J Surg 1996;172(5):546–50.

44. Buckley CJ, Arko FR, Lee S, et al. Intravascular ultrasound scanning improves long-term patency of iliac lesions treated with balloon angioplasty and primary stenting. J Vasc Surg 2002;35(2):316–23.

45. de Donato G, Setacci F, Galzerano G, et al. PS80. Safety and feasibility of intravascular optical coherence tomography to evaluate lesions of femoropopliteal arterial segment before and after endovascular treatment. J Vasc Surg 2014;59(6):54S.

46. Navarro F, Sullivan TM, Bacharach JM. Intravascular ultrasound assessment of iliac stent procedures 2000;7(4):315–9.

47. Shammas NW, Shammas WJ, Jones-Miller S, et al. Optimal vessel sizing and understanding dissections in infrapopliteal interventions: data from the idissection below the knee study. J Endovasc Ther 2020;27(4):575–80.

48. Nicolas WS. Intravascular ultrasound assessment and correlation with angiographic findings demonstrating femoropopliteal arterial dissections post atherectomy: results from the iDissection study. J Invasive Cardiol 2018;30(7). Available at: https://www.hmpgloballearningnetwork.com/site/jic/articles/intravascular-ultrasound-assessment-and-correlation-angiographic-findings-demonstrating. Accessed April 9, 2023.

49. Stefano GT, Mehanna E, Parikh SA. Imaging a spiral dissection of the superficial femoral artery in high resolution with optical coherence tomography-seeing is believing. Cathet Cardiovasc Interv 2013;81(3):568–72.

50. Singh T. Tissue removal by ultrasound evaluation (The TRUE Study): the jetstream G2 system postmarket peripheral vascular IVUS study. J Invasive Cardiol 2011;23(7). Available at: https://www.hmpgloballearningnetwork.com/site/jic/articles/tissue-removal-ultrasound-evaluation-true-study-jetstream-g2-system-post-market-peripheral. Accessed April 9, 2023.

51. Babaev AA, Zavlunova S, Attubato MJ, et al. Orbital atherectomy plaque modification assessment of the femoropopliteal artery via intravascular ultrasound (TRUTH Study). Vasc Endovasc Surg 2015;49(7):188–94.

52. Cilingiroglu M, Kilic ID, Hoyt T, et al. DIAMondback atherectomy with Oct visualization for calcified PAD lesions (DIAMOCT-PAD Study). J Invasive Cardiol 2022;34(2):E117–23.

53. Zhang J, Gao X, Kan J, et al. Intravascular ultrasound versus angiography-guided drug-eluting stent implantation: the ULTIMATE Trial. J Am Coll Cardiol 2018;72(24):3126–37.

54. Divakaran S, Parikh SA, Hawkins BM, et al. Temporal trends, practice variation, and associated outcomes with IVUS use during peripheral arterial intervention. JACC Cardiovasc Interv 2022;15(20):2080.

55. Setogawa N, Ohbe H, Matsui H, et al. Amputation after endovascular therapy with and without intravascular ultrasound guidance: a nationwide propensity score-matched study. Circ Cardiovasc Interv 2023;16(4):E012451.

56. Ko YG, Lee SJ, Ahn CM, et al. Intravascular ultrasound-guided drug-coated balloon angioplasty for femoropopliteal artery disease: a clinical trial. Eur Heart J 2024. https://doi.org/10.1093/EURHEARTJ/EHAE372.

57. Secemsky EA, Mosarla RC, Rosenfield K, et al. Appropriate use of intravascular ultrasound during arterial and venous lower extremity interventions. JACC Cardiovasc Interv 2022;15(15):1558–68.

58. Secemsky EA, Aronow HD, Kwolek CJ, et al. Intravascular ultrasound use in peripheral arterial and deep venous interventions: multidisciplinary expert opinion from SCAI/AVF/AVLS/SIR/SVM/SVS. J Soc Cardiovasc Angiogr Interv 2024;3(1):101205.

59. Panaich SS, Arora S, Patel N, et al. Intravascular ultrasound in lower extremity peripheral vascular interventions: variation in utilization and impact on in-hospital outcomes from the nationwide inpatient sample (2006-2011). J Endovasc Ther 2016;23(1):65–75.

Endovascular Abdominal Aortic Aneurysm Repair

Zafar Ali, MD[a], Luke Kim, MD[b], Kamal Gupta, MD[a],*

KEYWORDS

- Abdominal aortic aneurysm • Endovascular aortic repair • Endoleak

KEY POINTS

- A great majority of abdominal aortic aneurysm are treated with endovascular aortic repair (EVAR) in current practice and have lower peri-operative morbidity and mortality than open repair.
- Anatomic factors such as aneurysm neck morphology, iliac anatomy, and access vessel anatomy need careful assessment for the successful performance of EVAR.
- Regular and long-term follow-up with imaging is mandatory after EVAR and patients who are less likely to comply are not good EVAR candidates.
- Endoleaks are the most frequent complication of EVAR. Most can be managed with transcatheter or endovascular means.
- Evolving technology and techniques are allowing more patients to be treated with EVAR with better long-term outcomes.

INTRODUCTION

The treatment of abdominal aortic aneurysm (AAA) has evolved significantly over the past several decades. From the 1950s till the 90s, open surgical repair (OSR) had been the only treatment for AAA. Though OSR remains an important option in certain cases, it is no longer universally considered the gold standard due to its relatively high peri-procedural morbidity and mortality, with a mean operative mortality of about 4% for elective OSR.[1,2] In 1986, the first report of endovascular stent-graft based repair was published, and this paved the path for the evolution to minimally invasive endovascular aortic repair (EVAR).[1,3] Over the last 3 decades, EVAR has become the preferred treatment for AAA repair for most patients. In the USA, about 80% of all the AAA are treated with EVAR.[4]

INDICATIONS

Elective AAA repair is considered in asymptomatic patients with fusiform aneurysm with a diameter ≥5.5 cm and rapidly expanding sac (≥5 mm/6 months or 10 mm/year). Repair is also considered for a diameter ≥5 cm for women due to higher rupture risk and smaller aortas.[5,6] In addition, earlier repair is reasonable for those with a saccular aneurysm. Emergent repair of the AAA is recommended in patients with symptomatic AAA (evidence of distal embolization, abdominal/back pain, and/or rupture).

CONTRAINDICATIONS

The contraindications for an EVAR are primarily based on vessel anatomy.[7] Few absolute contraindications exist for EVAR. Even with adverse anatomy, new techniques or experimental devices often allow EVAR, but there is potentially an increased risk of future sac growth and rupture. Important relative contraindications include:

i. Adverse infrarenal aortic neck anatomy (Fig. 1)

---

[a] Department of Cardiovascular Medicine, University of Kansas School of Medicine, 3901 Rainbow Boulevard, Kansas City, KS 66209, USA; [b] Weill Cornell Medical College, 520 East 70th Street, Starr 4, F-441-B, New York, NY 10021, USA
* Corresponding author.
E-mail address: kgupta@kumc.edu

Intervent Cardiol Clin 14 (2025) 173–190
https://doi.org/10.1016/j.iccl.2024.11.005
2211-7458/25/© 2024 Elsevier Inc. All rights reserved, including those for text and data mining, AI training, and similar technologies.

ii. Suprarenal aneurysmal disease (unless using fenestrated devices)
iii. Bilateral iliac artery aneurysm
iv. Excessive iliac artery tortuosity especially with accompanying calcification and stenosis

Chronic kidney disease (CKD) is a relative contraindication due to the risk of contrast nephropathy. However, the use of intravascular ultrasound (IVUS) can minimize contrast use, mitigating this concern.[8,9] Further, OSR also carries a risk of worsening acute kidney injury and is associated with more frequent rates of adverse outcomes on renal function compared to EVAR in some studies.[10,11] Limited life expectancy is also considered a contraindication for both EVAR and OSR. To note, inability to comply with regular follow-up imaging for endoleak monitoring is an absolute contraindication for EVAR.

ENDOVASCULAR ANEURYSM REPAIR EVIDENCE BASE

There is a large body of evidence comparing both short-term and long-term outcomes of EVAR and OSR for AAA repair. The Dutch

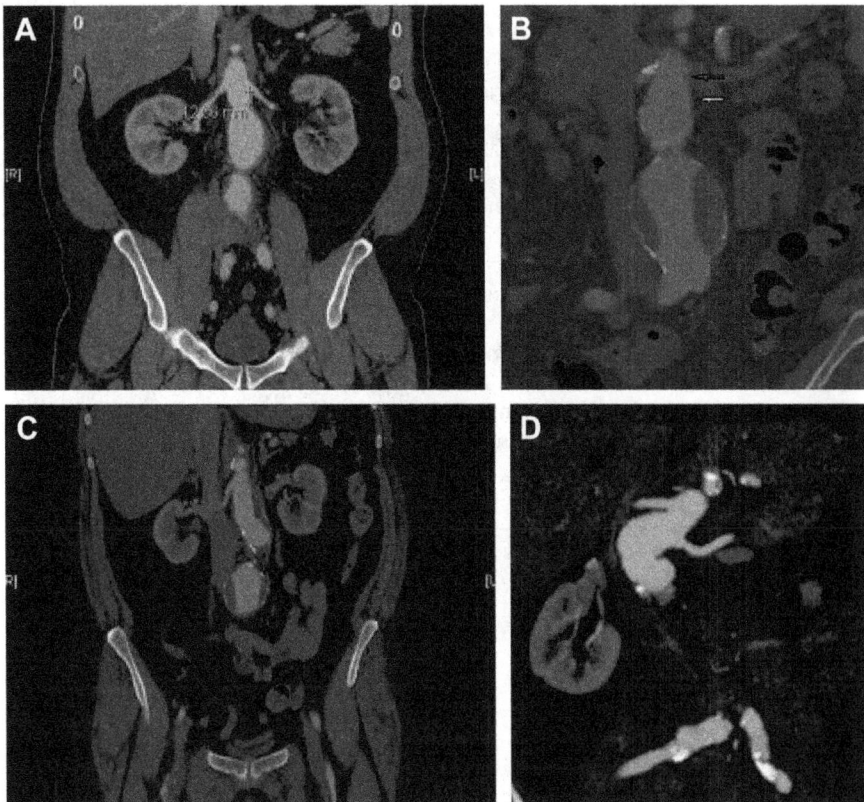

Fig. 1. Examples of adverse proximal neck anatomy. (A) Short (<15 mm) neck, (B) Reverse taper neck (*white and black arrow*), (C) Thick thrombus layer and dilated neck, (D) Tortuous and angulated neck.

Randomized Endovascular Aneurysm Management (DREAM) trial,[12,13] the UK Endovascular Aneurysm Repair versus Open Repair in Patients with Abdominal Aortic Aneurysm (EVAR -1) trial,[14] the U.S. Veterans Open versus Endovascular Repair (OVER) trial,[15] and the Anevrysme de L'aorte abdominale Chirugie versus Endoprosthe (ACE) trial[16] are the pivotal trials, which have helped establish EVAR as the standard-of-care for AAA repair. The key results of these trials are summarized in Table 1.

Meta-analysis shows that the EVAR cohort has lower short-term mortality (1.4% vs 4.2%), shorter hospital stays, and fewer complications compared to OSR. However, long-term mortality is similar, potentially due to patient comorbidities and late sac growth leading to rupture from endoleaks.[17–22] Notably, EVAR also has higher re-intervention rates due to endoleaks.[23] However, these studies are based on older technology and techniques, and the outcomes may change as endovascular graft technology and complication management continue to improve.[24]

ENDOVASCULAR ANEURYSM REPAIR DEVICES

Multiple EVAR devices are approved in the US[25,26] each with specific anatomic criteria in their instructions for use (IFU).[25] IFUs are based on device engineering, clinical trials, preclinical tests, and anatomic risk factors.[25] Anatomic factors include neck length, diameter, angle, and iliac diameter.[26] EVAR devices are categorized as suprarenal or infrarenal fixation based on proximal attachment site.

Infrarenal Fixation
These devices involve placement of the stent-graft in the infrarenal aorta without any graft or device material extending superior to the origin of the renal arteries. Most infrarenal fixation devices require a proximal sealing zone of at least 15 mm in length, aortic neck diameter less than 32 mm, and a neck angulation of less than 60°.[24]

Suprarenal Fixation
The suprarenal fixation devices have metallic stents (but not graft material) extending superior to the origin of the renal arteries.[26] Superior stent extensions may include hooks/barbs for suprarenal aortic wall attachment. While generally used routinely, some operators prefer them for unfavorable neck anatomy (shorter neck, significant angulation).[24] Bare metal struts crossing renal and visceral artery origins have shown safety comparable to infrarenal fixation devices

in observational studies.[27,28] A recent meta-analysis did not show significant differences in renal complications with the use of suprarenal devices compared to infrarenal devices.[29]

Device Innovations
While in current practice, EVAR is being performed in most patients who have an AAA large enough to be repaired, many of these patients do not meet the strict anatomic criterion for EVAR with currently available (US Food and Drug Administration-approved) devices in the USA. If one went strictly by IFU, greater than 60% of infrarenal AAA may be ineligible for EVAR.[26] Advancing technology and newer devices have been introduced to expand EVAR eligibility. For example, the Heli-FX EndoAnchor system (Aptus Endosystems, Sunnyvale, Calif) is FDA-approved to mimic surgical suture by applying endovascular stapling of graft to infrarenal aortic wall, thereby preventing leaks and graft slippage. Real-world registry and retrospective data have confirmed the safety and efficacy in preventing and treating proximal type 1 endoleaks in patients with unfavorable neck anatomy (Fig. 2).[30–32] In addition, Gore Excluder Conformable AAA Endoprosthesis allows for treating infrarenal AAA with neck angulations up to 90°, demonstrating high efficacy in aneurysm treatment at 1 year (Fig. 3).[33]

PATIENT SELECTION

AAA is classified based on its relation to renal arteries: suprarenal extends above, juxtarenal reaches up to, infrarenal occurs below, and pararenal sits at the level of the renal arteries.

Suitable aortic and access vessel anatomy are the key determinants of a successful endovascular repair.[34] AAA is classified based on its relation to renal arteries: suprarenal extends above, juxtarenal reaches up to, infrarenal occurs below, and pararenal sits at the level of the renal arteries.[35] Endovascular repair is best suited for infrarenal AAA where renal arteries are not involved. Technologic advances such as the use of fenestrated grafts, physician modified grafts and the use of advanced techniques such as snorkels/chimneys can allow endovascular repairs of more complex AAA types that encroaches the renal arteries.[36] However, there is a high incidence of late endoleaks and/or visceral vessel compromise.[37–40] A detailed discussion of this topic is beyond the scope of this article.[26]

Comorbid Factors
EVAR eligibility assessment includes comorbidities, such as CKD, cardiovascular disease, poor

Table 1
Summary of randomized controlled trials comparing the endovascular aortic repair and open surgical repair outcomes

| Study | Follow-up (Years) | Number of Patients | | Outcomes | | | | | |
| | | EVAR | OSR | 30-d Mortality | | | Long-Term Mortality | | |
				EVAR	OSR	RR (95% CI; P-Value)	EVAR	OSR	95% CI; P-Value
DREAM	Range: 5.1–8.2 Mean: 6.4	173	178	1.2%	4.6%	RR 3.9 (0.9–32.9; 0.10)	31.1%	30.1%	Difference 1% point (−8.8–10.8; 0.97)
EVAR-1	Median: 6.0	626	626	1.8%	4.3%	OR 0.39 (0.18–0.87; 0.02)	7.5/100-person y	7.7/100-person y	HR 1.03 (0.86–1.23; 0.72)
OVER	Mean: 5.2	444	437	0.5%	3.0%	HR and CI not reported (P = .004)	32.9%	33.4%	HR 0.97 (0.77–1.25; 0.81)
ACE	Median: 3.0	150	149	1.3%	0.6%	p = NS	11.3%	8%	p = NS

Abbreviations: ACE, Anevrysme de L'aorte abdominale Chirugie versus Endoprosthe; CI, confidence interval; DREAM, Dutch randomized endovascular aneurysm management trial; EVAR, endovascular aortic repair; EVAR -1, endovascular aneurysm repair versus open repair in patients with abdominal aortic aneurysm trial; HR, hazard ratio; NS, not significant; OR, odds ratio; OSR, open surgical repair; OVER, U.S. veterans open versus endovascular repair trial; RR, relative risk.

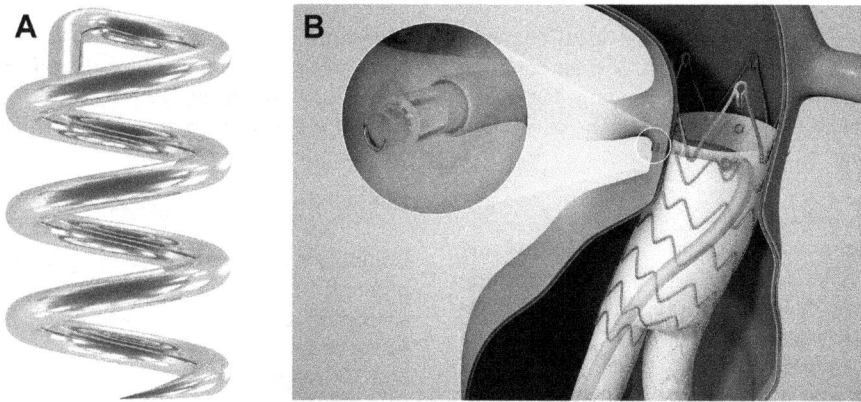

Fig. 2. Heli-FX Endoanchor endostapling system for proximal aortic neck type 1 Endoleak treatment and prophylaxis. (A) Individual endostaple, (B) delivery sheath deploying an endostaple to staple the graft material and aortic wall together. (*Reproduced with permission* of Medtronic, Inc.)

functional status, and chronic obstructive pulmonary disease. Bleeding diathesis and hematologic conditions, such as thrombocytopenia, may need to be factored in decision making as well. The 2018 Society of Vascular Surgery guidelines provide comprehensive information on these risk factors.[24]

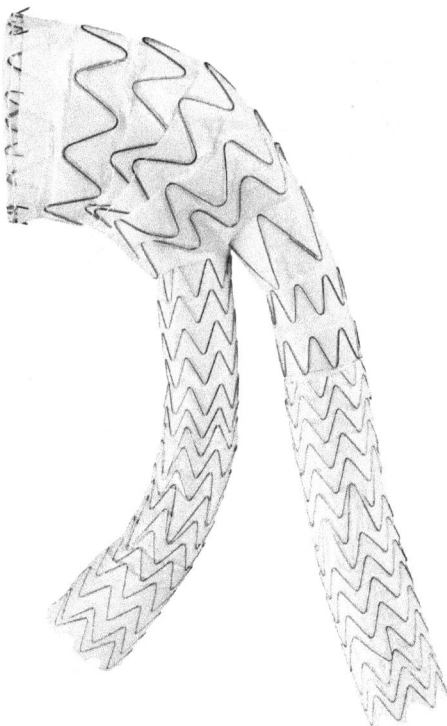

Fig. 3. Main body of the Gore Excluder Conformable bifurcated stent graft. The proximal body can be actively bent/curved during deployment to better conform to an angulated aortic neck. (GORE® EXCLUDER® Conformable AAA Endoprosthesis. See Instructions for Use for complete device information, including approved indications and safety information.)

Outcome in Elderly

Octogenarians comprise 25% of EVAR patients.[41] Although they face higher perioperative risks than younger cohort, studies demonstrate acceptable outcomes with EVAR.[41] EVAR is associated with improved 1-year mortality rates compared to OSR with similar 5-year mortality.[42] For patient with life expectancy of at least 5 years, there was a reintervention rate of 18%, emphasizing the importance of diligent follow-up even in this elderly population. However, major complication is associated with >2X mortality rate. Therefore, careful patient selection and evaluation is critical in this age group.

Anatomic Factors
Aortoiliac vessels

Access vessel anatomy is crucial for successful EVAR. Femoral and iliac arteries require adequate size with minimal tortuosity and calcification. Lower profile devices with the contemporary devices have increased wider application of EVAR procedures with decreased risk of access complication. Nevertheless, a distal aortic diameter ≥20 mm is recommended for bifurcated stent-graft placement.[43] AAA with small distal abdominal aorta may require either pretreatment of stenosis with angioplasty or conversion to aorto-uni-iliac graft with femoral to femoral bypass surgery. Iliac artery diameter, calcification, tortuosity, iliac angle, and common iliac artery length are important anatomic predictors for successful repair.[44] A minimum iliac diameter of 6 to 7 mm is usually needed for main body device delivery.[43] However, some lower-profile devices (14 F sheath compatible) can be delivered through even smaller vessels. Stenotic/occlusive iliac arteries may need intra-procedural treatment with angioplasty including lithotripsy if the vessel is heavily calcified. Aneurysmal common iliac artery may require graft extension to external iliac artery. Ideal common iliac length is greater than 3 cm. Shorter common iliac arteries may require extending the aortic stent-graft into the external iliac artery for successful distal fixation.[35]

Aneurysm neck
Suitable aortic neck anatomy is crucial for successful EVAR outcomes. Key factors include neck length, diameter, angle, shape, and presence of calcification or thrombus.[43,45,46]

Longer infrarenal aortic neck (>1.5 cm) and absence of significant calcification (especially protuberant calcific plaque) or thrombus are considered favorable factors.[35,43,45,46] Short neck length (<10 mm), neck angle greater than 60°, ≥ 50% circumferential proximal neck thrombus (≥2 mm thick), ≥50% calcified proximal neck, reverse taper neck, and a neck diameter greater than 31 mm are considered unfavorable for EVAR(see Fig. 1).[45,46]

Presence of a reverse tapered aortic neck is a strong predictor for early type I endoleak.[43] EVAR's long-term durability relies on a successful seal between the proximal aortic neck and stent-graft. Patients with larger aortic neck diameters face higher risks of type I endoleaks, more frequent reinterventions, increased aneurysmal sac expansion/rupture, and lower overall survival compared to those with smaller aortic necks undergoing EVAR.[34,45–47]

PREPROCEDURAL IMAGING

Computed tomography (CT) angiography is the primary imaging modality for preprocedural anatomic assessment and EVAR planning. Advanced software enabling centerline method and 3D image processing is crucial, especially for complex aortoiliac anatomy. The centerline method provides highly accurate measurements, critical for planning cases with challenging anatomy (Fig. 4).In addition to providing the anatomic extent of the aneurysm and aortoiliac vasculature, unenhanced CT images are often used to evaluate arterial wall calcification and evaluate for a possible intramural hematoma in the acute setting.[35] Alternatively, MRI provides an option for patients who are unable to receive iodinated contrast.

Aneurysm Morphology
Similar to aortic neck anatomy, aneurysm sac morphology may also influence the success of

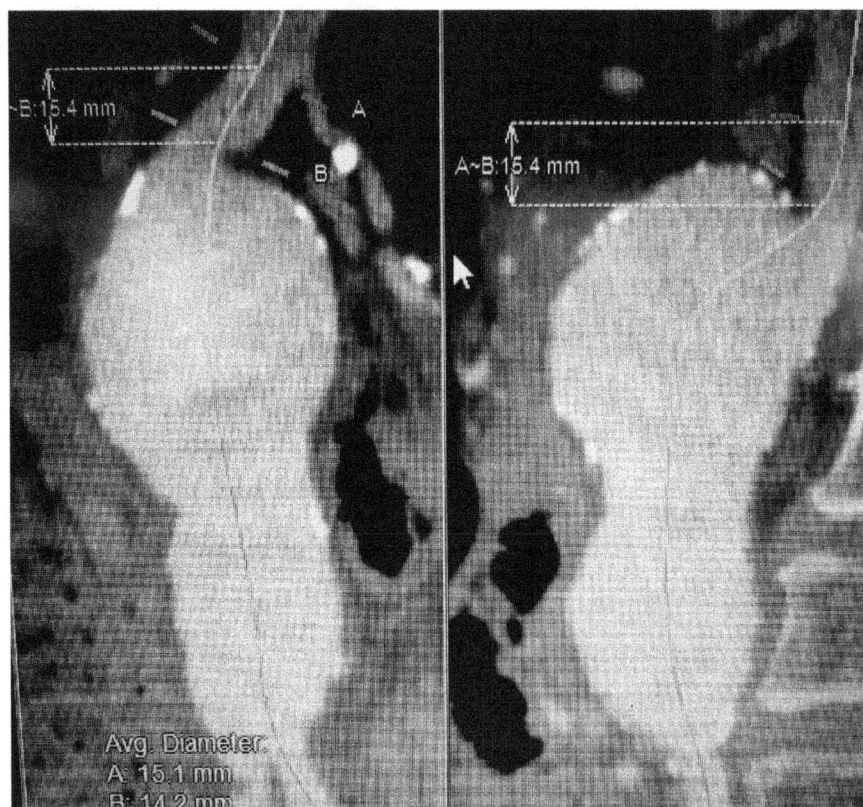

Fig. 4. The figure demonstrates how centerline method allows for accurate measurement of the proximal aortic neck and helps planning the case.

endovascular repair.⁴³ The aneurysmal angle, presence of branching vessels, and the presence of intramural thrombus are important anatomic factors. *Aortic aneurysm angle* is defined as the most acute angle in the line to the central lumen between the lowest renal artery and the aortic bifurcation.³⁵

Increased aneurysmal tortuosity is associated with challenging stent-graft delivery and deployment. Although rare, intra-luminal mural thrombus can cause distal embolization during device delivery. Aortic branches originating from the AAA, primarily inferior mesenteric (IMA) and lumbar arteries(LAs), serve as major collateral pathways and increase the risk of type II endoleaks post-EVAR.⁴³ It is important to note that majority of type II leaks do not lead to aneurysmal sac growth.

Stent-graft placement may occlude accessory renal arteries, potentially impairing renal function if these arteries perfuse a significant portion of the kidney. In addition, evaluation of the superior mesenteric artery is crucial, as the IMA is typically covered during EVAR. Patients with an occluded superior mesenteric artery face an increased risk of gut ischemia following the procedure.³⁵

PROCEDURE
Arterial Access
Historically, EVAR procedure has been performed with general anesthesia. However, the use of local anesthesia with moderate sedation is now widespread with contemporary EVAR procedures. Although surgical exposure via *cutdown* for common femoral arterial access is still occasionally performed for complex cases, a significant portion of cases are now being performed with percutaneous access with the advent of smaller devices and arterial closure devices. The Totally percutaneous access versus open femoral exposure for endovascular aortic aneurysm repair (PEVAR) Trial was a randomized, multicenter study that compared percutaneous access versus open femoral exposure for EVAR.⁴⁸ The study demonstrated that percutaneous EVAR was noninferior to the femoral cutdown, and was associated with reduced operative time, fewer wound complications, and shorter length-of-stay.⁴⁸

Ideally, percutaneous femoral access should be obtained by combining the use of fluoroscopy, ultrasound (US), micropuncture access, and femoral angiography. Targeted puncture of the anterior wall of common femoral artery (CFA) while avoiding calcified areas of the vessel can be performed with an US-guided access. Consequently, this leads to decreased risk

of access-related complications and facilitates the use of suture-based arterial site closure techniques. After the lower border of the femoral head is identified under fluoroscopy, US is used to visualize CFA and it's bifurcation. Subsequently, a micropuncture needle is inserted, under direct US guidance, to aim for anterior wall entry of the CFA. If the arterial stick is noted to be too high or too low, a repeat attempt can be made using the steps described earlier to target the middle third of the femoral head as the preferred needle entry point. Once a satisfactory wire position is achieved, a 6 or 7F sheath is advanced. A common femoral arteriogram could be obtained to confirm adequate sheath position prior to suture deployment. The standard method to perform percutaneous closure is to deploy 2 Perclose Proglide (Abbott Vascular) suture-mediated closure devices at 90° to each other. The sheath is then upsized sequentially to the desired sheath size to deliver the stent-graft. Similar technique of femoral arterial access is used to access contralateral CFA. Other newer devices for large bore closure are also in development or in early clinical use.

STENT-GRAFT DELIVERY

The decision for main body insertion side depends on several factors, including the caliber, tortuosity and calcification of common femoral and external iliac arteries, and aortic neck tortuosity and angulation. Another consideration in deciding which side serves as the main body side is the perceived ease of cannulating the *gate* of the contralateral limb. The final decision can be made with assistance of aortoiliac arteriogram as well. Once bilateral access is obtained, a digital subtraction aortogram (or limited arteriograms/IVUS in cases of renal insufficiency) is performed to confirm craniocaudal distance, aortic landmarks, and aneurysmal sac extent. Key measurements include the distance from the lower renal artery to the ipsilateral hypogastric artery and aortic bifurcation, proximal aortic neck diameter, and common iliac arteries diameters. The device is introduced over a stiff guidewire and positioned either for suprarenal or infrarenal fixation with the fabric-covered portion just distal to the lowest renal artery and the device is carefully deployed to expose the contralateral gate.²⁶,³⁵,⁴³

Thereafter, a guidewire and catheter are advanced in a retrograde fashion from contralateral side with careful cannulation of the gate. Extreme care is taken to ensure that this contralateral access did indeed occur through the gate and not anterior or posterior to the gate. This is usually done by advancing a curved catheter and rotating it to confirm intra-graft placement. Alternatively, IVUS can be used to confirm proper cannulation of the fate as well. At this stage, an angiogram may be obtained to determine the length of the contralateral limb from the gate to the distal attachment site (usually just proximal to the origin of the contralateral hypogastric artery). The contralateral iliac limb is then deployed over a stiff guidewire. Care is taken to ensure that there is adequate overlap between the main body at the gate and the contralateral limb (usually about 2–3 cm). An iliac extension limb can be used as needed in case of tall patients or an iliac bell-bottom extension limb can be used if the common iliac artery is ectatic. Using a compliant low-pressure balloon, the points of overlap and attachment sites are balloon dilated after stent-graft deployment. Occasionally high-pressure inflation with non-compliant balloons is needed to adequately expand the endograft, especially in the iliac arteries, in the presence of iliac artery stenosis or calcification. Completion angiography confirms renal and iliac artery patency, rules out proximal aortic dissection, and detects endoleaks.

STRATEGIES TO MANAGE COMMON ILIAC ARTERY ANEURYSM

EVAR devices are designed to seal distally in the common iliac arteries. However, dilatation and aneurysm of common iliac arteriess pose a technical challenge by preventing adequate distal seal and fixation. Various endovascular techniques are utilized in the contemporary era to overcome this challenge.[49] Two commonly used methods are discussed here.

Internal Iliac Artery Embolization

If the common iliac artery is too large to seal with an iliac limb graft, extension into the external iliac artery with a limb extender can be performed. However, this may result in an endoleak from the retrograde flow from the internal iliac artery (IIA). Therefore, the IIA needs to be occluded with either a placement of coils or a vascular plug followed by extension of the graft from the common iliac artery into the external iliac artery (Fig. 5). IIA exclusion can result in buttock claudication, erectile dysfunction, and rarely symptoms of pelvic ischemia such as pelvic or gluteal necrosis, colon ischemia, and spinal ischemia.[26,50,51] The complication rate is reported to be higher with bilateral IIA occlusion.[26,50,52] Unilateral embolization of the IIA carries a reported 26% to 41% risk of buttock claudication, but symptoms tend to improve with time.[24,53] Preservation of at least 1 IIA is recommended if possible. However, certain situations, such as bilateral iliac artery aneurysm, may require bilateral IIA occlusion. In such circumstances, technical considerations such as a staged-approach, embolization of only the proximal main trunk of IIA, preservation of collateral branches from the femoral arteries, and use of dedicated iliac branched endoprosthesis to maintain ipsilateral IIA perfusion should be considered.[24] Hybrid approaches to preserve one side IIA circulation such as bypass of IIA to the ipsilateral external iliac artery can also be considered in select cases.[54]

Iliac Branched Devices

Branch endoprosthesis have demonstrated high rates of technical success and excellent early patency.[26,55,56] Many versions of the branched devices have been developed, namely straight-branch iliac bifurcated device (IBD), Helical-

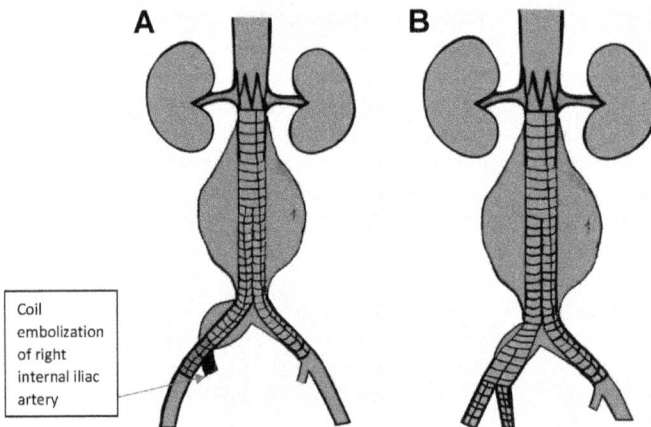

Coil embolization of right internal iliac artery

Fig. 5. Two common strategies to treat aneurysmal common iliac artery during EVAR. (A) Internal iliac artery occlusion (coils/plug) with iliac limb extension into external iliac artery. (B) Internal iliac flow preservation using bifurcated iliac stent graft to exclude iliac aneurysm.

branch IBD and bifurcated-bifurcated IBD.[57] The Gore Iliac Branch Endoprosthesis (Gore Medical, Flagstaff, AZ) is currently the only Iliac Branch device on the market and was approved for commercial use in 2016 (Fig. 6).[26] Bell-bottomed (flared) iliac endograft limbs, parallel endografting, and proximal endograft have been used to preserve antegrade IIA perfusion.[53,58,59] However, the addition of an Iliac branch limb to standard EVAR results in longer operative procedure time and increases the complexity of the procedure.[53] Long-term data on these iliac bifurcation devices now show a high rate of success in regards to sac exclusions and preservation of internal iliac flow with low rate of reintervention or complications.[60]

FOLLOW-UP

Long-term, clinical and radiologic follow-up is essential after EVAR to ensure continued successful exclusion of the AAA sac and to detect any problems such as graft limb kinking and thrombosis. Contrast-enhanced CT imaging is currently the preferred initial follow-up modality. CT allows for adequate visualization of the device location, limb patency, and endoleaks. However, CT use is associated with contrast use and radiation. If no endoleak is detected, then subsequent

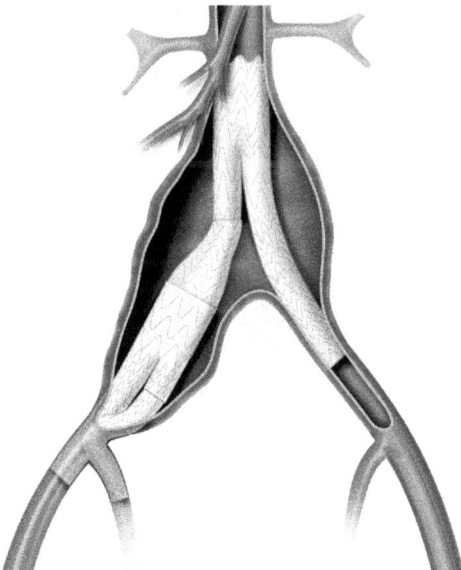

Fig. 6. Shows successful exclusion of an aortic and right common iliac aneurysm with a Gore Excluder Bifurcated stent graft with use of a Gore excluder iliac branched endoprosthesis attached into a bell-bottom right iliac limb of the aortic stent graft. (GORE® EXCLUDER® Iliac Branch Endoprosthesis. See Instructions for Use for complete device information, including approved indications and safety information.)

© 2006 W. L. Gore & Associates, Inc. Used with permission.

follow-ups can be performed with non-contrast CT scan (to monitor sac size) or with duplex US. Ultrasonic contrast-enhanced US is also being used in some centers to detect endoleaks.[61,62]

Current recommendations on post-procedure follow-up include CT angiography imaging at 1 month.[24] If any concerning findings are present (such as type 1), then the same imaging should be repeated at 6 months. If 1-month imaging does not show any endoleak (especially type I or III) or aneurysmal sac expansion, the 6-month follow-up can be omitted for a 1-year scan. Furthermore, if the 1-year imaging shows the absence of endoleak and stable aneurysmal sac, further imaging with duplex US can be considered to avoid contrast and radiation exposure.[24] If the patient had good anatomic features for EVAR, then it is reasonable to perform imaging every 5 years. However, if adverse features were present (such as the shorter neck) or if any endoleak is present, annual imaging should be considered. Prompt CT should be obtained for any new findings on surveillance duplex US.[24] The entire aorta should be imaged with CT every 5 years.

Patients should undergo complete lower extremity pulse examination and ankle-brachial index (ABI) at their follow-up.[24] Patients with new-onset lower extremity claudication, ischemia or reduction in ABIs should undergo a prompt evaluation to exclude graft limb occlusion.[24]

COMPLICATIONS

Early complications are mostly related to contrast use or access site complications. Access site complications after surgical cutdown include arterial dissection, perforation, arterial thrombosis, hematoma, lymphocele, embolization, infection, and pseudoaneurysm formation. The incidence has ranged from 1% to 2% (with a higher rate in earlier experience)[48,63,64] Access site complications have been reported to be significantly lower with the use of percutaneous access and closure.[64–66] Early graft limb thrombosis is rare but usually presents as an emergency with critical limb ischemia. It is more likely in patients with smaller, tortuous iliac arteries, external iliac stenosis causing limb kinking, or poor outflow due to distal arterial occlusive disease.[12,67] Inadequate high-pressure balloon angioplasty of narrowed iliac limbs is also a factor. Post-implantation syndrome, a self-limited inflammatory state, may occur, presenting with fever, flu-like symptoms, and leukocytosis. It must be distinguished from the more serious graft infection.[68,69] Endovascular graft infection is, fortunately, less common and in most studies is less than 1.0%.[70,71]

Ischemic colitis due to occlusion of the IMA or hypogastric artery or embolization is a rare event with an incidence of less than 1%.[72–75] This usually occurs in the presence of pre-existing visceral occlusive disease.

ENDOLEAKS

Endoleak refers to the persistence of blood flow in the aneurysmal sac after EVAR (Fig. 7).[24,26] Endoleaks are classified by the blood flow source into 4 major types, with some indeterminate cases referred to as type V.[2,24,76,77]

a. Type I: Occurs at the endovascular graft attachment site due to loss of seal with the aortic wall.

  i. Type IA: When leak or loss of seal occurs at the proximal end.
  ii. Type IB: When leak or loss of seal occurs at the distal end.

b. Type II: Occurs due to retrograde flow from the branch vessels arising from the AAA sac and now covered by the stent-graft (IMA, LAs, and median sacral artery). It is further subclassified into IIA (if the flow is from a single vessel) and IIB (if the flow is from multiple vessels).

c. Type III: Occurs due to lack of seal between stent-graft components (IIIA) or due to a defect/tear in the graft (IIIB).

d. Type IV: Occurs due to porosity of graft material (uncommon with most current generation devices).

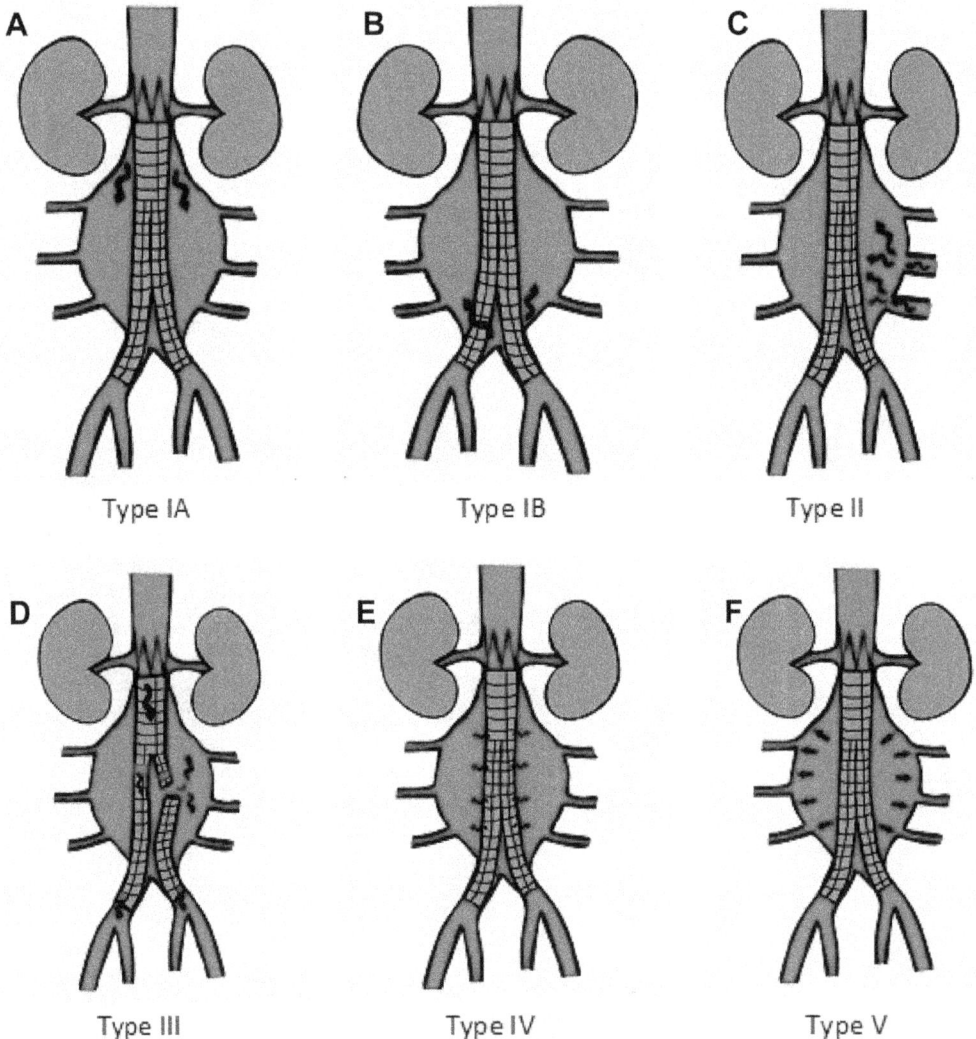

Type IA   Type IB   Type II

Type III   Type IV   Type V

Fig. 7. Different subtypes of endoleaks. (A) Type IA endoleak, (B) Type IB endoleak, (C) Type II endoleak, (D) Type III endoleak. (E) Type IV endoleak, (F) Type V endoleaks. Curved arrows indicate direction of blood flow. Straight arrows indicate direction of pressure transmission.

e. Type V: AAA sac growth without contrast material seen in the sac on imaging.

Endoleak is the most frequent complication following EVAR. Its incidence varies in literature, occurring in up to 25% of patients immediately after the procedure.[24,78] The OVER trial reported the combined incidence of endoleaks to be 30.5% (Type I 12.3%, Type II: 75.9%, Type III: 3.2%, Type IV: 2.7%, and Type V: 5.9%).[79] Buth and colleagues evaluated type I and III endoleaks from the EUROSTAR project, involving 110 European institutions. Patients with type I and III endoleaks had an average aneurysm diameter increase of 8 mm compared to those without. Significant infrarenal neck angulation, aneurysmal thrombus, and less center experience were linked to higher endoleak incidence.[80]

Abularrage and colleagues evaluated the incidence and predictors of persistent type II endoleaks. Patent IMA, multiple LAs, and a larger AAA sac size were significant predictors of persistent type II endoleaks with sac growth. Additional risk factors included increasing age and warfarin use.[81]

Management of Endoleaks
Majority of endoleaks are asymptomatic and are diagnosed on follow-up imaging. Type I and III usually require urgent action since these are relatively high-pressure endoleaks, which can lead to a rapid expansion of aneurysm and subsequent rupture.

Type I endoleaks
Traditionally, type I endoleaks were treated immediately, but recent evidence shows some early type IA endoleaks found at 1-month follow-up computed tomographic angiography may resolve spontaneously.[82]

Persistent type I endoleaks require treating the graft to ensure a proper seal of the endograft to the aortic wall. Initial approach is re-angioplasty at the aortic neck using a high-pressure balloon.[83] If this does not resolve the endoleaks, other options include placement of an aortic extension cuff (carefully avoiding covering the renal arteries) or a Palmaz type stent across the renal arteries.[84,85] More advanced techniques include use of endostaples (Heli-FX EndoAnchor system) (see Fig. 2), proximal extension with the use of chimney grafts, insertion of coils or glue (into the crevice between the graft material and aortic wall), conversion to fenestrated grafts, or to open repair.[30,86–91] Type IB endoleaks, often due to lack of apposition at the common iliac artery, are typically managed with iliac extension limbs if angioplasty fails. If there is no landing zone in the common iliac artery, the IIA may be coiled and the iliac limb extended, or a bifurcated iliac endoprosthesis may be used.

Type II endoleaks
Type II endoleaks, occurring in about 25% of EVAR cases, are typically benign with a low rupture risk. Half resolve spontaneously, but intervention is considered for persistent leaks causing ≥5 mm sac enlargement.[92,93] The goal of type II endoleak treatment is the elimination of aneurysm perfusing branch vessels. Both open and laparoscopic techniques have been described to eliminate side branch perfusion. However, endovascular methods are generally

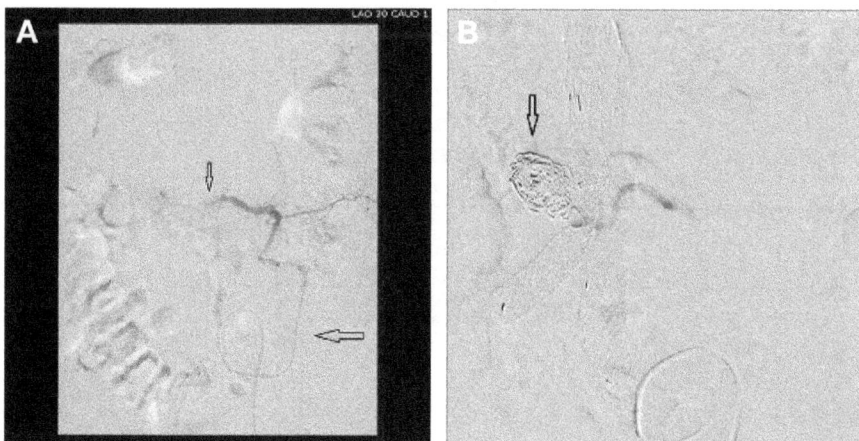

Fig. 8. Angiographic images of trans-arterial coil embolization of type 2 endoleak: (A) Microcatheter advanced via iliolumbar artery into lumbar branch (*horizontal arrow*). Lumbar branch emptying into aneurysm sac (*vertical arrow*). Bifurcated stent graft visible. (B) Microcatheter advanced into aneurysm sac. Coils inserted into aneurysm (*vertical arrow*).

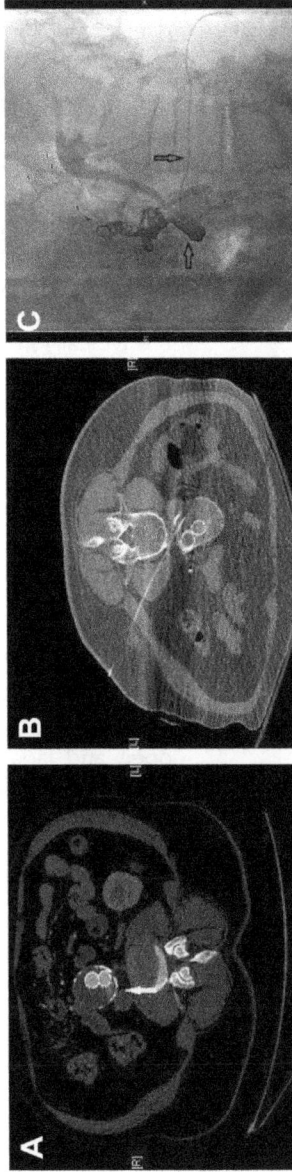

Fig. 9. This figure shows translumbar embolization for type 2 endoleak: (A) Axial computed tomography (CT): Aneurysm sac with bifurcated stent graft; arrow indicates endoleak contrast. (B) CT-guided needle placement into sac via translumbar approach; patient prone. (C) Fluoroscopy during embolization: Microcatheter entering sac (vertical arrow), injected embolic glue (horizontal arrow), visible coils superiorly.

preferred. Endovascular methods for side branch embolization include transarterial embolization (TAE), CT-guided translumbar embolization (TLE) and transcaval embolization (TCE). All these methods involve embolization of the feeding vessel (IMA or LAs) using coils, thrombin, gel foam, or onyx glue.[81,94] When direct catheterization of the feeding vessel is not possible, an alternative approach is used. In these cases, the embolic material is deployed within the aneurysm sac, specifically near the origin of the feeding vessels. These techniques use various embolic materials to block the feeding vessels. TAE is most common, accessed via transfemoral or trans-brachial approaches (Fig. 8). When this approach is not feasible due to inaccessible IMA, IIAs or prior failed transarterial approach due to vessel tortuosity, the alternative endovascular techniques such as TLE or TCE have been utilized to achieve successful embolization of the feeding vessels (Fig. 9).[95,96] TLE have shown safety, but their efficacy in halting AAA growth, particularly in larger aneurysms or those with Moyamoya leaks, remains limited.[97] TAE with neurointerventional materials shows promising 2-year outcomes.[98,99] A more recently, laser-assisted transgraft embolization has been described as an alternative methods.[100,101] Recent innovations in endoleak treatment have highlighted TCE as a promising option for type 2 endoleaks, boasting technical success rates of up to 90%.[102,103] This technique offers several advantages over traditional translumbar and transarterial methods. Unlike the TLE approach, TCE does not require CT guidance,[102] significantly simplifying the process. Given the high rate of reintervention for persistent endoleaks, TCE provides the additional benefit of preserving arterial access.[23] Regardless of the technique used, the long-term recurrence rate is relatively high with the need for reintervention.[104] When catheter-based techniques fail, open surgical sac resection is typically effective without endograft removal.

Persistent Type II endoleaks increase the risk of adverse events following EVAR for AAAs, including aneurysm enlargement, reintervention, ruptures, and mortality.[105] Imaging-based predictors, such as unsharp or blurred endoleak delineation on pre-interventional CT, may indicate persistent endoleaks and progressive aneurysm sac growth post-embolization.[106] Several risk factors for aneurysm sac enlargement post-EVAR have been identified, including advanced age, female sex, wide proximal neck,[105] CKD stage 4 or higher, patent IMA, and the number of patent LAs.[107] Preemptive embolization of

aneurysm sac side branches before EVAR reduces Type II endoleaks, promoting sac shrinkage and lowering postprocedure endoleak rates.[108–113] However, the efficacy of this approach remains debated, with some research indicating no benefit.[114]

Type III endoleaks
Type III endoleak is treated by addressing the defect involving the graft, typically with extension relining the disrupted zone. I.

Type IV endoleaks
Type IV endoleak is uncommon with current devices, occurs due to graft material porosity.

Type V endoleaks
Type V endoleaks likely result from pressure transmission through the graft or undetectable persistent flow. While their natural history is unclear, most can be observed unless sac growth occurs. Treatment options include endograft relining or, rarely, open repair.[115]

SUMMARY
EVAR is preferred for AAA repair due to lower perioperative risks than OSR. Endoleaks are common, with Type II often needing only observation, while Types I and III require prompt treatment. Most endoleaks are manageable via endovascular methods. Aortic neck and iliac artery anatomy strongly predict endoleak risk and complications. Advancing technology is expanding EVAR eligibility. Regular, long-term imaging follow-up is crucial post-EVAR; inability to comply contraindicates the procedure.

DISCLOSURE
Authors have no financial conflicts of interest to disclose.

REFERENCES
1. Eliason JL, Upchurch GR Jr. Endovascular abdominal aortic aneurysm repair. Circulation 2008; 117(13):1738–44.
2. Hirsch AT, Haskal ZJ, Hertzer NR, et al. ACC/AHA 2005 practice guidelines for the management of patients with peripheral arterial disease (lower extremity, renal, mesenteric, and abdominal aortic): a collaborative report from the American association for vascular surgery/society for vascular surgery, society for cardiovascular angiography and interventions, society for vascular medicine and biology, society of interventional radiology, and the ACC/AHA task force on practice guidelines (writing committee to develop guidelines

for the management of patients with peripheral arterial disease): endorsed by the American association of cardiovascular and pulmonary rehabilitation; National Heart, Lung, and blood Institute; Society for vascular nursing; TransAtlantic intersociety consensus; and vascular disease foundation. Circulation 2006;113(11):e463–654.

3. Volodos NL, Shekhanin VE, Karpovich IP, et al. A self-fixing synthetic blood vessel endoprosthesis. Vestn Khir Im I I Grekova 1986;137(11):123–5. Samofiksiruiushchiisia sinteticheskii protez dlia endoprotezirovaniia sosudov.

4. Dua A, Kuy S, Lee CJ, et al. Epidemiology of aortic aneurysm repair in the United States from 2000 to 2010. J Vasc Surg 2014;59(6):1512–7.

5. Heikkinen M, Salenius JP, Auvinen O. Ruptured abdominal aortic aneurysm in a well-defined geographic area. J Vasc Surg 2002;36(2):291–6.

6. Naylor AR, Forbes TL. Trans-Atlantic debate: whether evidence supports reducing the threshold diameter to 5 cm for elective interventions in women with abdominal aortic aneurysms. Eur J Vasc Endovasc Surg 2014;48(6):611.

7. Endovascular repair of abdominal aortic aneurysm: an evidence-based analysis. Ont Health Technol Assess Ser 2002;2(1):1–46.

8. von Segesser LK, Marty B, Ruchat P, et al. Routine use of intravascular ultrasound for endovascular aneurysm repair: angiography is not necessary. Eur J Vasc Endovasc Surg 2002;23(6):537–42.

9. Pecoraro F, Bracale UM, Farina A, et al. Single-center experience and preliminary results of intravascular ultrasound in endovascular aneurysm repair. Ann Vasc Surg 2019;56:209–15.

10. Wald R, Waikar SS, Liangos O, et al. Acute renal failure after endovascular vs open repair of abdominal aortic aneurysm. J Vasc Surg 2006;43(3):460–6 [discussion: 466].

11. Saratzis A, Sarafidis P, Melas N, et al. Comparison of the impact of open and endovascular abdominal aortic aneurysm repair on renal function. J Vasc Surg 2014;60(3):597–603.

12. De Bruin JL, Baas AF, Buth J, et al. Long-term outcome of open or endovascular repair of abdominal aortic aneurysm. N Engl J Med 2010;362(20):1881–9.

13. Prinssen M, Verhoeven EL, Buth J, et al. A randomized trial comparing conventional and endovascular repair of abdominal aortic aneurysms. N Engl J Med 2004;351(16):1607–18.

14. Greenhalgh RM, Brown LC, Powell JT, et al. Endovascular versus open repair of abdominal aortic aneurysm. N Engl J Med 2010;362(20):1863–71.

15. Lederle FA, Freischlag JA, Kyriakides TC, et al. Long-term comparison of endovascular and open repair of abdominal aortic aneurysm. N Engl J Med 2012;367(21):1988–97.

16. Becquemin JP, Pillet JC, Lescalie F, et al. A randomized controlled trial of endovascular aneurysm repair versus open surgery for abdominal aortic aneurysms in low- to moderate-risk patients. J Vasc Surg 2011;53(5):1167–73.e1.

17. Paravastu SC, Jayarajasingam R, Cottam R, et al. Endovascular repair of abdominal aortic aneurysm. Cochrane Database Syst Rev 2014;(1):Cd004178.

18. Doonan RJ, Girsowicz E, Dubois L, et al. A systematic review and meta-analysis of endovascular juxtarenal aortic aneurysm repair demonstrates lower perioperative mortality compared with open repair. J Vasc Surg 2019. https://doi.org/10.1016/j.jvs.2019.04.464.

19. Li B, Khan S, Salata K, et al. A systematic review and meta-analysis of the long-term outcomes of endovascular versus open repair of abdominal aortic aneurysm. J Vasc Surg 2019. https://doi.org/10.1016/j.jvs.2019.01.076.

20. Bulder RMA, Bastiaannet E, Hamming JF, et al. Meta-analysis of long-term survival after elective endovascular or open repair of abdominal aortic aneurysm. Br J Surg 2019;106(5):523–33.

21. Stather PW, Sidloff D, Dattani N, et al. Systematic review and meta-analysis of the early and late outcomes of open and endovascular repair of abdominal aortic aneurysm. Br J Surg 2013;100(7):863–72.

22. Kontopodis N, Antoniou SA, Georgakarakos E, et al. Endovascular vs open aneurysm repair in the young: systematic review and meta-analysis. J Endovasc Ther 2015;22(6):897–904.

23. Wanken ZJ, Barnes JA, Trooboff SW, et al. A systematic review and meta-analysis of long-term reintervention after endovascular abdominal aortic aneurysm repair. J Vasc Surg 2020;72(3):1122–31.

24. Chaikof EL, Dalman RL, Eskandari MK, et al. The Society for Vascular Surgery practice guidelines on the care of patients with an abdominal aortic aneurysm. J Vasc Surg 2018;67(1):2–77.e2.

25. de Vries JP. The proximal neck: the remaining barrier to a complete EVAR world. Semin Vasc Surg 2012;25(4):182–6.

26. Swerdlow NJ, Wu WW, Schermerhorn ML. Open and endovascular management of aortic aneurysms. Circ Res 2019;124(4):647–61.

27. O'Donnell ME, Sun Z, Winder RJ, et al. Suprarenal fixation of endovascular aortic stent grafts: assessment of medium-term to long-term renal function by analysis of juxtarenal stent morphology. J Vasc Surg 2007;45(4):694–700.

28. Antonello M, Menegolo M, Piazza M, et al. Outcomes of endovascular aneurysm repair on renal function compared with open repair. J Vasc Surg 2013;58(4):886–93.

29. Miller LE, Razavi MK, Lal BK. Suprarenal versus infrarenal stent graft fixation on renal complications after endovascular aneurysm repair. J Vasc Surg 2015;61(5):1340–9.e1.
30. Jordan WD Jr, Mehta M, Varnagy D, et al. Results of the ANCHOR prospective, multicenter registry of EndoAnchors for type Ia endoleaks and endograft migration in patients with challenging anatomy. J Vasc Surg 2014;60(4):885–92.e2.
31. Muhs BE, Jordan W, Ouriel K, et al. Matched cohort comparison of endovascular abdominal aortic aneurysm repair with and without EndoAnchors. J Vasc Surg 2018;67(6):1699–707.
32. Masoomi R, Lancaster E, Robinson A, et al. Safety of endoanchors in real-world use: a report from the manufacturer and user facility device experience database. Vascular 2019;1708538119844041.
33. Rhee R, Oderich G, Han S, et al. One-year results of the GORE EXCLUDER Conformable AAA Endoprosthesis system in the United States regulatory trial. J Vasc Surg 2022/10/01/2022;76(4):951–9.e2.
34. Antoniou GA, Georgiadis GS, Antoniou SA, et al. A meta-analysis of outcomes of endovascular abdominal aortic aneurysm repair in patients with hostile and friendly neck anatomy. J Vasc Surg 2013;57(2):527–38.
35. Bryce Y, Rogoff P, Romanelli D, et al. Endovascular repair of abdominal aortic aneurysms: vascular anatomy, device selection, procedure, and procedure-specific complications. Radiographics 2015;35(2):593–615.
36. Atkins AD, Atkins MD. Branched and fenestrated aortic endovascular grafts. Methodist Debakey Cardiovasc J 2023;19(2):15–23.
37. Ziegler P, Avgerinos ED, Umscheid T, et al. Fenestrated endografting for aortic aneurysm repair: a 7-year experience. J Endovasc Ther 2007;14(5):609–18.
38. Verhoeven EL, Katsargyris A, Oikonomou K, et al. Fenestrated endovascular aortic aneurysm repair as a first line treatment option to treat short necked, juxtarenal, and suprarenal aneurysms. Eur J Vasc Endovasc Surg 2016;51(6):775–81.
39. Roy IN, Millen AM, Jones SM, et al. Long-term follow-up of fenestrated endovascular repair for juxtarenal aortic aneurysm. Br J Surg 2017;104(8):1020–7.
40. Scali ST, Feezor RJ, Chang CK, et al. Critical analysis of results after chimney endovascular aortic aneurysm repair raises cause for concern. J Vasc Surg 2014;60(4):865–73 [discussion: 873–5].
41. Raju S, Eisenberg N, Montbriand J, et al. Endovascular repair of abdominal aortic aneurysm in octogenarians: clinical outcomes and complications. Can J Surg 2020;63(4):E329–e337.
42. Scallan O, Novick T, Power AH, et al. Long-term outcomes comparing endovascular and open abdominal aortic aneurysm repair in octogenarians. J Vasc Surg 2020;71(4):1162–8.
43. Kim HO, Yim NY, Kim JK, et al. Endovascular aneurysm repair for abdominal aortic aneurysm: a comprehensive review. Korean J Radiol 2019;20(8):1247–65.
44. Wyss TR, Dick F, Brown LC, et al. The influence of thrombus, calcification, angulation, and tortuosity of attachment sites on the time to the first graft-related complication after endovascular aneurysm repair. J Vasc Surg 2011;54(4):965–71.
45. Aburahma AF, Campbell JE, Mousa AY, et al. Clinical outcomes for hostile versus favorable aortic neck anatomy in endovascular aortic aneurysm repair using modular devices. J Vasc Surg 2011;54(1):13–21.
46. AbuRahma AF, Yacoub M, Mousa AY, et al. Aortic neck anatomic features and predictors of outcomes in endovascular repair of abdominal aortic aneurysms following vs not following instructions for use. J Am Coll Surg 2016;222(4):579–89.
47. Kouvelos GN, Antoniou G, Spanos K, et al. Endovascular aneurysm repair in patients with a wide proximal aortic neck: a systematic review and meta-analysis of comparative studies. J Cardiovasc Surg 2019;60(2):167–74.
48. Nelson PR, Kracjer Z, Kansal N, et al. A multicenter, randomized, controlled trial of totally percutaneous access versus open femoral exposure for endovascular aortic aneurysm repair (the PEVAR trial). J Vasc Surg 2014;59(5):1181–93.
49. Bekdache K, Dietzek AM, Cha A, et al. Endovascular hypogastric artery preservation during endovascular aneurysm repair: a review of current techniques and devices. Ann Vasc Surg 2015;29(2):367–76.
50. Bosanquet DC, Wilcox C, Whitehurst L, et al. Systematic review and meta-analysis of the effect of internal iliac artery exclusion for patients undergoing EVAR. Eur J Vasc Endovasc Surg 2017;53(4):534–48.
51. McGarry JG, Alenezi AO, McGrath FP, et al. How safe is internal iliac artery embolisation prior to EVAR? A 10-year retrospective review. Ir J Med Sci 2016;185(4):865–9.
52. Kouvelos GN, Katsargyris A, Antoniou GA, et al. Outcome after interruption or preservation of internal iliac artery flow during endovascular repair of abdominal aorto-iliac aneurysms. Eur J Vasc Endovasc Surg 2016;52(5):621–34.
53. Farivar BS, Abbasi MN, Dias AP, et al. Durability of iliac artery preservation associated with endovascular repair of infrarenal aortoiliac aneurysms. J Vasc Surg 2017;66(4):1028–36.e18.
54. Hosaka A, Kato M, Kato I, et al. Outcome after concomitant unilateral embolization of the internal iliac artery and contralateral external-to-internal iliac artery bypass grafting during endovascular aneurysm repair. J Vasc Surg 2011;54(4):960–4.

55. Karthikesalingam A, Hinchliffe RJ, Holt PJ, et al. Endovascular aneurysm repair with preservation of the internal iliac artery using the iliac branch graft device. Eur J Vasc Endovasc Surg 2010; 39(3):285–94.

56. Serracino-Inglott F, Bray AE, Myers P. Endovascular abdominal aortic aneurysm repair in patients with common iliac artery aneurysms–Initial experience with the Zenith bifurcated iliac side branch device. J Vasc Surg 2007;46(2):211–7.

57. Wong S, Greenberg RK, Brown CR, et al. Endovascular repair of aortoiliac aneurysmal disease with the helical iliac bifurcation device and the bifurcated-bifurcated iliac bifurcation device. J Vasc Surg 2013;58(4):861–9.

58. Malina M, Dirven M, Sonesson B, et al. Feasibility of a branched stent-graft in common iliac artery aneurysms. J Endovasc Ther 2006;13(4):496–500.

59. Ziegler P, Avgerinos ED, Umscheid T, et al. Branched iliac bifurcation: 6 years experience with endovascular preservation of internal iliac artery flow. J Vasc Surg 2007;46(2):204–10.

60. Schneider DB, Matsumura JS, Lee JT, et al. Five-year outcomes from a prospective, multicenter study of endovascular repair of iliac artery aneurysms using an iliac branch device. J Vasc Surg 2023;77(1):122–8.

61. Kapetanios D, Kontopodis N, Mavridis D, et al. Meta-analysis of the accuracy of contrast-enhanced ultrasound for the detection of endoleak after endovascular aneurysm repair. J Vasc Surg 2019;69(1):280–94.e6.

62. Jawad N, Parker P, Lakshminarayan R. The role of contrast-enhanced ultrasound imaging in the follow-up of patients post-endovascular aneurysm repair. Ultrasound 2016;24(1):50–9.

63. Cuypers P, Buth J, Harris PL, et al. Realistic expectations for patients with stent-graft treatment of abdominal aortic aneurysms. Results of a European multicentre registry. Eur J Vasc Endovasc Surg 1999;17(6):507–16.

64. Buck DB, Karthaus EG, Soden PA, et al. Percutaneous versus femoral cutdown access for endovascular aneurysm repair. J Vasc Surg 2015;62(1):16–21.

65. Malkawi AH, Hinchliffe RJ, Holt PJ, et al. Percutaneous access for endovascular aneurysm repair: a systematic review. Eur J Vasc Endovasc Surg 2010; 39(6):676–82.

66. Lee WA, Brown MP, Nelson PR, et al. Midterm outcomes of femoral arteries after percutaneous endovascular aortic repair using the Preclose technique. J Vasc Surg 2008;47(5):919–23.

67. Mehta M, Sternbach Y, Taggert JB, et al. Long-term outcomes of secondary procedures after endovascular aneurysm repair. J Vasc Surg 2010; 52(6):1442–9.

68. Arnaoutoglou E, Kouvelos G, Papa N, et al. Prospective evaluation of post-implantation inflammatory response after EVAR for AAA: influence on patients' 30 day outcome. Eur J Vasc Endovasc Surg 2015;49(2):175–83.

69. Moulakakis KG, Alepaki M, Sfyroeras GS, et al. The impact of endograft type on inflammatory response after endovascular treatment of abdominal aortic aneurysm. J Vasc Surg 2013;57(3):668–77.

70. Schermerhorn ML, O'Malley AJ, Jhaveri A, et al. Endovascular vs. open repair of abdominal aortic aneurysms in the Medicare population. N Engl J Med 2008;358(5):464–74.

71. Vogel TR, Symons R, Flum DR. The incidence and factors associated with graft infection after aortic aneurysm repair. J Vasc Surg 2008;47(2):264–9.

72. Dadian N, Ohki T, Veith FJ, et al. Overt colon ischemia after endovascular aneurysm repair: the importance of microembolization as an etiology. J Vasc Surg 2001;34(6):986–96.

73. Maldonado TS, Rockman CB, Riles E, et al. Ischemic complications after endovascular abdominal aortic aneurysm repair. J Vasc Surg 2004;40(4):703–9 [discussion: 709-10].

74. Miller A, Marotta M, Scordi-Bello I, et al. Ischemic colitis after endovascular aortoiliac aneurysm repair: a 10-year retrospective study. Arch Surg 2009;144(10):900–3.

75. Becquemin JP, Majewski M, Fermani N, et al. Colon ischemia following abdominal aortic aneurysm repair in the era of endovascular abdominal aortic repair. J Vasc Surg 2008;47(2):258–63 [discussion: 263].

76. Rooke TW, Hirsch AT, Misra S, et al. ACCF/AHA focused update of the guideline for the management of patients with peripheral artery disease (updating the 2005 guideline): a report of the American college of cardiology foundation/American heart association task force on practice guidelines. J Am Coll Cardiol 2011;58(19):2020–45.

77. Erbel R, Aboyans V, Boileau C, et al. 2014 ESC Guidelines on the diagnosis and treatment of aortic diseases: document covering acute and chronic aortic diseases of the thoracic and abdominal aorta of the adult. The task force for the diagnosis and treatment of aortic diseases of the European Society of Cardiology (ESC). Eur Heart J 2014;35(41):2873–926.

78. Abularrage CJ, Patel VI, Conrad MF, et al. Improved results using Onyx glue for the treatment of persistent type 2 endoleak after endovascular aneurysm repair. J Vasc Surg 2012;56(3):630–6.

79. Lal BK, Zhou W, Li Z, et al. Predictors and outcomes of endoleaks in the veterans affairs open versus endovascular repair (OVER) trial of abdominal aortic aneurysms. J Vasc Surg 2015;62(6):1394–404.

80. Buth J, Harris PL, van Marrewijk C, et al. The significance and management of different types of endoleaks. Semin Vasc Surg 2003;16(2):95–102.

81. Abularrage CJ, Crawford RS, Conrad MF, et al. Preoperative variables predict persistent type 2 endoleak after endovascular aneurysm repair. J Vasc Surg 2010;52(1):19–24.

82. O'Donnell TFX, Corey MR, Deery SE, et al. Select early type IA endoleaks after endovascular aneurysm repair will resolve without secondary intervention. J Vasc Surg 2018;67(1):119–25.

83. Thomas BG, Sanchez LA, Geraghty PJ, et al. A comparative analysis of the outcomes of aortic cuffs and converters for endovascular graft migration. J Vasc Surg 2010;51(6):1373–80.

84. Arthurs ZM, Lyden SP, Rajani RR, et al. Long-term outcomes of Palmaz stent placement for intraoperative type Ia endoleak during endovascular aneurysm repair. Ann Vasc Surg 2011;25(1):120–6.

85. Rajani RR, Arthurs ZM, Srivastava SD, et al. Repairing immediate proximal endoleaks during abdominal aortic aneurysm repair. J Vasc Surg 2011;53(5):1174–7.

86. de Vries JP, Ouriel K, Mehta M, et al. Analysis of EndoAnchors for endovascular aneurysm repair by indications for use. J Vasc Surg 2014;60(6):1460–7.e1.

87. Sheehan MK, Barbato J, Compton CN, et al. Effectiveness of coiling in the treatment of endoleaks after endovascular repair. J Vasc Surg 2004;40(3):430–4.

88. Maldonado TS, Rosen RJ, Rockman CB, et al. Initial successful management of type I endoleak after endovascular aortic aneurysm repair with n-butyl cyanoacrylate adhesive. J Vasc Surg 2003;38(4):664–70.

89. Kelso RL, Lyden SP, Butler B, et al. Late conversion of aortic stent grafts. J Vasc Surg 2009;49(3):589–95.

90. Martin Z, Greenberg RK, Mastracci TM, et al. Late rescue of proximal endograft failure using fenestrated and branched devices. J Vasc Surg 2014;59(6):1479–87.

91. Montelione N, Pecoraro F, Puippe G, et al. A 12-year experience with chimney and periscope grafts for treatment of type i endoleaks. J Endovasc Ther 2015;22(4):568–74.

92. Makaroun M, Zajko A, Sugimoto H, et al. Fate of endoleaks after endoluminal repair of abdominal aortic aneurysms with the EVT device. Eur J Vasc Endovasc Surg 1999;18(3):185–90.

93. Kray J, Kirk S, Franko J, et al. Role of type II endoleak in sac regression after endovascular repair of infrarenal abdominal aortic aneurysms. J Vasc Surg 2015;61(4):869–74.

94. Chen J, Stavropoulos SW. Management of endoleaks. Semin Intervent Radiol 2015;32(3):259–64.

95. Uthoff H, Katzen BT, Gandhi R, et al. Direct percutaneous sac injection for postoperative endoleak treatment after endovascular aortic aneurysm repair. J Vasc Surg 2012;56(4):965–72.

96. Giles KA, Fillinger MF, De Martino RR, et al. Results of transcaval embolization for sac expansion from type II endoleaks after endovascular aneurysm repair. J Vasc Surg 2015;61(5):1129–36.

97. Charitable JF, Patalano PI, Garg K, et al. Outcomes of translumbar embolization of type II endoleaks following endovascular abdominal aortic aneurysm repair. J Vasc Surg 2021;74(6):1867–73.

98. Iwakoshi S, Ogawa Y, Dake MD, et al. Outcomes of embolization procedures for type II endoleaks following endovascular abdominal aortic repair. J Vasc Surg 2023;77(1):114–21.e2.

99. Kalliafas S, Nana P, Spanos K, et al. Midterm outcomes of endoleak type 2 embolization after endovascular aortic aneurysm repair using a neurointerventional approach. Ann Vasc Surg 2023;92:178–87.

100. Mewissen MW, Jan MF, Kuten D, et al. Laser-assisted transgraft embolization: a technique for the treatment of type ii endoleaks. J Vasc Intervent Radiol 2017;28(11):1600–3.

101. Maitrias P, Belhomme D, Molin V, et al. Obliterative endoaneurysmorrhaphy with stent graft preservation for treatment of type ii progressive endoleak. Eur J Vasc Endovasc Surg 2016;51(1):38–42.

102. Burley CG, Kumar MH, Bhatti WA, et al. Transcaval embolization as the preferred approach. J Vasc Surg 2019;69(4):1309–13.

103. Nana P, Spanos K, Heidemann F, et al. Systematic review on transcaval embolization for type II endoleak after endovascular aortic aneurysm repair. J Vasc Surg 2022;76(1):282–91.e2.

104. Ultee KHJ, Buttner S, Huurman R, et al. Editor's choice - systematic review and meta-analysis of the outcome of treatment for type ii endoleak following endovascular aneurysm repair. Eur J Vasc Endovasc Surg 2018;56(6):794–807.

105. Seike Y, Matsuda H, Shimizu H, et al. Nationwide analysis of persistent type ii endoleak and late outcomes of endovascular abdominal aortic aneurysm repair in Japan: a propensity-matched analysis. Circulation 2022;145(14):1056–66.

106. Vandenbulcke R, Houthoofd S, Laenen A, et al. Embolization therapy for type 2 endoleaks after endovascular aortic aneurysm repair: imaging-based predictive factors and clinical outcomes on long-term follow-up. Diagn Intervent Radiol 2023;29(2):331–41.

107. Ide T, Masada K, Kuratani T, et al. Risk analysis of aneurysm sac enlargement caused by type II endoleak after endovascular aortic repair. Ann Vasc Surg 2021;77:208–16.

108. Branzan D, Geisler A, Steiner S, et al. Type II endoleak and aortic aneurysm sac shrinkage after

preemptive embolization of aneurysm sac side branches. J Vasc Surg 2021;73(6):1973–9.e1.

109. Yu HYH, Lindström D, Wanhainen A, et al. Systematic review and meta-analysis of prophylactic aortic side branch embolization to prevent type II endoleaks. J Vasc Surg 2020;72(5):1783–92.e1.

110. Li Q, Hou P. Sac embolization and side branch embolization for preventing type ii endoleaks after endovascular aneurysm repair: a meta-analysis. J Endovasc Ther 2020;27(1):109–16.

111. Nakai H, Iwakoshi S, Takimoto S, et al. Preemptive embolization of the lumbar arteries and inferior mesenteric artery to prevent abdominal aortic aneurysm enlargement associated with type 2 endoleak following endovascular aneurysm repair. Interv Radiol (Higashimatsuyama) 2023;8(3): 146–53.

112. Zhang H, Yang Y, Kou L, et al. Effectiveness of collateral arteries embolization before endovascular aneurysm repair to prevent type II endoleaks: a systematic review and meta-analysis. Vascular 2022; 30(5):813–24.

113. Nakayama H, Toma M, Kobayashi T, et al. Abdominal aortic aneurysm shrinkage up to 2 years following endovascular repair with pembolization for preventing type 2 endoleak: a retrospective single center study. Ann Vasc Surg 2023;88:308–17.

114. Kontopodis N, Galanakis N, Kiparakis M, et al. Pre-emptive embolization of the aneurysm sac or aortic side branches in endovascular aneurysm repair: meta-analysis and trial sequential analysis of randomized controlled trials. Ann Vasc Surg 2023;91:90–107.

115. Kougias P, Lin PH, Dardik A, et al. Successful treatment of endotension and aneurysm sac enlargement with endovascular stent graft reinforcement. J Vasc Surg 2007;46(1):124–7.

Carotid Disease and Management

Check for updates

Khawaja Hassan Akhtar, MD[a], David C. Metzger, MD[b], Faisal Latif, MD, FSCAI[c,d],*

KEYWORDS

- Carotid artery stenosis • Carotid endarterectomy • Carotid artery stenting
- Optimal medical therapy • Transcarotid artery revascularization • Stroke

KEY POINTS

- Carotid artery stenosis is a leading cause of stroke worldwide and optimal medical therapy is of paramount importance to improve clinical outcomes in these patients.
- Carotid endarterectomy or stenting can be considered based on patient's clinical characteristics, anatomic characteristics of aortic arch and carotid arteries, and the center's local expertise.
- Technical advancements and refined procedural techniques have helped CAS achieve parity to CEA in procedural success and stroke prevention.
- Randomized trials are needed to determine safety and efficacy of TCAR in comparison with CEA and CAS.
- Further refinement in carotid stent design, embolic protection will continue to enhance safety of stenting while reducing procedural risk.

INTRODUCTION

Stroke is the fifth major cause of death in the United States, and a leading cause of morbidity.[1,2] Carotid artery stenosis is a leading cause of stroke, transient ischemic attack (TIA), and neurocognitive decline.[3] Carotid artery stenosis is a marker of systemic atherosclerosis and frequently coexists with coronary artery disease (CAD) and peripheral artery disease.[3] Early detection and treatment is of paramount importance to reduce the risk of stroke, and treatment options include optimal medical therapy (OMT), carotid endarterectomy (CEA), and carotid artery stenting (CAS). The choice between CEA and CAS depends on the risk factors and patient characteristics, and improvements in catheter-based techniques have enabled patients to undergo CAS with outcomes similar to CEA.[2,4,5]

Prevalence

Stroke affects almost 795,000 people in the United States each year, and approximately 610,000 of these are first time strokes, whereas 185,000 are recurrent strokes.[1] Furthermore, it is estimated that 3.4 million adults over the age of 18 would suffer a stroke by 2030.[1,2] Carotid artery stenosis is deemed the culprit in approximately 8% to 15% of ischemic strokes, with an estimated 41,000 strokes per year in the United States.[6] Furthermore, carotid artery stenosis is associated with a high recurrence of stroke, with 25% of patients experiencing a recurrent stroke within 5 years.[7,8]

Another important consideration is asymptomatic carotid artery stenosis. The prevalence of moderate-to-severe carotid artery stenosis on carotid artery ultrasound in asymptomatic patients is estimated to be around 4% to 8%

[a] Department of Cardiovascular Diseases, University of Oklahoma Health Sciences Center, Oklahoma City, OK 73104, USA; [b] OhioHealth Vascular Institute, Columbus, OH 43214, USA; [c] University of Oklahoma Health Sciences Center, Oklahoma City, OK 73104, USA; [d] Cardiac Catheterization Laboratory, University of Oklahoma, SSM Health St. Anthony Hospital, Oklahoma City, OK
* Corresponding author. 608 NW 9th Street, Oklahoma City, OK 73104.
E-mail address: Faisal.Latif276@gmail.com

Intervent Cardiol Clin 14 (2025) 191–204
https://doi.org/10.1016/j.iccl.2024.11.006
2211-7458/25/© 2024 Elsevier Inc. All rights reserved, including for text and data mining, AI training, and similar technologies.

Abbreviations	
ARR	absolute risk reduction
CAD	coronary artery disease
CAS	carotid artery stenting
CDUS	carotid duplex ultrasound
CEA	carotid endarterectomy
CI	confidence interval
CMS	The centers for medicare & medicaid services
CTA	computed tomographic angiography
DAPT	dual antiplatelet therapy
DASH	dietary approaches to stop hypertension diet
DW-MRI	diffusion-weighted magnetic resonance imaging
ECAS	etracranial carotid artery stenosis
HR	hazard ratio
ICA	internal carotid artery
ICAS	intracranial carotid artery stenosis
LDL	low-density lipoprotein
MI	myocardial infarction
MRA	magnetic resonance angiography
NCD	National coverage determination
RCT	randomized clinical trial
RR	relative risk
TCAR	transcarotid artery revascularization
TF	transfemoral
TIA	transient ischemic attack

among adults in the United States.[9] Epidemiologic studies have suggested a prevalence of 1.5% (95% CI, 1.1–2.1) globally, which amounts to approximately 58 million people worldwide.[3,10] The incidence of carotid artery stenosis increases with age, and a study by de Weerd and colleagues showed that prevalence of asymptomatic severe stenosis (≥70%) was 0.1% in men below the age of 50, which increased to 3.1% among men above 80 years of age.[11]

Pathogenesis and Symptomatic Carotid Artery Stenosis

Atherosclerosis is the main precursor of developing carotid artery disease, and carotid artery stenosis and CAD share similar risk-factors (Fig. 1).[12,13] Carotid atherosclerosis leads to narrowing of the vessel lumen, and it most commonly involves the internal carotid artery (ICA). The vessel lumen gets progressively reduced leading to cerebral ischemia. In addition, an atheroma may embolize and cause distal infarct. Additionally, atherosclerotic plaque rupture leads to an acute thrombotic occlusion, or a thrombus can dislodge and cause embolic stroke.[2,14,15] Occasionally, a spontaneous or traumatic carotid artery dissection can lead to acute occlusion of the vessel.[2] Apart from this, fibromuscular dysplasia is an important cause of carotid artery stenosis particularly in women.[16]

Symptomatic carotid artery stenosis refers to an episode of focal neurologic ischemia in the distribution of carotid artery, in the past 6 months due to hemodynamically significant ICA stenosis (stenosis > 50%).[3] The symptoms typically involve anterior cerebral circulation and may include sudden onset of sensory or motor impairment, dysphagia, or monocular vision loss. Important fact to consider is that visual

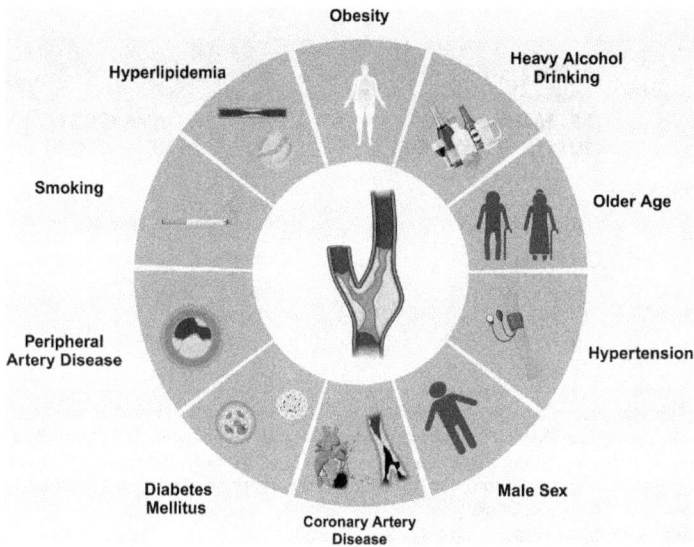

Fig. 1. Risk-factors for developing carotid artery stenosis. (Created in BioRender. Akhtar, K. (2025) https://BioRender.com/u41b288.)

symptoms are ipsilateral to the stenosis, whereas the cerebral symptoms are contralateral to the site of stenosis.[17] Ischemic neurologic symptoms that resolve completely within 24 hours after onset are classified as TIA, while symptoms persisting beyond 24 hours are classified as a stroke. The time period of 6 months after a neurologic event secondary to carotid artery stenosis is considered high-risk for recurrence of TIA/stroke.[12,17]

Extracranial and Intracranial Carotid Artery Stenosis

Carotid artery stenosis can involve both the extracranial and intracranial parts of ICA. The carotid canal is the landmark separating the extracranial segment of ICA from the intracranial segment.[17] Extracranial carotid artery stenosis (ECAS) and intracranial carotid artery stenosis (ICAS) can occur concurrently among patients and is associated with a higher risk of stroke. The estimated prevalence of concurrent ICAS among patients with ECAS is approximately 20% to 50%.[18] In a study by Lee and colleagues 48% of patients with significant ECAS also had significant ICAS. Presence of diabetes mellitus was found to be an independent predictor of developing concurrent ICAS and ECAS.[19] A study by Suo and colleagues shows that patients with concurrent ECAS and ICAS have a higher risk of recurrent stroke as compared to patients with either ECAS or ICAS alone (adjusted HR: 3.4; 95% CI: 1.15–10.04, P: 0.027).[20]

Diagnosis of Carotid Artery Stenosis

Carotid artery stenosis can be diagnosed by using 4 imaging modalities: carotid duplex ultrasound (CDUS), magnetic resonance angiography (MRA), computed tomographic angiography (CTA), and invasive cerebral angiography.[3] Guidelines recommend use of CDUS as the initial diagnostic test for evaluation of suspected stenosis.[12] CDUS is noninvasive and uses grayscale and doppler ultrasound to measure velocity of blood flow, which is translated into severity of stenosis. The peak systolic velocity, end-diastolic velocity, spectral waveform analysis, and the ratio of the peak internal carotid artery to common carotid artery (CCA) velocity (carotid index) are measured during a CDUS test. A peak velocity greater than 230 cm/sec, or the presence of a plaque filling more than 50% of the vessel diameter are used to identify severe stenosis.[3,21] The presence of a completely occluded contralateral carotid artery can lead to overestimation of stenosis due to increased flow velocity.[22] Invasive cerebral angiography is the gold standard imaging modality. Advantages include evaluation of other vessels and collateral flow, plaque morphology, and severity. The use of digital subtraction angiography allows for use of smaller catheters, reduces the dose of contrast used, and provides images of a higher quality. The main disadvantage is its invasive nature, with approximately 1% risk of neurologic complications.[3,23,24]

MRA and CTA are both validated as noninvasive imaging modalities. Both imaging modalities can provide anatomic details of the aortic arch, which can assist in planning treatment strategies. MRA can provide accurate assessment of vessel stenosis in the presence of extensive carotid artery calcifications and does not expose patients to radiation. However, MRA can overestimate the degree of stenosis and may not provide an accurate assessment of moderately

Table 1		
Comparison of society guidelines on revascularization of carotid artery stenosis		
Severity of Stenosis	U.S. Multisocietal (2011)[12] (Class/LOE)	SVS (2022)[32] (Class/LOE)
Symptomatic Carotid Artery Stenosis		
CEA (50%–99%)	Class I/LOE: A	Class I/LOE: A
CAS (50%–99%)	Class I/LOE: B	-
Asymptomatic Carotid Artery Stenosis		
CEA (70%–99%)	Class IIa/LOE: A	Class I/LOE: B
CAS (70%–99%)	Class IIa/LOE: B	-

US Multisocietal: American Stroke Association, American College of Cardiology Foundation, American Heart Association, American Association of Neuroscience Nurses, American Association of Neurologic Surgeons, American College of Radiology, American Society of Neuroradiology, Congress of Neurologic Surgeons, Society of Atherosclerosis Imaging and Prevention, Society for Cardiovascular Angiography and Interventions, Society of Interventional Radiology, Society of Neuro-Interventional Surgery, Society for Vascular Medicine, Society for Vascular Surgery.

    Abbreviations: LOE, level of evidence; SVS, society for vascular surgery.

stenotic lesions.[3,23] CTA provides an accurate assessment of the degree of stenosis and is particularly helpful in identifying completely occluded lesions. Significant arterial calcification can alter the accuracy of CTA. In addition, CTA exposes patients to radiation and iodinated contrast is relatively contraindicated in patients with chronic kidney disease.[3,23,25]

NATIONAL COVERAGE DETERMINATION

Treatment options for revascularization of carotid artery stenosis include CEA and CAS. The main role of revascularization in symptomatic disease is to prevent a recurrent stroke, and guidelines recommend revascularization to be performed within 2 weeks of index procedure.[26] Approximately 75% of carotid revascularization procedures are performed in asymptomatic patients to reduce the risk of future stroke.[27] CAS was developed as an alternative to CEA and has undergone rigorous evaluation in multiple clinical trials.[5,28,29] Technological advances, improved patient selection, and refined procedural techniques have helped CAS achieve parity to CEA in procedural success and stroke prevention.[27]

In view of this, the centers for medicare & medicaid services (CMS) updated the national coverage determination (NCD) for CAS in 2023. The NCD covers patients with symptomatic carotid artery stenosis of at least 50%, and asymptomatic carotid artery stenosis of at least 70%. The CMS has removed the requirement for facilities to be approved by CMS to perform CAS procedures. In addition, the NCD requires an independent neurologic assessment before and after CAS, along with

the use of CDUS as first-line imaging with the use of CTA or MRA as supplementary imaging modalities to confirm the degree of severity, and to evaluate the aortic arch along with extracranial and intracranial circulation. The NCD also places emphasis on a formal shared decision-making interaction with the patient before undergoing CAS including discussion of the risks and benefits of treatment options—CEA, CAS, or OMT. Furthermore, the NCD expanded coverage to patients with both the standard and high-surgical risk for revascularization.[30,31]

CURRENT SOCIETY GUIDELINES ON CAROTID ARTERY REVASCULARIZATION

The choice of revascularization strategy in patients with carotid artery stenosis depends on anatomic and clinical characteristics including surgical risk, and whether the revascularization is being performed for symptomatic or asymptomatic stenosis. The 2011 US Multisocietal guidelines provide detailed recommendations on the choice between CEA and CAS.[12] The guideline recommendations of various societies on carotid artery revascularization are summarized in Table 1.[12,32]

Symptomatic Carotid Artery Stenosis
CEA is recommended for patients with symptomatic carotid artery stenosis if the diameter of ipsilateral ICA is reduced more than 70% by non-invasive imaging (Level of Evidence: A) or reduced more than 50% by invasive cerebral angiography (Level of Evidence: B), and the anticipated risk of perioperative stroke or mortality is less than 6% (Class I). CAS is indicated as an alternative to CEA for symptomatic

patients when the risk of periprocedural stroke or mortality is less than 6% (Class I, Level of Evidence: B). Early revascularization within 2 weeks of index event is reasonable if there are no contraindications to early revascularization (Class IIa, Level of Evidence: B).[12]

Asymptomatic Carotid Artery Stenosis
Among patients with asymptomatic carotid artery stenosis, it is reasonable to perform CEA when the stenosis is more than 70% in the ICA and the risk of perioperative stroke, myocardial infarction (MI), and mortality is low (Class IIa, Level of Evidence: A). In addition, guidelines recommend CAS over CEA when revascularization is indicated among patients with neck anatomy unfavorable for CEA (Class IIa, Level of Evidence: B). In patients with asymptomatic carotid artery stenosis (stenosis of 60% by angiography, or 70% by doppler ultrasound), prophylactic CAS can be performed (Class IIb, Level of Evidence: B).[12]

MANAGEMENT OF CAROTID ARTERY STENOSIS

Treatment options for carotid artery stenosis include OMT, CEA and CAS. CAS can be performed via transfemoral (TF) or transradial (TR) route, and the choice between CAS and CEA depends on anatomic and clinical characteristics, operator experience, and shared decision-making.

Optimal Medical Therapy
All patients with carotid artery stenosis should receive OMT regardless of the need or strategy of revascularization.[3,33] The goal of OMT is to reduce the risk of stroke and cardiovascular events among patients. Hypertension remains the most important modifiable risk factor and treatment of hypertension reduces risk of both ischemic and hemorrhagic stroke. The guidelines recommend a target systolic blood pressure (BP) goal below 130 mm Hg. The use of angiotensin-converting enzyme inhibitors or angiotensin receptor blockers is preferred due to proven benefit in reduction of cardiovascular events.[3,12] Treatment of hyperlipidemia is of paramount importance, and guidelines recommend use of statins to reduce low-density lipoprotein (LDL) cholesterol below 100 mg/dL in all patients with carotid artery stenosis. Furthermore, among patients with symptomatic carotid artery disease, aggressive LDL reduction to below 70 mg/dL is recommended. Ezetimibe or proprotein convertase subtilisin kexin type 9

inhibitor can be used as additional therapy if target LDL is not achieved with the use of statin. Glycated hemoglobin should be reduced below 7% among patients with diabetes. Patients with atrial fibrillation should receive therapeutic anticoagulation per guideline recommendation. Antiplatelet therapy with aspirin is recommended in all patients with asymptomatic carotid artery stenosis. Aspirin can be substituted with clopidogrel in patients with aspirin intolerance. Among patients with symptomatic carotid artery stenosis, dual antiplatelet therapy (DAPT) with aspirin and clopidogrel can be used for 3 weeks and up to 3 months, followed by single antiplatelet therapy. The long-term use of DAPT is currently debated due to risk of hemorrhagic complications.[3,12,27]

Lifestyle modifications proven to reduce cardiovascular events should be encouraged. Drug therapy and counseling to discontinue smoking, and reduction or cessation of alcohol among heavy drinkers should be advised. Low sodium intake with dietary approaches to stop hypertension diet (DASH), weight-reduction among patients with body mass index above 30 kg/m^2, and moderate intensity exercise for a total of 150 minutes per week have been proven to reduce adverse cardiovascular events and should be encouraged.[3,27,34]

Carotid Endarterectomy
CEA was first reported by Eastcott and colleagues in 1954.[35] Since then, the advancements in surgical techniques have improved the periprocedural and postprocedural outcomes after CEA. Patients are placed in a supine position, and the neck is extended and turned away from the side of operation. Traditionally a longitudinal incision along the anterior border of the sternocleidomastoid muscle is placed; however, a transverse incision may be used based on operator experience for cosmetic effect. The ICA is clamped proximal and distal to the plaque and a bypass shunt is placed to temporarily shunt the blood around endarterectomy site. The ICA is dissected along the length of the ICA and plaque is surgically removed. ICA closure can either be performed by patch angioplasty or primary suture repair. Satisfactory blood flow is confirmed with angiography or doppler ultrasound.[36,37]

Carotid Endarterectomy for Symptomatic Patients
The North American symptomatic carotid endarterectomy trial was the first randomized clinical trial (RCT) evaluating role of CEA in symptomatic

patients.[8,38] The trial randomization was stratified according to the severity of stenosis. The high-grade stenosis was 70% to 99% diameter reduction and lower-grade stenosis was 30% to 69% diameter reduction. The trial was stopped earlier for high-grade stenosis group after 18 months of follow-up due to a significant benefit favoring CEA. At 2 years follow-up, patients included in the CEA group (328 patients) experienced a 9% cumulative risk of stroke, as compared to patients in the medical therapy group who experienced a 26% cumulative risk of stroke (absolute risk reduction [ARR] of 17% in favor of CEA).[12,38] Additionally, CEA showed benefit among patients with stenosis of 50% to 69%. At 5 years follow-up, the rate of stroke among patients included in the CEA group was 15.7% as compared to a risk of 22% in medical therapy arm (P: 0.045). Patients with less than 50% stenosis did not derive benefit in comparison to medical therapy (14.9% vs 18.7%, P =.16).[8]

Subsequently the veterans affairs cooperative studies trial was performed and compared CEA to medical therapy among patients with symptomatic carotid artery stenosis of greater that 50%. The trial enrolled 189 patients who were randomized to CEA (91 patients) or standard of care (98 patients). At a mean follow-up of 11.9 months, patients randomized to CEA experienced significant reduction in the risk of stroke/TIA (7.7% vs 19.4%; P: 0.011), corresponding to an absolute risk reduction of 11.7%. Furthermore, the benefit of CEA was more pronounced in patients with carotid stenosis more than 70% (ARR: 17.7%; P: 0.004).[39]

Carotid Endarterectomy for Asymptomatic Patients

The first major RCT comparing CEA to medical therapy in asymptomatic carotid artery stenosis was conducted in 10 US Veterans Affairs medical centers. The trial included 444 patients with angiographic stenosis of 50% or more and randomized to CEA (211 patients) versus medical therapy (233 patients). The primary outcome was incidence of ipsilateral stroke/TIA, and patients were followed for a mean duration of 47.9 months. Patients included in the CEA group experienced a significant reduction in the risk of ipsilateral stroke/TIA (8.0% vs 20.6%) as compared to patients in the medical therapy group (relative risk [RR]: 0.38; 95% confidence interval (CI): 0.22–0.67; P<.001).[40]

The symptomatic carotid atherosclerosis study was subsequently performed and randomized 1662 patients with asymptomatic carotid artery stenosis of 60% or more to CEA versus medical therapy. The primary outcome was stroke in the distribution of ipsilateral carotid artery or perioperative stroke or mortality. After a median follow-up of 2.7 years, patients in the CEA arm experienced a significant reduction in the risk of primary outcome (5.1% vs 11.0%) as compared to patients in medical therapy group (ARR of 53%; 95% CI: 22%–72%).[41]

Carotid Artery Stenting

CAS was developed as an alternative to CEA and has undergone rigorous evaluation in multiple clinical trials head to head against CEA.[5,28,29] Technical advancements and refined procedural techniques have helped CAS achieve parity to CEA in procedural success and stroke prevention.[27,42] CAS is mainly performed via TF approach.[27,43,44] TR and transcarotid access provide alternative access to perform CAS.[27] During TF-CAS, the common femoral artery is accessed percutaneously, and a 6 Fr sheath is placed in the artery over a 0.035 wire. Using an angled catheter and a left anterior oblique projection on the fluoroscopic system, the CCA is selectively cannulated and mapped using angiography including intracerebral angiography.

For CAS using distal protection, a 6 or 7 French sheath is advanced over a stiffer wire into the distal CCA. The lesion is traversed with a wire mounted embolic protection device (EPD), which is parked in the prepetrous position of ICA. The lesion is predilated with a small profile balloon, and an appropriately sized self-expanding stent is deployed across the stenosis. Postdilation can be performed for stent optimization in case of significant residual stenosis (greater than 30%). Carotid and cerebral angiogram is performed to confirm absence of distal embolization, followed by the removal of catheters and sheaths if the result is satisfactory. Hemostasis can be achieved by manual compression, or a closure device can be deployed at the arteriotomy site.[44]

While distal protection requires manipulation across the carotid stenosis before placement of EPD, CAS using proximal protection allows blocking antegrade blood flow before manipulation across the lesion. This procedure is reserved for patients who can tolerate blocking the antegrade blood flow.[45] In addition, 8 or 9 French sheath is required for this. Double balloon device has 2 balloons, 1 balloon in the CCA and the other balloon in the external carotid artery. Both the balloons are inflated to block antegrade flow; subsequently the lesion is crossed with a wire, followed by balloon inflation and stenting across the lesion. Following the stenting, the balloons are deflated leading to restoration of antegrade blood flow.

Single balloon devices can be used in patients with occluded external carotid artery.[44,45]

Transradial Carotid Artery Stenting

TR artery access for CAS provides an alternative arterial access when TF-CAS cannot be performed due to anatomic considerations (iliac artery occlusion or complex aortic arch anatomy, particularly right carotid stenting in the presence of a bovine arch).[27] TR access has improved procedural safety among patients undergoing coronary artery interventions.[46] Radial access for carotid artery stenting trial compared TR access with TF access among patients undergoing CAS. A total of 260 patients were randomized to either the TR group (130 patients) or the TF group (130 patients). The primary endpoint was combined major adverse cardiac and cerebral events, and rate of access site complications. Procedural success was achieved in all patients; however, the crossover rate was higher in the TR group, with 10% of the TR group crossing over to TF and 1.5% of the TF group crossing over to TR (P<.05). There was no significant difference between both groups in the primary endpoint (TR group: 0.9% vs TF group: 0.8%). A major vascular access complication occurred in 1 patient in each group. There was no difference between both groups in the procedural time and fluoroscopy time, but the radiation dose was significantly higher in the TR group (195 [25th and 75th percentile: 129–274] Gy/cm^2 vs 148 [25th and 75th percentile: 102–237] Gy/cm^2; P<.05).[47]

The TR access provides advantages over TF access among patients with difficult TF access (severe aortoiliac disease, morbid obesity, high bleeding risk), or unfavorable aortic arch anatomy (bovine aortic arches). Currently the evidence is lacking to support superiority of TR access and it may be best viewed as a complementary access rather than competing with femoral artery access.[27,48]

Carotid Artery Stenting for Symptomatic Patients

CAS has undergone rigorous comparative evaluation with CEA for the treatment of symptomatic carotid artery stenosis (Table 2). Carotid Revascularization Endarterectomy Versus Stenting Trial (CREST) is the largest study comparing CAS to CEA in average surgical risk patients.[5] The trial randomized symptomatic (53%) and asymptomatic (47%) patients to undergo CAS or CEA for carotid artery stenosis. Majority of the patients (86%) had severe stenosis of carotid artery. The primary composite end point was stroke, MI, or death from any cause during the peri-procedural period or any ipsilateral stroke within 4 years after randomization. The trial results did not show a significant difference in the primary outcome among symptomatic patients undergoing CAS (8.6% vs 8.4%) in comparison to CEA (hazard ratio [HR]: 1.08; 95% CI: 0.74–1.59, P: 0.69). In addition, there was no significant difference in the risk of stroke (periprocedural and post-procedural ipsilateral stroke) at 4 years between the groups (CAS: 7.6%, CEA: 6.4%; P: 0.25).[5] During long-term follow-up of 10 years, there was no significant difference in primary endpoint between both groups (HR: 1.17; 95% CI: 0.82–1.66, P: 0.40).[54] In the entire cohort (symptomatic and asymptomatic patients) patients undergoing CAS were found to have a higher risk of periprocedural stroke (4.1% vs 2.3%) (HR: 1.79; 95% CI: 1.14–2.82, P: 0.01). The higher risk of periprocedural stroke was mainly driven by minor stroke. Furthermore, patients undergoing CEA experienced a higher risk of periprocedural MI (CAS: 1.1%; CEA: 2.3%) (HR: 0.50; 95% CI: 0.26–0.94, P: 0.03).[5] Both of these peri-procedural complications were associated with a higher risk of late mortality.[55]

The Stenting and Angioplasty with Protection in Patients at High Risk for Endarterectomy (SAPPHIRE) trial enrolled 334 high surgical risk patients with a symptomatic stenosis of > 50% or an asymptomatic stenosis of > 80% to undergo CEA (167 patients) or CAS (167 patients).[29] The primary end point of death, stroke, or MI within 30 days after the intervention plus death or ipsilateral stroke between 31 days and 1 year occurred in 12.2% of patients in the CAS group and 20.1% of patients in the CEA group (P =.004 for non-inferiority).[27,29] In addition, long-term results at 3 year did not show a significant difference in outcomes between both the treatment arms.[56]

Carotid Artery Stenting for Asymptomatic Patients

The strongest evidence of revascularization in asymptomatic carotid artery stenosis comes from trials comparing CEA to medical therapy. Multiple trials have compared CEA to CAS in asymptomatic patients (Table 3). Recently published Second Asymptomatic Carotid Surgery trial (ACST – 2) enrolled 3625 average surgical risk patients with asymptomatic severe carotid artery stenosis (CAS: 1811 patients, CEA: 1814 patients). There was no significant difference in the risk of mortality, MI or stroke within 30 days (CAS: 3.9% vs CEA: 3.2%; P: 0.26). Additionally, Kaplan-Meier estimates of 5-year stroke

Table 2
Randomized clinical trials comparing carotid artery stenting to carotid endarterectomy in symptomatic patients

Study Title	Year	Patients	Surgical Risk	Primary Outcome	Results of Primary Outcome
CAVATAS[49]	2001	CAS: 251 CEA: 253	ASR	Death/Stroke within 30 d	CAS: 10%; CEA: 11% (P: NS)
Brooks et al,[50] 2001	2001	CAS: 53 CEA: 51	ASR	Death/Stroke/ TIA within 30 d	CAS: 1 TIA CEA: 1 Death
SAPPHIRE[29] (Symptomatic Stenosis: ~ 30%)	2004	CAS: 167 CEA: 167	HSR	Death/Stroke/ MI at 30 d plus Death/Stroke within 1 y	CAS: 12.2% CEA: 20.1% (P = .004 for non-inferiority)
EVA-3S[51]	2006	CAS: 261 CEA: 259	ASR	Death/Stroke within 30 d	CAS: 9.6% CEA: 3.9% (P: 0.01)
SPACE[52]	2006	CAS: 599 CEA: 584	ASR	Death/Stroke within 30 d	CAS: 6.8% CEA: 6.3% (P = .09 for non-inferiority)
CREST[5]	2010	CAS: 668 CEA: 653	ASR	Periprocedural Stroke/MI/Death or Stroke within 4 y	CAS: 8.6% CEA: 8.4% (P: 0.69)
ICSS[53]	2010	CAS: 855 CEA: 858	ASR	Fatal and disabling Stroke within 5 y	CAS: 6.4% CEA: 6.5% (P: 0.77)

Abbreviations: ASR, average surgical risk; CAVATAS, carotid and vertebral artery transluminal angioplasty study; CREST, carotid revascularization endarterectomy versus stenting trial; EVA-3S, endarterectomy versus angioplasty in patients with symptomatic severe carotid stenosis; HSR, high surgical risk; ICSS, international carotid stenting study; MI, myocardial infarction; NS, non-significant; SAPPHIRE, stenting and angioplasty with protection in patients at high risk for endarterectomy; SPACE, Stent- Protected Angioplasty versus Carotid Endarterectomy

was 5·3% with CAS and 4·5% with CEA (RR: 1·16; 95% CI: 0.86–1.57, P =.33).[58]

Stent-Protected Angioplasty versus Carotid Endarterectomy – 2 trial (SPACE -2) included 3 arms; OMT alone, CAS with OMT, and CEA with OMT.[57] The trial was terminated prematurely due to poor enrollment after 513 patients had been randomized. There was no difference in the 30-day risk of stroke or mortality between CAS (2.5%) and CEA (2.5%). Patients in the OMT group did not experience any stroke within 30 days. Trial results showed no difference in the cumulative rates of any stroke or death from any cause within 30 days plus ipsilateral ischemic stroke within 1 year of follow-up (2.5% for CAS, 3.0% for CEA, and 0.9% for OMT; P: non-significant). Of note, the 1-year incidence of TIA was 5.3% in the OMT group, which was numerically twice as high as in the CAS (2.0%) and CEA (2.5%) groups.[27,57]

In asymptomatic high-surgical risk patients enrolled in the SAPPHIRE trial, the cumulative incidence of the primary endpoint (composite of death, stroke, or MI within 30 days after the intervention or death or ipsilateral stroke between 31 days and 1 year) was lower among those who received CAS (9.9% vs 21.5%, P: 0.02) than among those who received CEA.[27,29]

Transcarotid Artery Revascularization

TCAR is a hybrid approach to CAS where a surgical incision is performed to gain access to the CCA in order to insert an arterial sheath to deliver a carotid stent. Flow-reversal EPD is usually used during this procedure. The advantages over CEA include less invasive nature and reduced recovery time. In addition, TCAR avoids excessive catheter manipulation in the aortic arch with direct CCA access. TCAR should be avoided in small (<6 mm) and severely diseased carotid artery (presence of thrombus or severe tortuosity and calcifications). In addition, stenotic lesions lesser than 5 cm cranial to the clavicle are relative contraindications to TCAR.

There are no RCTs comparing TCAR to CAS or CEA. Galyfos and colleagues performed a systematic review and meta-analysis of observational

Table 3
Randomized clinical trials comparing carotid artery stenting to carotid endarterectomy in asymptomatic patients

Study Title	Year	Patients	Surgical Risk	Primary Outcome	Results
SAPPHIRE[29] (Asymptomatic Stenosis: ~ 70%)	2004	CAS: 167 CEA: 167	HSR	Death/Stroke/MI at 30 d plus Death/Stroke within 1 y	CAS: 12.2% CEA: 20.1% (P =.004 for non-inferiority)
CREST[5]	2010	CAS: 594 CEA: 587	ASR	Peri-procedural Stroke/MI/Death or Stroke within 4 y	CAS: 5.6% CEA: 4.9% (P: 0.56)
ACT-1[28]	2016	CAS: 1,089 CEA: 364	ASR	Death/Stroke/MI at 30 d plus Death /Stroke within 1 y	CAS: 3.8% CEA: 3.4% (P: NS)
SPACE-2[57]	2020	CAS: 197 CEA: 203	ASR	Death/Stroke at 30 d plus Stroke within 1 y	CAS: 2.5% CEA: 3.0% (P: NS)
ACST-2[58]	2021	CAS: 1811 CEA: 1814	ASR	Death/MI/Stroke within 30 d	CAS: 3.9% CEA: 3.2% (P: 0.26)

Abbreviations: ACST-2, second asymptomatic carotid surgery trial; ACT-1, Asymptomatic Carotid Trial-1; ASR, average surgical risk; CAS, carotid artery stenting; ; CREST, carotid revascularization endarterectomy versus stenting trial; HSR, high surgical risk; NS, non-significant; SAPPHIRE, stenting and angioplasty with protection in patients at high risk for end-arterectomy; SPACE, Stent- Protected Angioplasty versus Carotid Endarterectomy-2 trial

studies including a total of 4,852 patients comparing TCAR. Technical success was achieved in 97.6% patients, and 30-day pooled mortality was 0.7%. Patients with symptomatic stenosis had a higher risk of early stroke/TIA than asymptomatic patients (2.5% vs 1.2%).[59] Another retrospective observational study by Mehta and colleagues compared clinical outcomes between patients undergoing CEA, TF-CAS, or TCAR. The study included 33,115 patients, and majority of patients had CEA (80%), followed by TF-CAS, (11%) and TCAR (9.1%). Patients receiving TCAR experienced a similar risk of 30-day stroke/mortality as compared to CEA (HR:1.10; 95% CI: 0.75–1.62).[60] TCAR is a promising therapy for revascularization in patients with carotid artery stenosis, but randomized comparative studies are warranted to evaluate the safety and efficacy of TCAR in comparison to CEA and TF-CAS.[61]

CHOICE OF REVASCULARIZATION PROCEDURE

The choice between revascularization strategies for carotid artery stenosis should incorporate assessment of surgical risk, indication for revascularization, clinical and anatomic factors, and shared decision making (Fig. 2). The clinical factors associated with a high risk of periprocedural complications during CEA include left ventricular ejection fraction < 30%, CAD with left main coronary artery disease, recent MI within 30 days, severe renal and pulmonary disease. The anatomic features associated with a high complication risk during CEA include surgically inaccessible lesion (above C2 or below the clavicle), contralateral carotid artery occlusion, and previous ipsilateral CEA or neck surgery.

The clinical factors imparting a high risk of periprocedural complications with CAS include advanced age (>75 years), severe aortic stenosis, severe renal disease, and bleeding disorder. Additionally, the anatomic features associated with a high periprocedural complication risk during CAS include high-grade aortic arch atheroma, stenosis at the origin of great vessels, lack of femoral access, inability to deploy EPD, and thrombotic lesion (Table 4).

CAROTID STENT DESIGN

Carotid stents can be classified as open-cell, closed-cell, or dual-layered (covered) stent. Open-cell stents have a free cell area of greater than 5 mm^2 and adapt well to the contour of vessel. Theoretically, stents with higher free cell area may result in plaque protrusion through

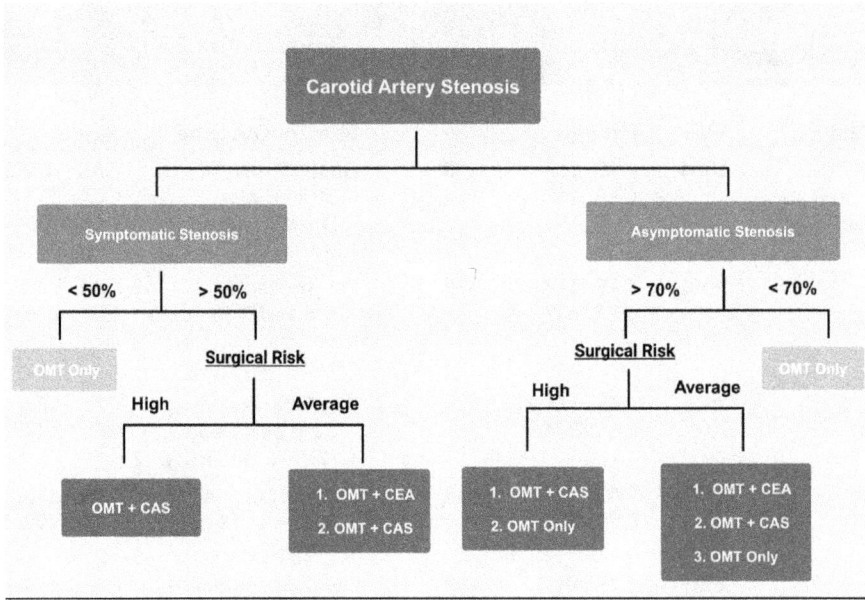

Fig. 2. A Treatment Algorithm for Management of CAS, CEA; OMT. (Created in BioRender. Akhtar, K. (2025) https://BioRender.com/r19b887.)

struts and embolization, particularly in thrombotic lesions and symptomatic patients. Closed-cell stents may not conform well to vessel contour and have a small risk of kinking the vessel if placed inappropriately, but the risk of plaque protrusion through the struts is lower.[27,42] The evidence comparing open-cell stents to closed-cell stents is conflicting. Stabile and colleagues performed an analysis of registry data including 1,604 patients and compared closed-cell stents to open-cell stents. The use of open-cell stent with free cell area greater than 7.5 mm^2 was associated with a higher risk of 30-day stroke as compared to closed-cell stent (3.05% vs 1.12%, P: 0.045).[62] A small RCT of 40 patients compared the risk of subclinical

Table 4
High-risk features for periprocedural complications between carotid endarterectomy and carotid artery stenting

Carotid Artery Stenting (High-Risk Features)[27,43]		Carotid Endarterectomy (High-Risk Features)[27,43]	
Clinical	Anatomic	Clinical	Anatomic
Age > 75 y	Severe aortic arch atheroma	Unstable angina	Neck irradiation
Severe aortic stenosis	Type II/III aortic arch	Left main/ multivessel severe CAD	Contralateral carotid artery occlusion
Severe renal disease	Inability to use EPD	Congestive heart failure	Previous ipsilateral CEA or neck surgery
Dementia	Thrombotic lesion	LVEF < 30%	Lesion above C2
Bleeding disorder	Circumferential lesion calcification	Severe pulmonary disease	Lesion below the clavicle
	Lack of femoral access	Severe renal disease	Spinal immobility

Abbreviations: LVEF, left ventricular ejection fraction

cerebral embolization measured by diffusion-weighted magnetic resonance imaging (DW-MRI) among patients undergoing CAS with either open-cell stent (20 patients) or closed-cell stent (20 patients). New acute cerebral emboli occurred in 53% and 47% of patients undergoing CAS with open-cell and closed-cell stents, respectively (P=1.0).[63]

Dual-layered carotid stents have been developed to reduce the risk of plaque protrusion. There are 3 types of dual-layered stents Scaffold (W.L. Gore and Associates), Roadsaver (Microvention), and CGuard (Inspire-MD).[27] These stents are being evaluated in pivotal trials and are yet not commercially available. A recent single-center RCT of 100 patients treated with CAS compared an open-cell stent (Acculink; Abbott Vascular) to a covered stent (CGuard; Inspire-MD) and demonstrated significantly higher periprocedural embolic events for the open-cell stent group (RR: 7.8; 95% CI: 1.3–14.9, P=.021). In addition, there were 2 strokes in patients with open-cell stent design in comparison to 0 strokes in the covered-stent group.[27,64] These findings may influence the choice of stent design for CAS; however; further evidence is warranted to establish safety and efficacy of dual-layered stent design.

EMBOLIC PROTECTION DEVICE

The 2 classes of EPDs used commonly include proximal protection with flow-reversal and distal umbrella-like filters to capture downstream particles. The embolic risk during CAS is highest during the stent deployment and postdilation phase. As the risk of stroke during CAS is relatively low, clinical efficacy of EPD has been difficult to demonstrate in individual clinical trials.[27] A large meta-analysis of 24 studies compared risk of stroke among patients undergoing CAS with EPD versus no protection device. The use of EPD was associated with significant reduction in the risk of stroke (RR: 0.62; 95% CI: 0.54–0.72). Study results further support the use of EPD with benefit in stroke reduction in both symptomatic carotid artery stenosis (RR: 0.67; 95% CI: 0.52–0.56, P<.05) and asymptomatic carotid artery stenosis (RR: 0.61; 95% CI: 0.41–0.90, P<.05).[65]

There is no convincing clinical evidence that proximal EPD is superior to distal EPD in terms of clinical efficacy. A large meta-analysis of 18 studies with 12,281 patients compared CAS with distal EPD versus proximal EPD. There was no significant difference between the 2 modalities in terms of the risk of stroke (risk difference (RD): 0.0; 95% CI: −0.01–0.01) or mortality (RD: 0.0; 95% CI: −0.01–

0.01).[45] A single-center study by Kajihara and colleagues performed dual protection (combined proximal EPD and distal EPD) and compared it to distal EPD. A total of 78 patients undergoing CAS were analyzed (dual protection: 54 patients, distal EPD: 24 patients). Hyperintensity lesions on DW-MRI and perioperative complications were compared between both the strategies. Imaging showed hyperintensity lesions among 54.2% (13/24 patients) in the distal EPD group and in 27.8% (15/54 patients) in the dual protection group (P=.024).[66] Further RCTs are required to evaluate the superiority of dual protection strategy among patients undergoing CAS.

SUMMARY

Carotid artery stenosis is a major cause of stroke worldwide. OMT should be ensured in these patients. For patients with severe stenosis, CEA or CAS can be considered based on patient's clinical characteristics, symptomatic status, anatomic characteristics of aortic arch and carotid arteries, and the center's local expertise. Further refinement of equipment including stent design, use of EPDs, and techniques for stenting are in development and would continue to enhance options available to patients while reducing procedural risks. We recognize that the recommendations on treatment of carotid stenosis particularly among asymptomatic patients rests on clinical studies performed well before current medical standards, and there is an unmet need to evaluate the efficacy of revascularization procedures in comparison to OMT in asymptomatic patients. Further high-quality RCTs are warranted to address these concerns and improve the evidence base for treatment of this vulnerable patient population.

CLINICS CARE POINTS

- Use imaging appropriately to identify patients with significant carotid stenosis, whether symptomatic or asymptomatic.
- Patients with significant carotid stenosis should be started on optimal medical therapy.
- Carefully, choose revascularization strategy using clinical and anatomic characteristics and shared decision making.

REFERENCES

1. Martin SS, Aday AW, Almarzooq ZI, et al. 2024 Heart disease and stroke statistics: a report of US

and global data from the American Heart association. Circulation 2024;149(8):e347–913.

2. Krawisz AK, Carroll BJ, Secemsky EA. Risk stratification and management of extracranial carotid artery disease. Cardiol Clin 2021;39(4):539–49.

3. Hackam DG. Optimal medical management of asymptomatic carotid stenosis. Stroke 2021;52(6): 2191–8.

4. Mohd AB, Alabdallat Y, Mohd OB, et al. Medical and surgical management of symptomatic and asymptomatic carotid artery stenosis: a comprehensive literature review. Cureus 2023;15(8): e43263. https://doi.org/10.7759/cureus.43263.

5. Brott TG, Hobson RW, Howard G, et al. Stenting versus endarterectomy for treatment of carotid-artery stenosis. N Engl J Med 2010;363(1):11–23.

6. Flaherty ML, Kissela B, Khoury JC, et al. Carotid artery stenosis as a cause of stroke. Neuroepidemiology 2013;40(1):36–41.

7. Marnane M, Ni Chroinin D, Callaly E, et al. Stroke recurrence within the time window recommended for carotid endarterectomy. Neurology 2011;77(8): 738–43.

8. Barnett HJ, Taylor DW, Eliasziw M, et al. Benefit of carotid endarterectomy in patients with symptomatic moderate or severe stenosis. North American Symptomatic Carotid Endarterectomy Trial Collaborators. N Engl J Med 1998;339(20):1415–25.

9. Suri MFK, Ezzeddine MA, Lakshminarayan K, et al. Validation of two different grading schemes to identify patients with asymptomatic carotid artery stenosis in general population. J Neuroimaging 2008;18(2):142–7.

10. Song P, Fang Z, Wang H, et al. Global and regional prevalence, burden, and risk factors for carotid atherosclerosis: a systematic review, meta-analysis, and modelling study. Lancet Glob Health 2020;8(5):e721–9.

11. de Weerd M, Greving JP, Hedblad B, et al. Prevalence of asymptomatic carotid artery stenosis in the general population: an individual participant data meta-analysis. Stroke 2010;41(6):1294–7.

12. Brott TG, Halperin JL, Abbara S, et al. 2011 ASA/ACCF/AHA/AANN/AANS/ACR/ASNR/CNS/SAIP/SCAI/SIR/SNIS/SVM/SVS guideline on the management of patients with extracranial carotid and vertebral artery disease: executive summary: a report of the American College of Cardiology foundation/American Heart association task force on practice guidelines, and the American stroke association, American association of neuroscience Nurses, American association of neurological Surgeons, American College of Radiology, American society of Neuroradiology, congress of neurological Surgeons, society of atherosclerosis imaging and prevention, society for cardiovascular angiography and interventions, society of interventional Radiology, society of NeuroInterventional surgery, society for vascular medicine, and society for vascular surgery. J Am Coll Cardiol 2011;57(8): 1002–44.

13. Woo SY, Joh JH, Han S-A, et al. Prevalence and risk factors for atherosclerotic carotid stenosis and plaque: a population-based screening study. Medicine (Baltim) 2017;96(4):e5999.

14. Gonzalez NR, Liebeskind DS, Dusick JR, et al. Intracranial arterial stenoses: current viewpoints, novel approaches, and surgical perspectives. Neurosurg Rev 2013;36(2):175–84. discussion 184-185.

15. Lee DK, Kim JS, Kwon SU, et al. Lesion patterns and stroke mechanism in atherosclerotic middle cerebral artery disease: early diffusion-weighted imaging study. Stroke 2005;36(12):2583–8.

16. Olin JW, Gornik HL, Bacharach JM, et al. Fibromuscular dysplasia: state of the science and critical unanswered questions: a scientific statement from the American Heart Association. Circulation 2014; 129(9):1048–78.

17. Arasu R, Arasu A, Muller J. Carotid artery stenosis: an approach to its diagnosis and management. Aust J Gen Pract 2021;50(11):821–5.

18. Kappelle LJ, Eliasziw M, Fox AJ, et al. Importance of intracranial atherosclerotic disease in patients with symptomatic stenosis of the internal carotid artery. The North American Symptomatic Carotid Endarterectomy Trail. Stroke 1999;30(2):282–6.

19. Lee SJ, Cho S-J, Moon H-S, et al. Combined extracranial and intracranial atherosclerosis in Korean patients. Arch Neurol 2003;60(11):1561–4.

20. Suo Y, Jing J, Pan Y, et al. Concurrent intracranial and extracranial artery stenosis and the prognosis of transient ischaemic symptoms or imaging-negative ischaemic stroke. Stroke Vasc Neurol 2021;6(1):33–40.

21. Grant EG, Benson CB, Moneta GL, et al. Carotid artery stenosis: gray-scale and Doppler US diagnosis–society of radiologists in ultrasound consensus conference. Radiology 2003;229(2):340–6.

22. Fujitani RM, Mills JL, Wang LM, et al. The effect of unilateral internal carotid arterial occlusion upon contralateral duplex study: criteria for accurate interpretation. J Vasc Surg 1992;16(3):459–67. discussion 467-468.

23. Adla T, Adlova R. Multimodality imaging of carotid stenosis. Int J Angiol 2015;24(3):179–84.

24. Heiserman JE, Dean BL, Hodak JA, et al. Neurologic complications of cerebral angiography. AJNR Am J Neuroradiol 1994;15(8):1401–7. discussion 1408-1411.

25. Wardlaw JM, Chappell FM, Best JJK, et al. Noninvasive imaging compared with intra-arterial angiography in the diagnosis of symptomatic carotid stenosis: a meta-analysis. Lancet 2006;367(9521): 1503–12.

26. Kleindorfer DO, Towfighi A, Chaturvedi S, et al. 2021 guideline for the prevention of stroke in patients with stroke and transient ischemic attack: a guideline from the American Heart association/American stroke association. Stroke 2021;52(7):e364–467.

27. White CJ, Brott TG, Gray WA, et al. Carotid artery stenting: JACC state-of-the-art review. J Am Coll Cardiol 2022;80(2):155–70.

28. Rosenfield K, Matsumura JS, Chaturvedi S, et al. Randomized trial of stent versus surgery for asymptomatic carotid stenosis. N Engl J Med 2016;374(11):1011–20.

29. Yadav JS, Wholey MH, Kuntz RE, et al. Protected carotid-artery stenting versus endarterectomy in high-risk patients. N Engl J Med 2004;351(15):1493–501.

30. Nca - percutaneous transluminal angioplasty (PTA) of the carotid artery concurrent with stenting (CAG-00085R8) - proposed decision memo. Available at: https://www.cms.gov/medicare-coverage-database/view/ncacal-decision-memo.aspx?proposed=Y&ncaid=311. Accessed September 22, 2024.

31. Paraskevas KI, Zeebregts CJ, AbuRahma AF, et al. Implications of the Centers for Medicare and Medicaid Services decision to expand indications for carotid artery stenting. J Vasc Surg 2024;80(3):599–603.

32. AbuRahma AF, Avgerinos ED, Chang RW, et al. Society for Vascular Surgery clinical practice guidelines for management of extracranial cerebrovascular disease. J Vasc Surg 2022;75(1S):4S–22S.

33. Aday AW, Beckman JA. Medical management of asymptomatic carotid artery stenosis. Prog Cardiovasc Dis 2017;59(6):585–90.

34. Meschia JF, Bushnell C, Boden-Albala B, et al. Guidelines for the primary prevention of stroke: a statement for healthcare professionals from the American Heart Association/American Stroke Association. Stroke 2014;45(12):3754–832.

35. Eastcott HH, Pickering GW, Rob CG. Reconstruction of internal carotid artery in a patient with intermittent attacks of hemiplegia. Lancet 1954;267(6846):994–6.

36. Uno M, Takai H, Yagi K, et al. Surgical technique for carotid endarterectomy: current methods and problems. Neurol Med Chir (Tokyo) 2020;60(9):419–28.

37. Findlay JM, Marchak BE, Pelz DM, et al. Carotid endarterectomy: a review. Can J Neurol Sci 2004;31(1):22–36.

38. Barnett HJM, Taylor DW, Peerless SJ, et al, North American Symptomatic Carotid Endarterectomy Trial Collaborators. Beneficial effect of carotid endarterectomy in symptomatic patients with high-grade carotid stenosis. N Engl J Med 1991;325(7):445–53.

39. Mayberg MR, Wilson SE, Yatsu F, et al. Carotid endarterectomy and prevention of cerebral ischemia in symptomatic carotid stenosis. Veterans Affairs Cooperative Studies Program 309 Trialist Group. JAMA 1991;266(23):3289–94.

40. Hobson RW, Weiss DG, Fields WS, et al. Efficacy of carotid endarterectomy for asymptomatic carotid stenosis. The Veterans Affairs cooperative study group. N Engl J Med 1993;328(4):221–7.

41. Endarterectomy for asymptomatic carotid artery stenosis. Executive committee for the asymptomatic carotid atherosclerosis study. JAMA 1995;273(18):1421–8.

42. Lamanna A, Maingard J, Barras CD, et al. Carotid artery stenting: current state of evidence and future directions. Acta Neurol Scand 2019;139(4):318–33.

43. White CJ. Carotid artery stenting. J Am Coll Cardiol 2014;64(7):722–31.

44. Saleem T, Baril DT. Carotid artery stenting. StatPearls. Treasure island (FL): StatPearls Publishing; 2024.

45. Omran J, Mahmud E, White CJ, et al. Proximal balloon occlusion versus distal filter protection in carotid artery stenting: a meta-analysis and review of the literature. Catheter Cardiovasc Interv 2017;89(5):923–31.

46. Brueck M, Bandorski D, Kramer W, et al. A randomized comparison of transradial versus transfemoral approach for coronary angiography and angioplasty. JACC Cardiovasc Interv 2009;2(11):1047–54.

47. Ruzsa Z, Nemes B, Pintér L, et al. A randomised comparison of transradial and transfemoral approach for carotid artery stenting: RADCAR (RADial access for CARotid artery stenting) study. EuroIntervention 2014;10(3):381–91.

48. Jaroenngarmsamer T, Bhatia KD, Kortman H, et al. Procedural success with radial access for carotid artery stenting: systematic review and meta-analysis. J Neurointerv Surg 2020;12(1):87–93.

49. Endovascular versus surgical treatment in patients with carotid stenosis in the Carotid and Vertebral Artery Transluminal Angioplasty Study (CAVATAS): a randomised trial. Lancet 2001;357(9270):1729–37.

50. Brooks WH, McClure RR, Jones MR, et al. Carotid angioplasty and stenting versus carotid endarterectomy: randomized trial in a community hospital. J Am Coll Cardiol 2001;38(6):1589–95.

51. Mas J-L, Chatellier G, Beyssen B, et al. Endarterectomy versus stenting in patients with symptomatic severe carotid stenosis. N Engl J Med 2006;355(16):1660–71.

52. SPACE Collaborative Group, Ringleb PA, Allenberg J, et al. 30 day results from the SPACE trial of stent-protected angioplasty versus carotid endarterectomy in symptomatic patients: a randomised non-inferiority trial. Lancet 2006;368(9543):1239–47.

53. Bonati LH, Dobson J, Featherstone RL, et al. Long-term outcomes after stenting versus endarterectomy

for treatment of symptomatic carotid stenosis: the International Carotid Stenting Study (ICSS) randomised trial. Lancet 2015;385(9967):529–38.

54. Brott TG, Howard G, Roubin GS, et al. Long-term results of stenting versus endarterectomy for carotid-artery stenosis. N Engl J Med 2016;374(11):1021–31.

55. Jones MR, Howard G, Roubin GS, et al. Periprocedural stroke and myocardial infarction as risks for long-term mortality in CREST. Circ Cardiovasc Qual Outcomes 2018;11(11):e004663.

56. Gurm HS, Yadav JS, Fayad P, et al. Long-term results of carotid stenting versus endarterectomy in high-risk patients. N Engl J Med 2008;358(15):1572–9.

57. Reiff T, Eckstein HH, Mansmann U, et al. Angioplasty in asymptomatic carotid artery stenosis vs. endarterectomy compared to best medical treatment: one-year interim results of SPACE-2. Int J Stroke 2019;15(6). 1747493019833017.

58. Halliday A, Bulbulia R, Bonati LH, et al. Second asymptomatic carotid surgery trial (ACST-2): a randomised comparison of carotid artery stenting versus carotid endarterectomy. Lancet 2021; 398(10305):1065–73.

59. Galyfos GC, Tsoutsas I, Konstantopoulos T, et al. Editor's choice - early and late outcomes after transcarotid revascularisation for internal carotid artery stenosis: a systematic review and meta-analysis. Eur J Vasc Endovasc Surg 2021;61(5):725–38.

60. Mehta A, Patel PB, Bajakian D, et al. Transcarotid artery revascularization versus carotid endarterectomy and transfemoral stenting in octogenarians. J Vasc Surg 2021;74(5):1602–8.

61. Zarrintan S, Malas MB. What is the role of transcarotid artery revascularization? Adv Surg 2023;57(1): 115–40.

62. Stabile E, Giugliano G, Cremonesi A, et al. Impact on outcome of different types of carotid stent: results from the European Registry of Carotid Artery Stenting. EuroIntervention 2016;12(2):e265–70.

63. Timaran CH, Rosero EB, Higuera A, et al. Randomized clinical trial of open-cell vs closed-cell stents for carotid stenting and effects of stent design on cerebral embolization. J Vasc Surg 2011;54(5): 1310–6.e1. discussion 1316.

64. Karpenko A, Bugurov S, Ignatenko P, et al. Randomized controlled trial of conventional versus MicroNet-covered stent in carotid artery revascularization. JACC Cardiovasc Interv 2021;14(21): 2377–87.

65. Garg N, Karagiorgos N, Pisimisis GT, et al. Cerebral protection devices reduce periprocedural strokes during carotid angioplasty and stenting: a systematic review of the current literature. J Endovasc Ther 2009;16(4):412–27.

66. Kajihara Y, Sakamoto S, Kiura Y, et al. Comparison of dual protection and distal filter protection as a distal embolic protection method during carotid artery stenting: a single-center carotid artery stenting experience. Neurosurg Rev 2015;38(4): 671–6.

Renal and Mesenteric Artery Intervention

Jose D. Tafur, MD[a], Khanjan B. Shah, MD[b],
Christopher J. White, MD, MACC, MSCAI, FAHA, FESC, FACP[a,c,d,e],*

KEYWORDS

- Renal artery stent • Mesenteric artery stent • Renal artery stenosis • Chronic mesenteric ischemia
- Renovascular hypertension

KEY POINTS

- Uncontrolled hypertension on 3 antihypertensive medications (including a diuretic), ischemic nephropathy, and cardiac destabilization syndromes with hemodynamically significant renal artery stenosis are likely to benefit from stenting.
- Radial access, embolic protection devices, and intravascular ultrasound-guided stenting increase the safety and success rate of interventions.
- Symptomatic chronic mesenteric ischemia usually results from significant stenosis affecting 2 or more vessels. Endovascular revascularization has largely replaced open surgery as the initial treatment.

RENAL AND MESENTERIC ARTERY INTERVENTION

Introduction

Atherosclerotic disease of the abdominal aorta and its visceral branches poses significant health risks because of its potential to cause severe complications. This condition is primarily driven by risk factors such as age, smoking, hypertension, dyslipidemia, and diabetes mellitus. It is prevalent among older adults, with increasing incidence in those with multiple risk factors. The disease's significance lies in its potential to lead to critical outcomes such as abdominal aortic aneurysm, thromboembolism, and acute mesenteric ischemia. Atherosclerosis can also affect renal and mesenteric vessels, contributing to renal hypoperfusion and mesenteric ischemia, respectively, both of which can result in organ damage if left untreated. Management involves aggressive risk factor modification and revascularization procedures when indicated.

Percutaneous renal artery stenting has been shown to be safe and effective for atherosclerotic renal artery stenosis (ARAS), however, several randomized controlled trials (RCTs) have not shown superior outcomes when compared with guideline-directed medical therapy (GDMT).[1-3] Additionally, meta-analyses demonstrate that a high technical success rate (>95%) for renal stenting is accompanied by a modest clinical improvement (~70%). This discrepancy in procedural success and clinical effectiveness exists due to suboptimal patient selection by stenting nonhemodynamically significant lesions or patients with essential hypertension.

---

[a] Department of Cardiovascular Diseases, John Ochsner Heart & Vascular Center, Ochsner Medical Center, The Ochsner Clinical School, Univ of Queensland, New Orleans, LA, USA; [b] Division of Cardiovascular Disease, University of Florida College of Medicine, Gainesville, FL, USA; [c] Department of Cardiology, 3rd Floor, 1514 Jefferson Highway, New Orleans, LA 70121, USA; [d] Department of Cardiology, Ochsner Medical Center, 1514 Jefferson Highway, New Orleans, LA 70121, USA; [e] Value Based Care
* Corresponding author. Department of Cardiology, Ochsner Medical Center, 1514 Jefferson Highway, New Orleans, LA 70121.
E-mail address: cwhite@ochsner.org

Intervent Cardiol Clin 14 (2025) 205–223
https://doi.org/10.1016/j.iccl.2024.11.007
2211-7458/25/© 2024 Elsevier Inc. All rights reserved, including those for text and data mining, AI training, and similar technologies.

Abbreviations	
ACC	American College of Cardiology
ACS	acute coronary syndrome
AHA	American Heart Association
AP	antero-posterior
ARAS	atherosclerotic renal artery stenosis
AUS	Appropriate Use Criteria
BMS	bare-metal stent
CCS	Canadian Cardiovascular Society
CHF	congestive heart failure
CKD	chronic kidney disease
CMI	chronic mesenteric ischemia
CS	covered stent
CTA	computed tomographic angiography
DES	drug eluting stent
DSA	digital subtraction angiography
DUS	Doppler ultrasound
EPD	embolic protection device
EVT	endovascular therapy
FMD	fibromuscular dysplasia
GDMT	guideline-directed medical therapy
GFR	glomerular filtration rate
HTN	hypertension
ISR	in-stent restenosis
IVUS	intravascular ultrasound
LAT	lateral
LOE	level of evidence
MRA	magnetic resonance angiography
NIS	National Inpatient Sample
NYHA	New York Heart Association
OSR	open surgical repair
PSV	peak systolic velocity
RCT	randomized controlled trial
RFFR	renal fractional flow reserve
SMA	superior mesenteric artery
SRF	split renal function

For chronic mesenteric ischemia (CMI), open surgical repair (OSR) was historically the standard of treatment, but surgery has been largely supplanted by endovascular therapy (EVT), due to the significant morbidity and mortality associated with OSR in these often frail and undernourished patients. EVT is associated with a high technical success rate with a low rate of complications in properly selected patients. However, mesenteric artery stenting is associated with 1 year restenosis rates of 30% to 40%.[4]

We will review this literature and supporting evidence base, indications, contraindications, procedural technique, complications, and follow-up for renal and mesenteric artery interventions.

RENAL ARTERY INTERVENTIONS

It is of paramount importance that the clinician understands clearly which patients are likely to benefit from renal artery revascularization. Appropriate patient selection combined with safe technique can result in excellent clinical outcomes. We will review the main indications for renal artery stenting in light of the current evidence.

Supporting Evidence Base

Renovascular Hypertension: The safety and efficacy of renal stenting has been demonstrated in clinical trials have shown significant decrease in systolic and diastolic blood pressure. Renal stents have excellent long-term patency rates, with cumulative primary patency of 79% to 85% and a secondary patency of 92% to 98% at 5 years.[5,6] Secondary interventions for renal in-stent restenosis (ISR) have higher target lesion revascularization versus de novo renal stents (21% vs 11%; P=.003).[7]

There have been 3 recent RCTs that have failed to demonstrate superiority of renal stents with GDMT over GDMT alone in patients with mild to moderate ARAS (Table 1). The Stent Placement in Patients with Atherosclerotic Renal Artery Stenosis and Impaired Renal Function: A Randomized Trial (STAR) enrolled patients with ARAS stenoses greater than 50% and a creatinine clearance less than 80 mL/min per 1.73 m^2.[3] GDMT alone compared with GDMT with renal artery stenting had no effect on progression of chronic kidney disease (CKD). A major limitation of this study was that 30% of the patients randomized to the renal stenting arm had ARAS less than 50% and as such would not be candidates for revascularization.

The Angioplasty and Stenting for Renal Artery Lesions (ASTRAL) trial reported no benefit of revascularization over medical therapy with regard to blood pressure, renal function, cardiovascular events, or mortality.[3] However, the revascularization group were on fewer antihypertensive medications than the medical group (2.77 vs 2.97, P=.03). The major criticisms of this trial include only 60% of the patients had a greater than 70% ARAS (by

Table 1
Summary of recent renal stent trials

Trial	STAR[62]	ASTRAL[3]	CORAL[2]
Year	2009	2009	2014
Number of patients	140	806	947
Inclusion criteria	• Impaired renal function (CrCl < 80) • Ostial ARAS of 50% or more (CTA, MRA, DSA) • Controlled BP < 140/90	• Renal artery atherosclerotic disease in ≥1 renal artery amenable to revascularization • Clinician unsure if revascularization would provide clear benefit	• Severe RAS (angiograpically defined as > 60% but < 100%, AND • HTN with systolic BP ≥ 155 on 2 or more agents OR • CKD defined as GFR < 60
Exclusion criteria	• Renal size < 8 cm • Renal artery < 4 mm • CrCl < 15 • Diabetes with proteinuria > 3 g/d • Malignant HTN	• Disease needing surgical revascularization • High likelihood of needing revascularization in 6 mo • Nonatheromatous disease • Prior ARAS revascularization • Lack of informed consent	• FMD • CKD from causes other than ischemic nephropathy • Cr > 4 • Kidney size <7 cm • Lesions that could not be treated with one stent
Primary end point	• Worsening renal function > 20% decrease of CrCl	• Slope of the reciprocal of Cr over 5 y	• Time to major renal or cardiovascular event (stroke, heart attack, CHF hospitalization, progressive renal insufficiency, need for dialysis)
Limitations	• Patients had controlled blood pressure • Considerable number of patients had < 50% stenoses	• Rate of complications much higher than reported • Lower number of antihypertensives used in intervention group • Diagnosis of ARAS made with noninvasive imaging without functional studies • Patients with kidney size < 6 cm included in study • Patients with nonsignificant lesions included	• Patients were not optimized on antihypertensive therapy • Inclusion of patients with mild stenosis • Only moderate correlation between angiography and hemodynamically significant stenoses.

Abbreviations: ARAS, atherosclerotic renal artery stenosis; BP, blood pressure; CHF, congestive heart failure; CKD, chronic kidney disease; Cr, creatinine; CrCl, creatinine clearance; CTA, computerized tomographic angiography; DSA, digital subtraction angiography; FMD, fibromuscular dysplasia; GFR, glomerular filtration rate; HTN, hypertension; MRA, magnetic resonance angiography.

ultrasound, not angiographic measurement), so that many of the patients in the trial may not have had an indication for revascularization. Additionally, the complication rate by the trial operators was very high (9%).

The Cardiovascular Outcomes in Renal Atherosclerotic Lesions (CORAL) trial enrolled patients with hypertension (HTN) defined as a systolic blood pressure of ≥155 mm Hg despite taking ≥2 antihypertensive medications, which by definition included patients without refractory hypertension.[2] Because the hemodynamic severity of moderate (50%–70% diameter stenosis) lesions was not hemodynamically confirmed, it is very likely that patients with nonobstructive ARAS were enrolled in the trial and would be unlikely to benefit from revascularization.

Because randomization requires clinical equipoise for GDMT, patients with the most severe ARAS and most severe symptoms were underrepresented in these trials. This paradox is humorously illustrated by the parachute study, where a RCT found no difference in preventing death or major trauma between parachutes and empty backpacks when jumping from a low height (about 2 feet). This demonstrates the limitations of RCTs. The study's conclusion that parachutes were no more effective than empty backpacks only applies to short falls, not high-altitude jumps, highlighting that the study did not directly address the efficacy of parachutes at higher altitudes.[8]

The 3 RCTs mentioned above all enrolled patients with mild to moderate ARAS, in whom the benefit of renal stents was uncertain, and with equipoise allowing the investigators to enroll "low risk" patients to justify the option of GDMT alone. These trials failed to document the hemodynamic significance of the mild to moderate ARAS (ie, trans-lesional gradient). They did not include patients with the most severe ARAS, in whom observational data would justify renal stenting, and whom investigators would be unwilling to randomize to GDMT alone. The population tested in the 3 RCTs, similar to the parachute trial, were at low risk for adverse events with mild to moderate ARAS, and therefore, it was "safe" to withhold renal stenting.

The publication of these studies showing little to no benefit of revascularization in ARAS patients has led to a significant reduction in annual renal angiography and ARAS detection rates in major hospitals across Europe and the United States, as shown in Fig. 1.[9]

True resistant hypertension defined as systolic blood pressure (SBP) greater than 160 mm Hg,

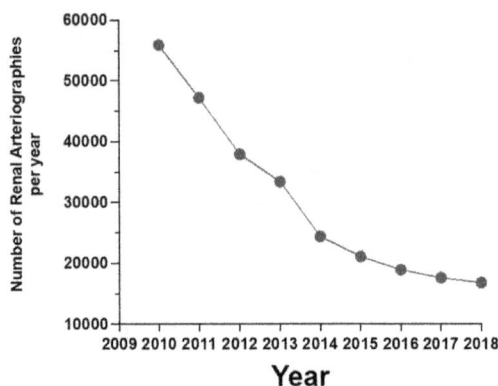

Fig. 1. Temporal trends of renal artery angiography.[9]

DBP greater than 90 mm Hg despite the use of 3 or more antihypertensive medications at maximally tolerated doses including a diuretic, remains an indication for renal artery revascularization when unilateral or bilateral stenosis is present. Long-term follow-up studies have shown sustained blood pressure reduction and decreased antihypertensive medication use after renal artery stenting (RAS) in appropriately selected patients.[10]

Ischemic Nephropathy: Multiple trials have demonstrated that renal artery stent placement improves or stabilizes renal function in patients with atherosclerotic renovascular renal insufficiency. Harden and coworkers reported on a series of 32 patients (33 kidneys) with unexplained renal insufficiency and hemodynamically significant renal artery stenosis treated with renal artery stent placement.[11] The majority of patients had bilateral or solitary renal artery stenoses, although unilateral disease was present in 7 patients. The authors concluded that stent placement slows the progression of renal artery insufficiency.

A second study examined 33 patients undergoing successful renal artery stent placement for bilateral or solitary renal artery stenosis (≥70%) with a baseline serum creatinine between 1.5 and 4.0 mg/dL.[12] Follow-up (≥8 months) data were available in 25 patients, all of whom had either improvement or stabilization of renal function. One of the strongest predictors of improvement in renal function after intervention for RAS is rapidly progressing renal failure.[13] The slope of the reciprocal serum creatinine plot before renal intervention was associated with a favorable change in renal function. Three prospective trials have established renal function benefit after successful stent treatment of unilateral RAS.[14–16] They all consistently demonstrate that hyperfiltration

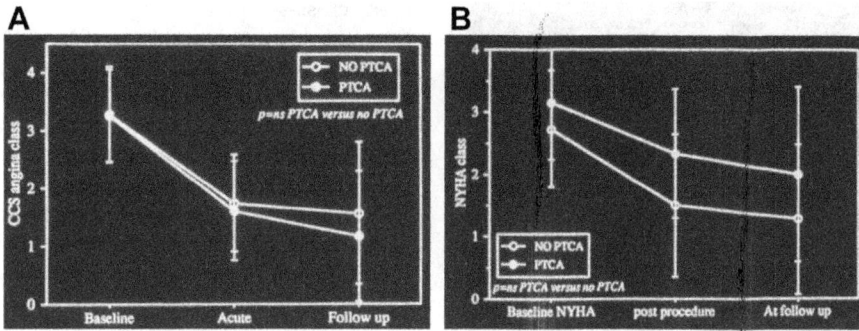

Fig. 2. (A) Graph demonstrating improvement in CCS Angina Classification in patients with renal stenting showing no difference for those with and without coronary interventions. (B) Graph demonstrating improvement in NYHA Classification of heart failure in patients with renal stenting showing no difference for those with and without coronary interventions.

of the normal kidney returns toward normal, and glomerular filtration rate (GFR) of the treated kidney increases with net stabilization of total GFR after successful revascularization.

Cardiac Destabilization Syndromes: Patients with ARAS can suffer acutely decompensated heart failure (ie, flash pulmonary edema), refractory heart failure, or exacerbations of acute coronary syndrome (ACS), the so-called cardiac destabilization syndromes. Often patients with a solitary functioning kidney or bilateral RAS will manifest volume overload as decompensated heart failure. This can result in increased myocardial oxygen consumption leading to unstable angina.

The importance of renal artery stent placement in the treatment of cardiac destabilization syndromes has been described in a series of patients with presenting with either congestive heart failure or an ACS.[17] Successful renal stent placement resulted in a significant decrease in blood pressure and control of symptoms in 88% (42 of 48) of the patients (Fig. 2A, B). Some patients underwent both coronary and renal intervention, while others had only renal artery stent placement due to no coronary lesions suitable for revascularization. Assessment of the treatment effects acutely and at 8 months using the Canadian Cardiovascular Society (CCS) angina classification and the New York Heart Association (NYHA) functional classification were not different between the combined coronary and renal revascularization group compared with those who had only renal stent placement, suggesting that renal revascularization was the most significant intervention.

In another study, 39 patients underwent renal artery stent implantation for control of heart failure which represented 19% of the renal artery stent population.[18] Eighteen (46%) patients had bilateral RAS and 21 (54%) patients had stenosis of a solitary functioning kidney. Renal artery stent implantation was successful in all patients. Hypertension responded to the successful renal stent placement in 72% of the patients. Renal function improved in 51% and remained stable in an additional 26% of patients. The mean number of hospitalizations for heart failure prior to stenting was 2.37 + 1.42 (range 1–6) and after renal stenting was 0.30 + 0.65 (range 0–3) ($P<.001$). Three-quarters of patients had no further hospitalizations after renal artery stenting over a 2-year follow-up.

In a literature review of 87 cases of bilateral RAS and flash pulmonary edema (ie, Pickering Syndrome), 35% were treated with unilateral and 22% with bilateral stenting.[19] In 43% of patients, in earlier reports, surgical revascularization was performed. Renal function improved in 81% of patients and the mean creatinine on follow-up was 1.6 mg/dL (141 mol/L) after the procedure. Importantly, in 92% of all patients, there were no further episodes of flash pulmonary edema after revascularization. The diagnosis of Pickering Syndrome is feasible even when administration of iodine contrast medium quantity would seem to be contraindicated because of severely reduced renal function. Revascularization with RAS with little use of contrast medium can help these patients avoid dialysis and recurrent episodes of life-threatening pulmonary edema.

The American College of Cardiology/American Heart Association (ACC/AHA) Guidelines make renal stenting for hemodynamically significant RAS and recurrent, unexplained congestive heart failure, or sudden unexplained pulmonary edema a Class I, level of evidence (LOE) B indication. Renal stenting for unstable angina earned a Class IIa, LOE B indication.[20]

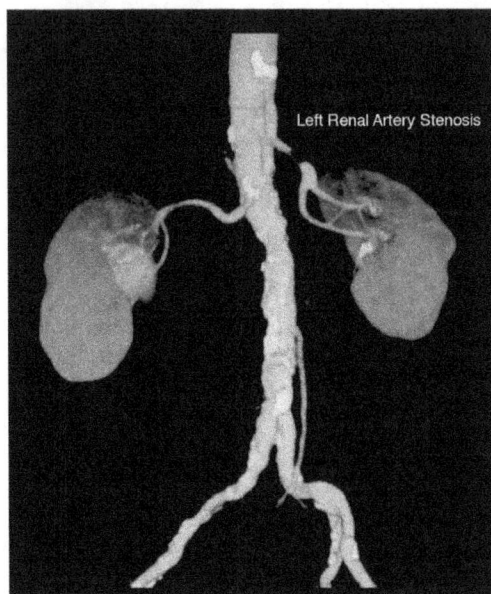

Fig. 3. Abdominal CTA angiogram showing left renal artery stenosis[17]; with permission.

Diagnostic Methods

Noninvasive: Renal Doppler ultrasound (DUS) imaging is an excellent tool for the diagnosis of ARAS. A peak systolic velocity (PSV) of greater than 200 cm/s is very sensitive and specific for greater than 50% stenosis. A ratio of renal artery PSV to the PSV of the aorta of greater than 3.5 has 92% sensitivity for greater than 60% diameter stenosis.[21] If DUS is unable to confirm the hemodynamic severity of ARAS,

then cross-sectional imaging with computed tomographic angiography (CTA) or magnetic resonance angiography (MRA) is the next option (Fig. 3). The sensitivity and specificity of CTA have been shown to be 90% to 100% and 97% for stenosis greater than 50%. The sensitivity of MRA is 92% to 97% with a specificity of 73% to 93%; however, patients with acute or chronic renal dysfunction may not be candidates for these modalities.[22]

Split renal function (SRF) is a nuclear imaging technique to assess the impact of hemodynamically significant unilateral ARAS on overall renal function. SRF using [99m]Technetium Tc-diethylene-triamine-pentaacetate renal scintigraphy was performed before and after renal stenting for unilateral ARAS. Following successful stenting, ambulatory systolic and diastolic blood pressures significantly decreased from 145 to 138 mm Hg and diastolic BP decreased from 80 to 77 mm Hg (*P*=.005) and the estimated glomerular filtration rate increased in the stented kidney from 22 to 26, and normalized in the hyperfiltering, nonstenotic kidney from 37 to 34 (*P*<.026).[23] This technique may be helpful in determining who may benefit from revascularization when a significant unilateral stenosis is detected but GFR is normal.

Invasive: Digital subtraction angiography (DSA) is a 2-dimensional imaging modality that suffers from relatively poor discrimination of renal artery lesion severity because these stenoses are often located in tortuous, overlapping arteries. By consensus of experts an angiographic ARAS greater than 70% diameter stenosis is

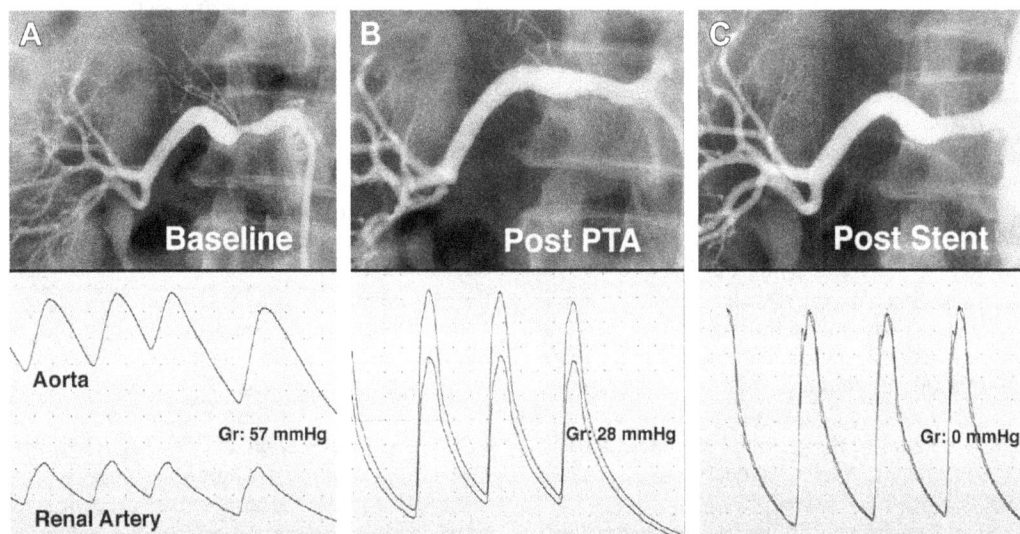

Fig. 4. Angiogram and proximal and distal pressure tracing. (*A*) Baseline angiogram with 57 mm Hg trans-lesional gradient. (*B*) Following balloon angioplasty with improvement in stenosis, but residual 28 mm Hg gradient. (*C*) After renal stent with slight angiographic improvement, but no residual trans-lesional gradient.

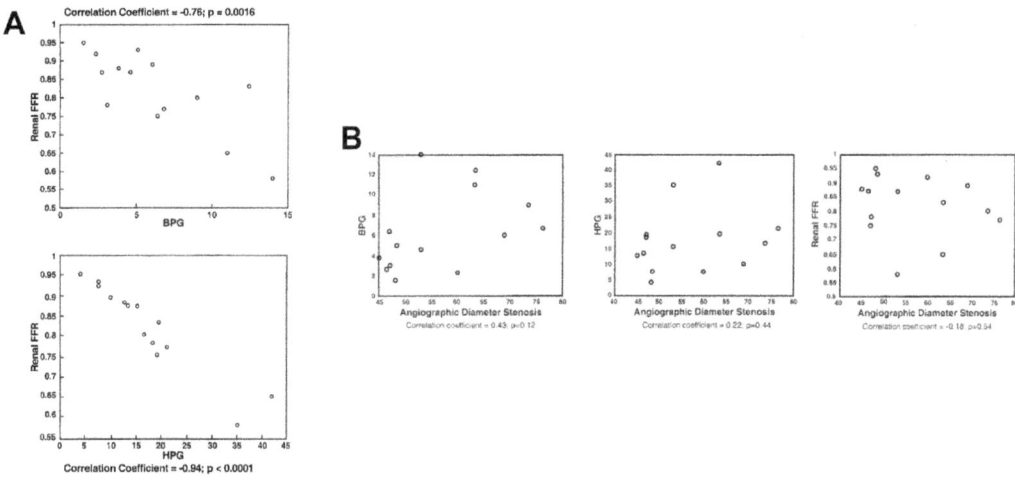

Fig. 5. (A) Left: The correlation of quantitative angiographic diameter stenosis (angiographic diameter stenosis) with baseline mean trans-lesional pressure gradient (BPG); Center: hyperemic mean trans-lesional pressure gradient (HPG); and Right: RFFR. (B) The correlation of RFFR with the baseline mean trans-lesional pressure gradient (BPG; top) and hyperemic mean trans-lesional pressure gradient (HPG; bottom). Reproduced with permission.[26]

severe/significant and diameter stenoses of 50% to 69% are considered moderately severe, of uncertain hemodynamic significance.[20] For moderately severe stenoses (50%–69%), confirmation of the hemodynamic severity of the RAS is recommended prior to stenting.[24,25]

A resting or hyperemic trans-lesional systolic gradient of ≥20 mm Hg, a resting or hyperemic mean trans-lesional gradient of ≥10 mm Hg or a renal fractional flow reserve (RFFR) ≤ 0.8 will confirm hemodynamically severe ARAS (Fig. 4A–C).[24,25] We compared conventional angiography to RFFR and to trans-lesional pressure gradients to determine ARAS stenosis severity. There was a poor correlation between the angiographic stenosis, and RFFR (r = −0.18; P=.54) as well as to the trans-lesional pressure gradient (r = 0.22; P=.44). However, the correlation between RFFR and the trans-lesional pressure gradient was excellent (r = 0.76; P=.0016) (Fig. 5A, B).[26]

The trans-lesional pressure gradient should be measured with a nonobstructive catheter or with a 0.014-inch pressure wire. Hyperemia may be induced with an intrarenal bolus of papaverine at a dose of 40 mg or an intrarenal bolus of 50 µg/kg dopamine.[26,27] It is important to note that papaverine will precipitate in heparinized saline solutions commonly used for catheterization laboratory flush solutions.

Indications and Contraindications

The ACC/AHA Guidelines[20] and Appropriate Use Criteria (AUC) recommend that patients most likely to benefit from renal artery stenting have hemodynamically significant ARAS [moderate (50% −70%) ARAS with a resting/hyperemic trans-lesional mean gradient of ≥10 mm Hg, systolic gradient ≥20 mm Hg/or angiographically severe (>70%) ARAS] and (1) recurrent congestive heart failure, or sudden onset, "flash," pulmonary edema. Patients with hemodynamically significant ARAS with refractory ACS (2) those with refractory HTN who fail or are intolerant of GDMT and (3) patients with progressive CKD due to bilateral/solitary ARAS, or with unilateral ARAS (Table 2).

There is no indication for the treatment of ARAS in asymptomatic patients.[24,25] The initial treatment of symptomatic ARAS, as demonstrated in the CORAL trial, is GDMT.[2] When evaluating a patient with ARAS, it is important to determine whether their symptoms are caused by renal hypoperfusion, or if ARAS is an innocent bystander. ARAS may be found on routine abdominal imaging when evaluating a patient for other problems. However, if ARAS is not causing a clinical problem, there is no role for revascularization. Also, not likely to benefit from renal artery stenting are patients that have uncontrolled blood pressure but are not on maximally tolerated GDMT including a total of 3 antihypertensives with a diuretic. Lastly, ischemic nephropathy patients unlikely to benefit from revascularization include those with chronic CKD stage III to stage IV and a pole-to-pole kidney size of ≤7 cm or patients on hemodialysis ≥3 months.[20,24,25]

Table 2
Renal artery stenting and appropriate use criteria (AUC) and guidelines

Scenario	AUC[25]	AHA/ACC Guideline[20]
Cardiac Disturbance Syndromes (Flash pulmonary edema, unstable angina or ACS) with hypertension and significant ARAS.	Appropriate	Class I, LOE B (CHF) Class IIa, LOE B (unstable angina)
CKD IV with bilateral significant ARAS with a with a kidney size > 7 cm in pole-to-pole length.	Appropriate	Class IIa, LOE B
CKD IV and global renal ischemia (unilateral significant ARAS with a solitary kidney or bilateral significant ARAS) without another explanation.	Appropriate	Class IIb, LOE B
Resistant hypertension (uncontrolled hypertension having failed maximally tolerated doses of at least 3 antihypertensive agents, one of which a diuretic) and bilateral or solitary significant ARAS.	Appropriate	Class IIa, LOE B
Recurrent CHF with unilateral significant ARAS.	May be appropriate	Class IIa, LOE B
Resistant hypertension (uncontrolled hypertension having failed maximally tolerated doses of at least 3 antihypertensive agents, one of which a diuretic) and unilateral significant ARAS.	May be appropriate	Class IIa, LOE B
Asymptomatic, unilateral, bilateral, or solitary kidney with hemodynamically significant ARAS.	Rarely appropriate	Class III, LOE C

Abbreviations: ACC, American College of Cardiology; ACS, acute coronary syndrome; AHA, American Heart Association; ARAS, atherosclerotic renal artery stenosis; AUC, appropriate use criteria; CHF, congestive heart failure; CKD, chronic kidney disease; Significant ARAS, moderate (50%–70%) ARAS with a resting/hyperemic trans-lesional mean gradient of $\geq$ 10 mm Hg, systolic gradient $\geq$ 20 mm Hg/or severe (>70%) ARAS.

Procedural Technique

Preprocedural Imaging: A nonselective renal angiogram (aortography) should be performed prior to renal intervention unless prior noninvasive imaging is available (CTA or MRA) to delineate the anatomy of the aorta and renal arteries (Fig. 6).

The catheter-in-catheter or no-touch techniques: This technique should be used to minimize contact with the aortic wall and prevent injury to the renal ostium during guiding catheter manipulation (Fig. 7A–C). Ostial atherosclerotic plaque usually extends to the aortic wall and manipulation of this can result in distal embolization. The no-touch technique requires a 0.035-inch J-wire resting on the suprarenal wall of the aorta during engagement of the renal artery. This 0.035-inch J-wire prevents the tip of

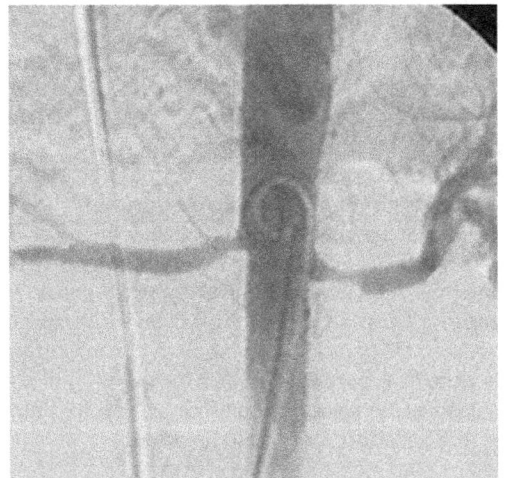

Fig. 6. Abdominal aortogram showing mild to moderate renal artery stenosis of uncertain hemodynamic significance.

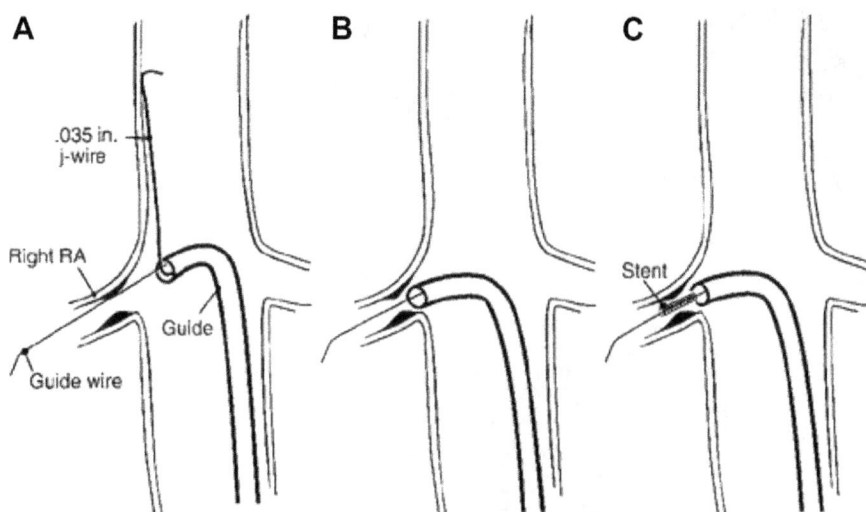

Fig. 7. (A) Baseline angiography using right radial artery access of a 90% stenosis of right renal artery using a 6 Fr multipurpose (125 cm) guide catheter. Note the landing zone prior to the bifurcation, suitable for a filter device (off-label use). (B) The filter device has been deployed and the undeployed stent is being positioned across the lesion. (C) Final angiography following stent deployment and filter retrieval. (From White CJ. Optimizing outcomes for renal artery intervention. Circulation Cardiovascular interventions. 2010;3(2):184-192; with permission.)

the guide catheter from scraping the wall of the aorta during maneuvering. Once the artery is engaged, a 0.014-inch guidewire is advanced into the renal artery.[28]

Radial access: Radial artery access with a 6 Fr sheath, or sheathless with a 6 or 7 Fr guiding catheter is the preferred route for percutaneous diagnostic and interventional renal artery procedures to reduce access site bleeding complications, improve postprocedural patient comfort, and to facilitate renal artery ostial engagement (Fig. 8A–F).

For renal interventions, there is an operator learning curve for catheter manipulation, catheter guide selection, and stent placement. The left radial artery may provide a shorter route to the renal arteries. The use of longer guiding catheters (125–135 cm) and balloon shafts (150 cm) in taller patients is often necessary with the radial technique. It is important to confirm the compatibility of the locally available stents with the radial equipment. Larger diameter stents usually require larger guiding catheters which may favor femoral access in some cases.

Embolic Protection Devices (EPDs): Atheroembolism likely plays a role in postprocedural deterioration of renal function seen in about one-quarter of successful renal artery stent patients. EPDs may prevent embolic injury during renal stenting and have been shown to be safe.[29,30] A randomized study (100 patients) looking at patients with chronic kidney disease undergoing renal artery stenting suggested

there was preservation of renal function with embolic protection when combined with IIb/IIIa antiplatelet inhibitors.[31]

More data are needed to evaluate the impact of EPDs in patients with normal and abnormal renal function undergoing renal stenting. EPDs may be considered in high-risk patients with baseline renal insufficiency as a strategy to prevent worsening renal function related to atheroembolism resulting from stent placement.

Stent sizing with intravascular ultrasound (IVUS): In renal interventions, it is harder to visually estimate vessel diameter in these larger arteries (5–8 mm). IVUS can help operators with better lesion measurement, appropriate stent sizing, appropriate stent expansion, and achieve better outcomes measured by decrease in blood pressure and a lower incidence of angiographic restenosis. Restenosis in renal artery stenting with bare-metal stents (BMSs) is largely driven by the acute gain in lumen area, placing a premium on delivery of the largest stent that is safely possible. While undersizing renal stents is safe, it is associated with significantly higher restenosis rates.[32] The judicious use of IVUS can assist the operator to safely place optimally sized stents.

Drug eluting stents (DESs) vs BMS: A prospective trial that compared BMS to DES in ARAS found no difference in the restenosis rate for sirolimus-eluting stents compared with the BMS.[33] At 6 months and 1 year, the target lesion revascularization rate was not different between the 2 types of stents. There has been

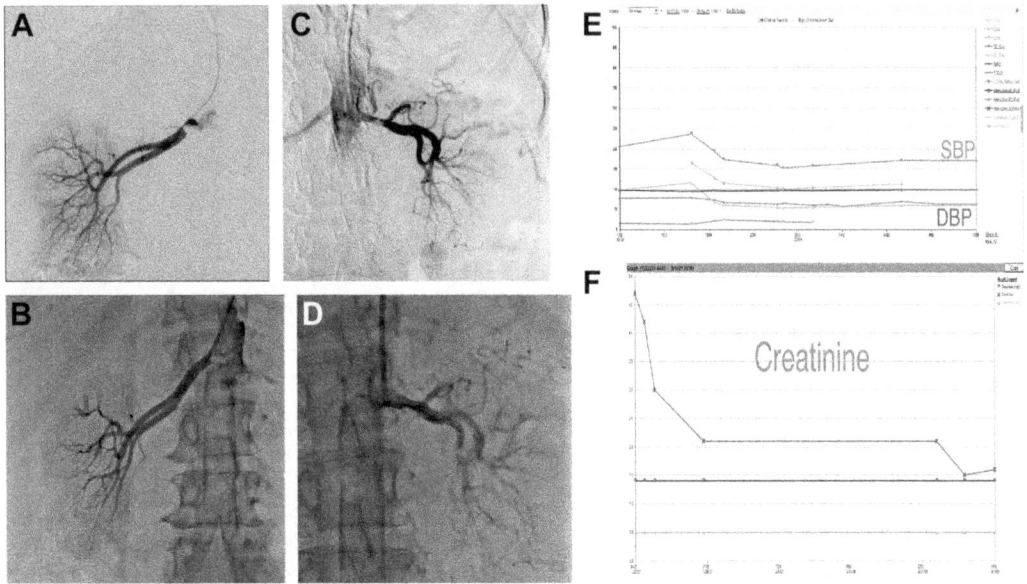

Fig. 8. Bilateral renal artery stenosis (*A, C*) and results after renal artery stenting from radial access (*B, D*). The graph in (*E*) shows the trends in the blood pressure and the graph in (*F*) shows the stabilization of renal function.

data published that did not compare DES to BMS head-to-head reporting outcomes favoring the DES in renal stenting, but it relied on a hybrid technique of placing a BMS within the DES.[34] These results are hypothesis generating and need to be more rigorously studied. A major problem with coronary DES in the renal arteries is their lack of radial strength due to their thin struts, resulting in stent recoil due to the bulky renal plaque exerting external compression. The largest diameter DES available is 6 mm, which may be undersized for some renal arteries.

ISR lesions: The best treatment of renal artery ISR has not been established due to a lack of comparative trials. Multiple options include balloon angioplasty, DES-in-BMS, BMS-in-BMS, covered stent (CS) placement, and brachytherapy.

Repeat renal artery BMS placement demonstrated improved patency compared with balloon angioplasty alone with a 58% reduction in recurrent ISR (29.4% vs 71.4%, $P=.02$).[35] The repeat BMS group also had better secondary patency ($P=.05$) and a greater freedom from repeat ISR ($P=.01$) when compared with balloon angioplasty alone. There was a trend favoring repeat BMS placement for cumulative freedom from target vessel revascularization ($P=.08$). In a small series of patients having at least their second ISR following BMS, CS had 17% (1/6) ISR at a mean follow-up of 36 months while coronary DES were free of ISR (0/10).[36] There is no evidence supporting a role for the use of debulking devices or cutting balloons in the management of

renal artery ISR. Studies have demonstrated acceptable long-term patency rates and clinical outcomes for CS in renal arteries.[37,38] Balloon-expandable CS have been successfully used to treat various indications, including unstable atheromatous lesions and recurrent ISR.[37] In a long-term follow-up study, CS effectively excluded renal artery aneurysms while maintaining vessel patency and improving blood pressure control and renal function.[38] Notably, CS has been associated with a lower incidence of in-stent stenosis compared with uncovered stents in renal arteries.[39]

CSs in coronary circulation are linked to higher adverse event rates, such as ISR, reinfarction, and thrombosis, compared with regular stents.[40] Despite their critical role in addressing arterial perforations, they pose ongoing risks of thrombosis and restenosis.[41] Conversely, CSs have shown excellent results in treating visceral artery aneurysms and pseudoaneurysms, with high technical success rates of 96% to 97% and long-term patency rates up to 88% over a mean follow-up of 32.8 months.[42,43] CSs seem generally effective and safe for use in visceral vessels, though further research is needed to understand long-term risks and the role of antithrombotic therapy.

Complications and Their Management

Vascular access: The most common complications in renal artery interventions are related to femoral access (hematoma, pseudoaneurysm, arteriovenous fistula, retroperitoneal bleed).[44,45] All are minimized or eliminated if radial artery access is utilized. Management of femoral access complications include use of CS placement, thrombin injection for pseudoaneurysms, and vascular surgical repair when necessary.

Vessel rupture and dissections: Fortunately, catastrophic complications during renal artery stenting are very uncommon. The overall incidence of major complications with renal artery stenting is near 2%.[45] The cause for significant dissection of the renal artery is typically the subintimal passage of the guidewire, excess catheter manipulations, over dilation prior to stent deployment, oversizing the stent, or aggressive balloon dilatation of the stent. The use of hydrophilic guidewires is to be discouraged because of the higher risk of vessel perforation.

It is critical to maintain guidewire access across the lesion. With a guidewire in place, the dissection flap may be sealed with prolonged balloon inflation or the placement of an additional stent. If complete arterial thrombosis occurs, this can be managed with a local infusion of a thrombolytic agent but reestablishing a patent lumen is essential for fibrinolytic agents to be successful.

If vessel perforation occurs, reversal of anticoagulation and prolonged balloon inflation is the first steps to control the hemorrhage. CS has been used for intraprocedural complications such as perforation or vessel rupture. If bleeding cannot be controlled, nephrectomy may be required.

Follow-up and Surveillance

The current AUC recommendations for DUS follow-up after renal intervention are that it is "appropriate" to perform a poststent baseline study within 30 days of the procedure.[46] It "may be appropriate" to perform additional DUS studies at 6 months and/or 9 months. It is "appropriate" to perform a follow-up DUS at 12 months and annually thereafter.

When duplex imaging is performed after renal stent placement, it is important to make adjustments to the velocity parameters poststenting compared with a native vessel, as decreased compliance due to the stent will result in higher velocities.[21] Therefore, obtaining a postprocedure DUS is reasonable to establish a new baseline PSV. If anatomic renal ISR is detected with surveillance, the patient must still meet the clinical requirements for reintervention, that is, refractory hypertension despite GDMT, progressive CKD, or develop a cardiac destabilization syndrome. Many patients can be followed with serial DUS and GDMT with stable ISR for years.

MESENTERIC ARTERY INTERVENTIONS
Supporting Evidence Base

There are no large RCTs comparing EVT to OSR for CMI. However, there are multiple retrospective studies supporting EVT for CMI especially in older, higher surgical risk patients.

The National Inpatient Sample (NIS) from 1988 to 2006 was used to compare 6342 EVT and 16,071 OSR for CMI, with EVT surpassing OSR for annual volume in 2002.[47] The mortality rate was lower after EVT than after OSR for CMI (3.7% vs 13%, $P<.01$) and acute mesenteric ischemia was less prevalent after EVT (16% vs 28%, $P<.01$)[48,49] (Fig. 9). Bowel resection was more common after OSR than EVT for CMI (7% vs 3%, $P<.01$).

A more modern sample of the NIS was used to retrospectively examine 4150 patients treated

Chronic Mesenteric Ischemia

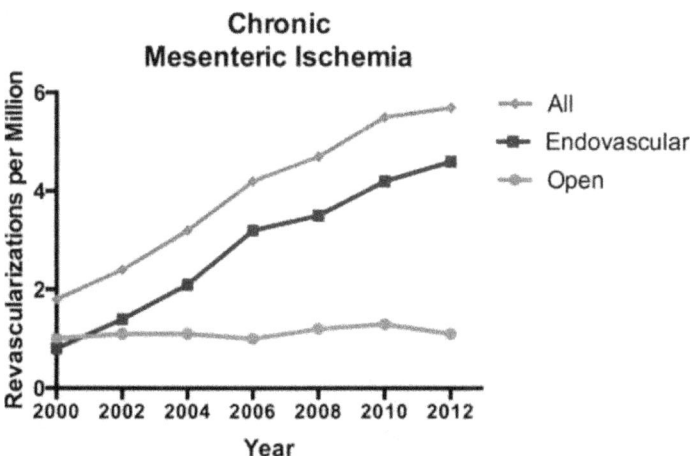

Fig. 9. Over time, the total number of revascularizations among patients with chronic mesenteric ischemia has increased (1.8–5.6 per million, $P<.01$) (Fig. 1). However, the volume of open revascularizations remained stable (1–1.1 per million), thus the rise in chronic mesenteric ischemia interventions was driven by endovascular treatment (0.8–4.6 per million, $P<.01$), which surpassed open surgery as the dominant method of revascularization in 2002(49).

Table 3
Results of revascularization for chronic mesenteric ischemia

Study	N	Study Details	Technical Success	Outcomes	Primary Patency
Matsumoto et al,[52] 2002	33 EVT	Retrospective	81.3	Complications = 13.8%	89% at 2 y
Sharafuddin et al,[53] 2003	25 EVT	Retrospective	96%	Major complication = 12%	85% at 11 mo
Landis et al,[54] 2005	29 EVT	Retrospective	97%	Major complication = 3.4%	70% 1 y
Silva et al,[4] 2006	59 EVT	Retrospective	96%	81% 3-y survival	71% at 14
Oderich et al,[48] 2009	229 (OSR = 146 vs EVT = 83)	Retrospective	95%	OSR patients had more complications (36% vs 18%; P<.001)	3 y: OSR 93% vs EVT 52% (P<.05).
Oderich et al,[55] 2013	225 EVT (164 BMS 61 CS)	Retrospective	CS = 95% BMS = 98%	Complications: BMS = 21% vs CS = 12%	3 y: CS = 92% vs BMT = 52% (P = .003)

Abbreviations: EVT, endovascular therapy; OSR, open surgical repair; BMS, bare-metal stent; CS, covered stent.

for CMI between 2007 and 2014 comparing OSR to EVT.[50] In this propensity-matched cohort, major adverse cardiovascular and cerebrovascular events and composite in-hospital complications occurred significantly less often after EVT than OSR (8.6% vs 15.9%; P<.001; and 15.3% vs 20.3%; P<.006). EVT was also associated with lower median hospital costs ($20,807.00 vs $31,137.00; P<.001, respectively) and a shorter length of stay (5 vs 10 days, respectively; P<.001) compared with OSR.

A 2015 meta-analysis of 8 CMI studies compared EVT to OSR and found no difference in 30-day mortality or 3-year cumulative survival rate. Compared with OSR, EVT resulted in a significantly lower rate of in-hospital complications (P=.002), while the recurrence rate within 3 years after revascularization was significantly greater for EVT (P<.00001).[51] A listing of studies reporting outcomes for CMI treatment by EVT and/or OSR is available in Table 3.[4,48,52–55] A comparative effectiveness and cost-effectiveness comparison of EVT versus OSR demonstrated that EVT was the preferred treatment of CMI patients despite more reinterventions.[56]

Recent studies have shown that EVT is increasingly used for treating CMI, offering high technical and clinical success rates with low mortality and complications.[57] While EVT outcomes have remained consistent over time, high-intensity preoperative statins have been associated with improved superior mesenteric artery (SMA) patency.[58] CTA or contrast-enhanced MRA is now preferred for CMI diagnosis.[59] A large Danish cohort study reported a 3-year mortality rate of 25% for CMI patients treated endovascularly, with low risk of symptomatic ischemia recurrence.[60]

Diagnosis of chronic mesenteric ischemia
CMI is defined as insufficient blood supply to the gastrointestinal tract resulting in ischemic symptoms with a duration of at least 3 months. The diagnosis of CMI is a clinical one, based on the symptoms and consistent anatomic findings.[61] The clinical presentation is often vague and nonspecific; chronic abdominal pain (often postprandial and described as "crampy"), diarrhea, fear of eating, and significant weight loss/malnutrition (Fig. 10). The majority of the patients are female, have a history of cardiovascular disease, and have had prior revascularization. A broad differential diagnosis is necessary for nonatherosclerotic etiologies such as fibromuscular dysplasia, median arcuate ligament syndrome, vasculitis, malignancy, and postradiation stenoses.[62]

Once clinical suspicion for CMI is high, imaging with DUS is the first choice, followed by

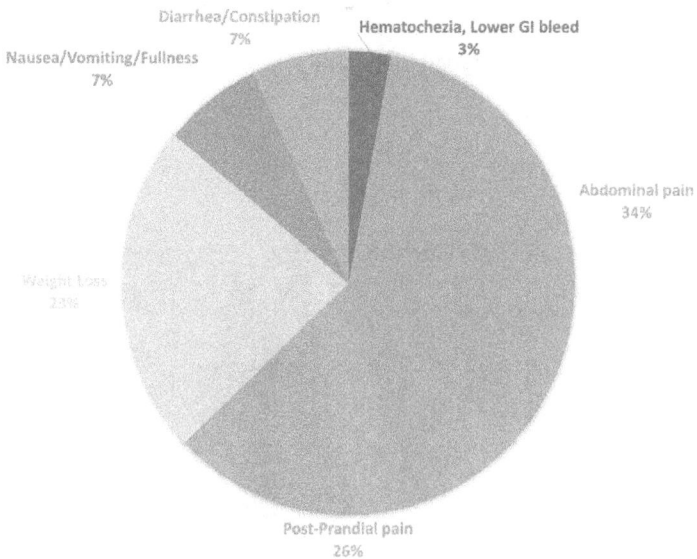

Fig. 10. Distribution of presenting symptoms for CMI.

Diarrhea/Constipation 7%

Hematochezia, Lower GI bleed 3%

Nausea/Vomiting/Fullness 7%

Abdominal pain 34%

Weight loss 23%

Post-Prandial pain 26%

cross-sectional noninvasive imaging with CTA or MRA.[63] The reported accuracy for DUS in identifying significant stenoses of the celiac and SMA approaches 90% with the caveat that ultrasound velocities will be higher for stented arteries than native arteries, making the diagnosis of ISR more difficult. DUS success is heavily influenced by technician expertise, the patient's body habitus, and the presence of bowel gas.

CTA is the favored cross-sectional noninvasive angiographic imaging modality of choice due to its higher resolution compared with MRA.[64] MRA has the advantage of better imaging in heavily calcified vessels without exposure to radiation or iodinated contrast.[65]

Selective mesenteric DSA remains the gold standard for diagnosing CMI, especially for the detection of distal vessel disease, or when a concurrent intervention is planned. It is important to perform both antero-posterior (AP) and lateral (LAT) views to delineate the visceral vessels which arise anteriorly from the aorta (Fig. 11A, B).

Indications and Contraindications for Revascularization

Percutaneous endovascular treatment of mesenteric arterial stenosis is indicated in patients with symptomatic CMI not amenable to conservative therapy. (Class I, LOE B).[20] The reported recurrence rates (30%–40%) mandate careful follow-

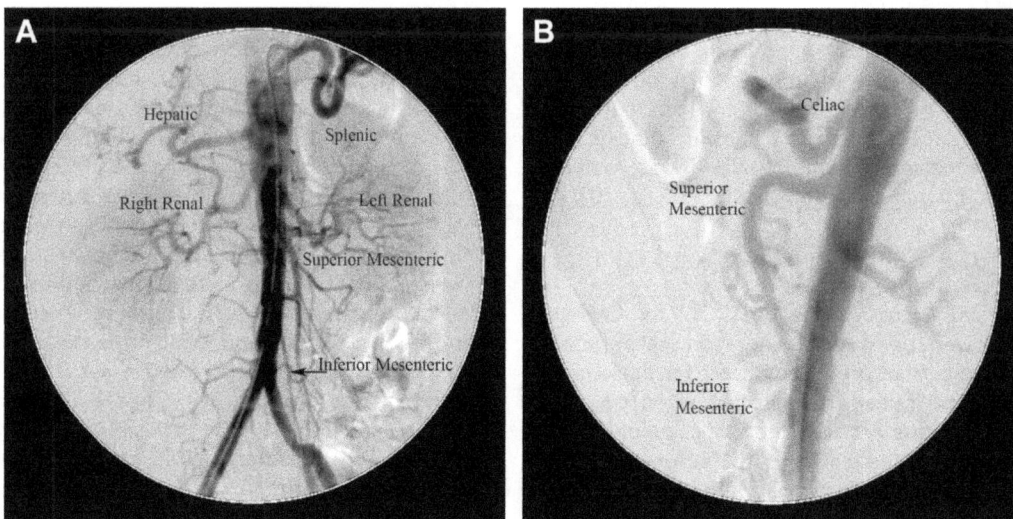

Fig. 11. (A) AP abdominal angiogram. (B) LAT abdominal angiogram.

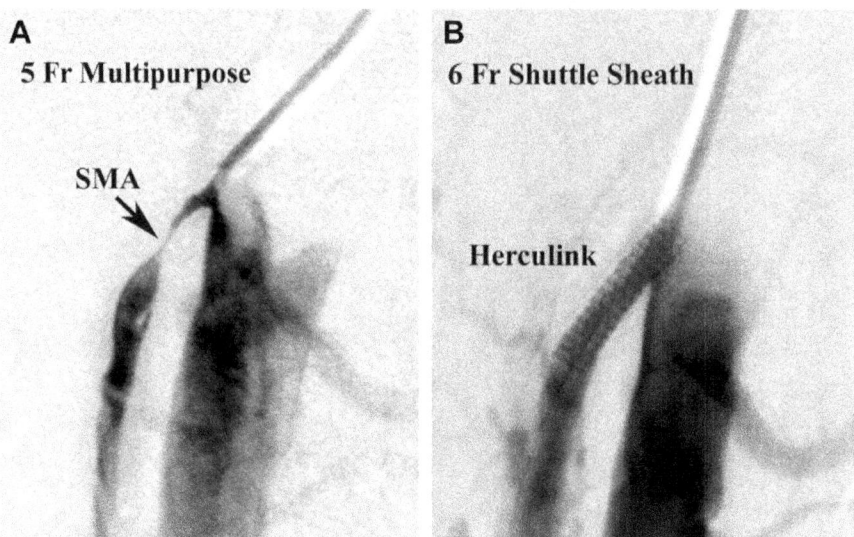

Fig. 12. (A) Baseline selective angiogram of the SMA with a 5 Fr multipurpose catheter from right radial access. (B) Stent delivery to the SMA using a 6 Fr shuttle sheath over a 0.014-inch guidewire.

up of patients treated with EVT. Revascularization of intestinal arterial stenosis that is discovered incidentally in an asymptomatic patient is "rarely appropriate" (Class III harm).[20]

Procedural Technique

Stenting atherosclerotic aorto-ostial obstructions of the visceral vessels is similar to that of the renal arteries, and the technical skills necessary for EVT are similar to those for renal stenting (Fig. 12A, B). Some considerations before EVT include adequate operator experience and surgical backup to rescue acute treatment failure. Meticulous case selection and procedure planning are necessary as some lesion(s) may not be amenable to an endovascular approach and may be better surgical candidates due to calcification, angulation of vessel or lesion, number or recurrence of stenoses. The patient and physician must make a joint and informed decision to proceed with EVT knowing that despite high initial success rates (88%–100%), patency rates at 1 year may decrease to 60% to 70%.[66]

Technical Aspects of Endovascular Intervention

Vascular Access: In the past, EVT for CMI patients were performed using a femoral approach but the current preferred access for these cases should be radial artery access when possible. Radial access reduces the difficulty of coaxial alignment of the guiding catheter for stent delivery as these vessels typically arise in a caudal direction, making delivery of stents from the femoral access more difficult. The delivery of

CS may require larger equipment (8 Fr), and thus necessitate femoral access.

Recommended equipment for EVT: Equipment choices for CMI EVT parallels renal stent placement. From the radial artery, a multipurpose shaped guide is ideal. From the femoral artery, a shepherd's crook shape (ie, Simmons) is often helpful. The use of 6 Fr guides requires a 0.014″ inch platform, while larger catheters from the femoral access may accommodate 0.018″ or 0.035″ inch systems. As in the case for renal stenting, we strongly discourage the use of hydrophilic guidewires, as the risk of vessel perforation is increased.

Recent evidence suggests that CS may be superior to BMS for treating CMI. The covered versus bare-metal stenting of the mesenteric arteries in patients with chronic mesenteric ischemia (CoBaGI) trial; a Danish RCT suggested superiority of CS over BMS in CMI treatment. In 94 patients with CMI, patency at 24 months was 84% in the CS group and 49% in the BMS group ($P<.00001$).[67] A systematic review and meta-analysis also indicated that CS may reduce or delay ISR compared with BMS.[68] These studies have not reported an increased incidence of stent thrombosis with either group. A single arm study of 86 patients with mesenteric disease treated with CS reported 2 cases of stent thrombosis at 2 years.[69] The CoBaGI trial also aims to compare quality of life and cost-effectiveness outcomes.[70] This has not been published at the time of this review. These studies collectively suggest that CS may offer improved outcomes in CMI treatment, although further research is needed to confirm these findings.

Peri-procedural Issues, Complications, and Their Management

Complications: In a series of 156 EVT patients reported from Mayo Clinic, serious complications occurred in 7% of cases, including branch perforation, distal embolization, vessel dissection, and stent embolization.[48] The use of antiplatelet therapy reduced the risk of embolization, and smaller platform equipment (0.014 inch vs 0.035 inch) reduced the risk of vessel complications.[48]

Restenosis in the mesenteric vessels has been one of the major pitfalls of mesenteric stenting occurring in 30% to 40% of patients.[71] Reinterventions are associated with low mortality (0%–3%) but significant morbidity (15%–27%).[71,72] Treatment options include balloon angioplasty and restenting, with restenting showing superior 1-year durability and symptom resolution compared with balloon angioplasty alone.[73] CS may reduce the need for reintervention compared with BMS. However, even after reintervention, about one-third of patients had restenosis.[71] Despite these challenges, endovascular reinterventions remain the first-line therapy for restenosis due to their lower mortality and acceptable morbidity.

Follow-up

The current recommendations for DUS follow-up after CMI intervention are that it is "appropriate" to perform a poststent baseline study within 30 days of the procedure.[46] It "may be appropriate" to perform additional DUS surveillance at 6 months or 9 months. It is "appropriate" to perform a follow-up DUS at 12 months and annually thereafter. When DUS is performed after stent placement, it is important to make adjustments to the velocity parameters poststenting compared with a native vessel, as decreased compliance due to the stent will result in higher velocities.[74,75] Therefore, obtaining a postprocedure DUS is reasonable to establish a new baseline PSV. Clinical symptoms are required even in the setting of ISR before repeat intervention.

ISR can be seen in 30% to 40% of EVT patients within 2 years after EVT. Independent predictors of restenosis after mesenteric revascularization are prior mesenteric intervention, female gender, and small vessel (<6 mm) diameter.[76] Severe mesenteric calcification, occlusions, longer lesions, and small vessel diameter are associated with an increased risk of distal embolization, restenosis, and reinterventions after endovascular revascularization.

SUMMARY

Renal Stenting: Significant ARAS is caused by the narrowing of arteries transporting blood to the kidney(s) most often caused by atherosclerosis and increases the risk of developing resistant hypertension, ischemic nephropathy, as well as cardiac destabilization syndromes (acute decompensated heart failure, specifically flash pulmonary edema, and ACS) (see Fig. 8).

Patients with refractory, uncontrolled renovascular hypertension despite maximally tolerated GDMT (including a diuretic), progressive ischemic nephropathy, and cardiac destabilization syndromes who have hemodynamically severe ARAS are likely to benefit from renal stenting. Radial access is preferred to avoid access-related complications and to facilitate stent delivery. Use of IVUS-guided stenting and EPDs may reduce the risk of complications. Surveillance poststenting can be done with periodic clinic visits, laboratory testing, and DUS.

Mesenteric Artery Stenting: CMI is an unusual, but serious condition. A high index of clinical suspicion is necessary for the diagnosis. In most cases, the cause is atherosclerotic stenosis or occlusion involving the mesenteric arteries. Because there is significant mesenteric collateral circulation, multivessel visceral stenosis is usually present in symptomatic patients. The limited comparative evidence available suggests that EVT is the preferred cost-effective choice in selected patients over OSR. The current treatment recommendation is that patients who are candidates for either OSR or EVT should receive percutaneous therapy with stent placement.

CLINICS CARE POINTS

- Renal Artery Interventions: Avoid renal artery stenting for mild to moderate atherosclerotic renal artery stenosis (ARAS) without hemodynamic significance.

- Use embolic protection devices (EPDs) in patients with chronic kidney disease to minimize postprocedural renal deterioration.

- Radial artery access is preferred for reducing complications, but operator experience and patient anatomy should guide the access decision.

- Use intravascular ultrasound (IVUS) for accurate lesion sizing and optimal stent placement to minimize restenosis risk.

- Revascularization is indicated for patients with true resistant hypertension despite maximally tolerated guideline-directed medical therapy (GDMT).

- Mesenteric Artery Interventions: Chronic mesenteric ischemia (CMI) with symptoms unresponsive to conservative therapy warrants endovascular intervention (Class I, LOE B).
- Radial artery access is often preferred for mesenteric stenting due to better alignment for stent delivery.
- Covered stents (CS) may offer better patency rates than bare-metal stents (BMS) for mesenteric artery interventions.
- Reinterventions for restenosis are associated with low mortality but should aim for durability with stenting rather than balloon angioplasty alone.
- Routine duplex ultrasound surveillance post-intervention is critical for identifying in-stent restenosis (ISR) early.

DISCLOSURE

The authors have no financial disclosures.

REFERENCES

1. Bax L, Woittiez AJ, Kouwenberg HJ, et al. Stent placement in patients with atherosclerotic renal artery stenosis and impaired renal function: a randomized trial. Ann Intern Med 2009;150(12):840–8. W150-1.
2. Cooper CJ, Murphy TP, Cutlip DE, et al. Stenting and medical therapy for atherosclerotic renal-artery stenosis. N Engl J Med 2014;370(1):13–22.
3. Wheatley K, Ives N, Gray R, et al. Revascularization versus medical therapy for renal-artery stenosis. N Engl J Med 2009;361(20):1953–62.
4. Silva JA, White CJ, Collins TJ, et al. Endovascular therapy for chronic mesenteric ischemia. J Am Coll Cardiol 2006;47(5):944–50.
5. Blum U, Krumme B, Flügel P, et al. Treatment of ostial renal-artery stenoses with vascular endoprostheses after unsuccessful balloon angioplasty. N Engl J Med 1997;336(7):459–65.
6. Henry M, Amor M, Henry I, et al. Stents in the treatment of renal artery stenosis: long-term follow-up. J Endovasc Surg 1999;6(1):42–51.
7. Stone PA, Campbell JE, Aburahma AF, et al. Ten-year experience with renal artery in-stent stenosis. J Vasc Surg 2011;53(4):1026–31.
8. Yeh RW, Valsdottir LR, Yeh MW, et al. Parachute use to prevent death and major trauma when jumping from aircraft: randomized controlled trial. BMJ 2018;363:k5094.
9. Lee P, Reeves RA, Leung SS, et al. Updated trends in percutaneous renal arteriography among radiologists and other specialties. Clin Imaging 2023;102: 14–8.
10. Khan Z, Tolia S, Sanam K, et al. Is there still a role for renal artery stenting in the management of renovascular hypertension - a single-center experience and where do we stand? Cardiovasc Revascularization Med 2019;20(3):202–6.
11. Harden PN, MacLeod MJ, Rodger RS, et al. Effect of renal-artery stenting on progression of renovascular renal failure. Lancet 1997;349(9059):1133–6.
12. Watson PS, Hadjipetrou P, Cox SV, et al. Effect of renal artery stenting on renal function and size in patients with atherosclerotic renovascular disease. Circulation 2000;102(14):1671–7.
13. Muray S, Martín M, Amoedo ML, et al. Rapid decline in renal function reflects reversibility and predicts the outcome after angioplasty in renal artery stenosis. Am J Kidney Dis 2002;39(1):60–6.
14. Batide-Alanore A, Azizi M, Froissart M, et al. Split renal function outcome after renal angioplasty in patients with unilateral renal artery stenosis. J Am Soc Nephrol 2001;12(6):1235–41.
15. Leertouwer TC, Derkx FH, Pattynama PM, et al. Functional effects of renal artery stent placement on treated and contralateral kidneys. Kidney Int 2002;62(2):574–9.
16. Coen G, Moscaritolo E, Catalano C, et al. Atherosclerotic renal artery stenosis: one year outcome of total and separate kidney function following stenting. BMC Nephrol 2004;5:15.
17. Khosla S, White CJ, Collins TJ, et al. Effects of renal artery stent implantation in patients with renovascular hypertension presenting with unstable angina or congestive heart failure. Am J Cardiol 1997;80(3): 363–6.
18. Gray BH, Olin JW, Childs MB, et al. Clinical benefit of renal artery angioplasty with stenting for the control of recurrent and refractory congestive heart failure. Vasc Med 2002;7(4):275–9.
19. Messerli FH, Bangalore S. The Pickering Syndrome–a pebble in the mosaic of the cardiorenal syndrome. Blood Press 2011;20(1):1–2.
20. Hirsch AT, Haskal ZJ, Hertzer NR, et al. ACC/AHA 2005 guidelines for the management of patients with peripheral arterial disease (lower extremity, renal, mesenteric, and abdominal aortic): executive summary a collaborative report from the American association for vascular surgery/society for vascular surgery, society for cardiovascular angiography and interventions, society for vascular medicine and biology, society of interventional radiology, and the ACC/AHA task force on practice guidelines (writing committee to develop guidelines for the management of patients with peripheral arterial disease) endorsed by the American association

of cardiovascular and pulmonary rehabilitation; national heart, lung, and blood institute; society for vascular nursing; TransAtlantic inter-society consensus; and vascular disease foundation. J Am Coll Cardiol 2006;47(6):1239–312.

21. Chi YW, White CJ, Thornton S, et al. Ultrasound velocity criteria for renal in-stent restenosis. J Vasc Surg 2009;50(1):119–23.

22. Tan KT, van Beek EJ, Brown PW, et al. Magnetic resonance angiography for the diagnosis of renal artery stenosis: a meta-analysis. Clin Radiol 2002; 57(7):617–24.

23. Saeed A, Fortuna EN, Jensen G. Split renal function in patients with unilateral atherosclerotic renal artery stenosis-effect of renal angioplasty. Clin Kidney J 2017;10(4):496–502.

24. Klein AJ, Jaff MR, Gray BH, et al. SCAI appropriate use criteria for peripheral arterial interventions: an update. Cathet Cardiovasc Interv 2017;90(4):E90–110.

25. Bailey SR, Beckman JA, Dao TD, et al. ACC/AHA/SCAI/SIR/SVM 2018 appropriate use criteria for peripheral artery intervention: a report of the American College of Cardiology appropriate use criteria task force, American heart association, society for cardiovascular angiography and interventions, society of interventional radiology, and society for vascular medicine. J Am Coll Cardiol 2019;73(2):214–37.

26. Subramanian R, White CJ, Rosenfield K, et al. Renal fractional flow reserve: a hemodynamic evaluation of moderate renal artery stenoses. Cathet Cardiovasc Interv 2005;64(4):480–6.

27. Mangiacapra F, Trana C, Sarno G, et al. Translesional pressure gradients to predict blood pressure response after renal artery stenting in patients with renovascular hypertension. Circ Cardiovasc Interv 2010;3(6):537–42.

28. Safian RD, Madder RD. Refining the approach to renal artery revascularization. JACC Cardiovasc Interv 2009;2(3):161–74.

29. Holden A, Hill A, Jaff MR, et al. Renal artery stent revascularization with embolic protection in patients with ischemic nephropathy. Kidney Int 2006; 70(5):948–55.

30. Laird JR, Tehrani F, Soukas P, et al. Feasibility of FiberNet® embolic protection system in patients undergoing angioplasty for atherosclerotic renal artery stenosis. Cathet Cardiovasc Interv 2012; 79(3):430–6.

31. Cooper CJ, Haller ST, Colyer W, et al. Embolic protection and platelet inhibition during renal artery stenting. Circulation 2008;117(21):2752–60.

32. Lederman RJ, Mendelsohn FO, Santos R, et al. Primary renal artery stenting: characteristics and outcomes after 363 procedures. Am Heart J 2001; 142(2):314–23.

33. Zähringer M, Sapoval M, Pattynama PM, et al. Sirolimus-eluting versus bare-metal low-profile stent for renal artery treatment (GREAT Trial): angiographic follow-up after 6 months and clinical outcome up to 2 years. J Endovasc Ther 2007;14(4):460–8.

34. Bradaric C, Eser K, Preuss S, et al. Drug-eluting stents versus bare metal stents for the prevention of restenosis in patients with renovascular disease. EuroIntervention 2017;13(2):e248–55.

35. N'Dandu ZM, Badawi RA, White CJ, et al. Optimal treatment of renal artery in-stent restenosis: repeat stent placement versus angioplasty alone. Cathet Cardiovasc Interv 2008;71(5):701–5.

36. Patel PM, Eisenberg J, Islam MA, et al. Percutaneous revascularization of persistent renal artery in-stent restenosis. Vasc Med 2009;14(3):259–64.

37. Giles H, Lesar C, Erdoes L, et al. Balloon-expandable covered stent therapy of complex endovascular pathology. Ann Vasc Surg 2008;22(6):762–8.

38. Gandini R, Morosetti D, Chiocchi M, et al. Long-term follow-up of endovascular treatment of renal artery aneurysms with covered stent deployment. J Cardiovasc Surg 2016;57(5):625–33.

39. Mohabbat W, Greenberg RK, Mastracci TM, et al. Revised duplex criteria and outcomes for renal stents and stent grafts following endovascular repair of juxtarenal and thoracoabdominal aneurysms. J Vasc Surg 2009;49(4):827–37 [discussion 37].

40. Harnek J, James SK, Lagerqvist B. Very long-term outcome of coronary covered stents: a report from the SCAAR registry. EuroIntervention 2019; 14(16):1660–7.

41. Grines CL, Tummala PE. Covered stents: initially life-saving but long-term consequences persist. Cathet Cardiovasc Interv 2021;98(5):882–3.

42. Venturini M, Marra P, Colombo M, et al. Endovascular treatment of visceral artery aneurysms and pseudoaneurysms in 100 patients: covered stenting vs transcatheter embolization. J Endovasc Ther 2017;24(5):709–17.

43. Qiu C, Liu Z, Huang L, et al. Covered stents for treatment of visceral artery aneurysms: a multicenter study. J Vasc Intervent Radiol 2022;33(6): 640–7.

44. Ivanovic V, McKusick MA, Johnson CM, et al. Renal artery stent placement: complications at a single tertiary care center. J Vasc Intervent Radiol 2003; 14(2 Pt 1):217–25.

45. Rocha-Singh K, Jaff MR, Rosenfield K, et al. Evaluation of the safety and effectiveness of renal artery stenting after unsuccessful balloon angioplasty: the ASPIRE-2 study. J Am Coll Cardiol 2005;46(5):776–83.

46. Mohler ER, Gornik HL, Gerhard-Herman M, et al. ACCF/ACR/AIUM/ASE/ASN/ICAVL/SCAI/SCCT/SIR/SVM/SVS/SVU [corrected] 2012 appropriate use criteria for peripheral vascular ultrasound and physiological testing part I: arterial ultrasound and

physiological testing: a report of the American College of Cardiology foundation appropriate use criteria task force, American College of radiology, American institute of ultrasound in medicine, American society of echocardiography, American society of nephrology, intersocietal commission for the accreditation of vascular laboratories, society for cardiovascular angiography and interventions, society of cardiovascular computed tomography, society for interventional radiology, society for vascular medicine, society for vascular surgery, [corrected] and society for vascular ultrasound. [corrected]. J Am Coll Cardiol 2012;60(3):242–76.

47. Schermerhorn ML, Giles KA, Hamdan AD, et al. Mesenteric revascularization: management and outcomes in the United States, 1988-2006. J Vasc Surg 2009;50(2):341–8.e1.

48. Oderich GS, Bower TC, Sullivan TM, et al. Open versus endovascular revascularization for chronic mesenteric ischemia: risk-stratified outcomes. J Vasc Surg 2009;49(6):1472–9.e3.

49. Zettervall SL, Lo RC, Soden PA, et al. Trends in treatment and mortality for mesenteric ischemia in the United States from 2000 to 2012. Ann Vasc Surg 2017;42:111–9.

50. Lima FV, Kolte D, Kennedy KF, et al. Endovascular versus surgical revascularization for chronic mesenteric ischemia: insights from the National Inpatient Sample Database. JACC Cardiovasc Interv 2017; 10(23):2440–7.

51. Cai W, Li X, Shu C, et al. Comparison of clinical outcomes of endovascular versus open revascularization for chronic mesenteric ischemia: a meta-analysis. Ann Vasc Surg 2015;29(5):934–40.

52. Matsumoto AH, Angle JF, Spinosa DJ, et al. Percutaneous transluminal angioplasty and stenting in the treatment of chronic mesenteric ischemia: results and longterm followup. J Am Coll Surg 2002;194(1 Suppl):S22–31.

53. Sharafuddin MJ, Olson CH, Sun S, et al. Endovascular treatment of celiac and mesenteric arteries stenoses: applications and results. J Vasc Surg 2003;38(4):692–8.

54. Landis MS, Rajan DK, Simons ME, et al. Percutaneous management of chronic mesenteric ischemia: outcomes after intervention. J Vasc Intervent Radiol 2005;16(10):1319–25.

55. Oderich GS, Erdoes LS, Lesar C, et al. Comparison of covered stents versus bare metal stents for treatment of chronic atherosclerotic mesenteric arterial disease. J Vasc Surg 2013;58(5):1316–23.

56. Hogendoorn W, Hunink MG, Schlösser FJ, et al. A comparison of open and endovascular revascularization for chronic mesenteric ischemia in a clinical decision model. J Vasc Surg 2014;60(3): 715–25.e2.

57. Ali AA, Farahat MS, Elmaleh HM, et al. Role of endovascular intervention in management of chronic mesenteric ischemia. QJM 2023;116(Supplement_ 1):hcad069–281.

58. Alnahhal KI, Sorour AA, Lyden SP, et al. Management of patients with chronic mesenteric ischemia across three consecutive eras. J Vasc Surg 2023; 78(5):1228–12238 e1.

59. Miklosh B. Diagnostic and therapeutic approaches in chronic mesenteric ischemia have improved. United European Gastroenterol J 2020;8(4):369–70.

60. Altintas Ü, Lawaetz M, de la Motte L, et al. Endovascular treatment of chronic and acute on chronic mesenteric ischaemia: results from a National Cohort of 245 cases. Eur J Vasc Endovasc Surg 2021;61(4):603–11.

61. Clair DG, Beach JM. Mesenteric ischemia. N Engl J Med 2016;374(10):959–68.

62. Escárcega RO, Mathur M, Franco JJ, et al. Nonatherosclerotic obstructive vascular diseases of the mesenteric and renal arteries. Clin Cardiol 2014;37(11):700–6.

63. Biri S, Biri İ, Gultekin Y, et al. Doppler ultrasonography criteria of superior mesenteric artery stenosis. J Clin Ultrasound 2019;47(5):267–71.

64. Schaefer PJ, Pfarr J, Trentmann J, et al. Comparison of noninvasive imaging modalities for stenosis grading in mesenteric arteries. Röfo 2013;185(7): 628–34.

65. Hohenwalter EJ. Chronic mesenteric ischemia: diagnosis and treatment. Semin Intervent Radiol 2009;26(4):345–51.

66. Rawat N, Gibbons CP, Group JVR. Surgical or endovascular treatment for chronic mesenteric ischemia: a multicenter study. Ann Vasc Surg 2010;24(7):935–45.

67. Terlouw LG, van Dijk LJD, van Noord D, et al. Covered versus bare-metal stenting of the mesenteric arteries in patients with chronic mesenteric ischaemia (CoBaGI): a multicentre, patient-blinded and investigator-blinded, randomised controlled trial. Lancet Gastroenterol Hepatol 2024;9(4):299–309.

68. Cerecedo Lopez CD, Feliz J, Heindel P, et al. Covered versus bare metal stents for chronic mesenteric ischemia: systematic review and meta-analysis. J Vasc Surg 2022;75(6):e292–3.

69. Girault A, Pellenc Q, Roussel A, et al. Midterm results after covered stenting of the superior mesenteric artery. J Vasc Surg 2021;74(3):902–909 e3.

70. van Dijk LJD, Harki J, van Noord D, et al. Covered stents versus Bare-metal stents in chronic atherosclerotic Gastrointestinal Ischemia (CoBaGI): study protocol for a randomized controlled trial. Trials 2019;20(1):519.

71. Zhou Y, Ryer EJ, Garvin RP, et al. Outcomes of endovascular treatments for in-stent restenosis in patients with mesenteric atherosclerotic disease. J Vasc Surg 2019;69(3):833–42.

72. Tallarita T, Oderich GS, Macedo TA, et al. Reinterventions for stent restenosis in patients treated for

atherosclerotic mesenteric artery disease. J Vasc Surg 2011;54(5):1422–9.e1.

73. Taaffe J, Alexander A, Smith A, et al. Superior one-year durability of restenting for mesenteric artery in-stent restenosis. J Vasc Surg 2023;78(4):e94–5.

74. AbuRahma AF, Scott Dean L. Duplex ultrasound interpretation criteria for inferior mesenteric arteries. Vascular 2012;20(3):145–9.

75. AbuRahma AF, Stone PA, Srivastava M, et al. Mesenteric/celiac duplex ultrasound interpretation criteria revisited. J Vasc Surg 2012;55(2):428, 436. e6; [discussion 35-6].

76. Sivamurthy N, Rhodes JM, Lee D, et al. Endovascular versus open mesenteric revascularization: immediate benefits do not equate with short-term functional outcomes. J Am Coll Surg 2006;202(6):859–67.

Renal Denervation
A Review of Current Devices, Techniques, and Evidence

Monica Tung, MD[a], Taisei Kobayashi, MD[b,c],
Rajesh V. Swaminathan, MD[d,e], Debbie L. Cohen, MD[f],
Dmitriy N. Feldman, MD[g], Brian Fulton, MD[a,h],*

KEYWORDS

- Renal denervation • Hypertension • Blood pressure • Transcatheter therapy

---

KEY POINTS

- Renal denervation is an additive treatment modality to medical antihypertensive therapy that aims to disrupt overactive sympathetic afferent and efferent activity.
- There are currently 2 devices for transcatheter renal denervation approved for commercial use in the United States.
- Multiple, randomized, sham-controlled trials have demonstrated significant blood pressure lowering without device-related safety concerns.

INTRODUCTION

Hypertension (HTN) is a leading cause of cardiovascular (CV) morbidity and mortality in the United States and worldwide, yet among patients who carry the diagnosis, it is estimated that approximately 40% to 50% of patients in the United States are failing to meet blood pressure goals.[1] Furthermore, approximately one-third of patients with hypertension in the United States are nonadherent to their antihypertensive medications.[2]

Renal denervation (RDN) is a catheter-based therapy for HTN that targets the sympathetic afferent and efferent nerves in the kidneys along the renal arteries, which are implicated in contributing to development of systemic HTN.[3,4] These nerve bundles run along the adventitia in the renal arteries. Renal sympathetic nerve efferents terminate in glomerular arterioles. There, activation of adrenergic alpha and beta receptors, which are increased in number in hypertensive patients, leads to sodium and water retention, renal vasoconstriction, reduction of renal blood flow and glomerular filtration rate (GFR), and renin secretion, thus activating the angiotensin-aldosterone system.[3] Renal afferents are activated by ischemic stimuli in the renal pelvis and increase sympathetic efferent activity locally and systemically.[3] Sympathetic nervous system overactivity increases cardiac output, heart rate, and systemic vascular resistance. Disruption of these afferent and efferent signals is designed to restore autonomic balance. RDN models show that after denervation, there is a corresponding decrease in overall

---

[a] Division of Cardiovascular Medicine, Hospital of the University of Pennsylvania, Philadelphia, PA 19104, USA; [b] Division of Cardiovascular Medicine, Cardiovascular Medicine, Cardiac Catheterization Laboratory, Hospital of the University of Pennsylvania, Philadelphia, PA 19104, USA; [c] Cardiovascular Outcomes, Quality and Evaluative Research Center, Philadelphia, PA 19104, USA; [d] Department of Medicine, Duke University School of Medicine, Durham, NC, USA; [e] Durham VA Medical Center, Durham, NC 27710, USA; [f] Division of Renal, Electrolyte and Hypertension, Hospital of the University of Pennsylvania, Philadelphia, PA 19104, USA; [g] Division of Cardiology, Interventional Cardiac and Endovascular Laboratory, Weill Cornell Medical College, New York Presbyterian Hospital, New York, NY 10021, USA; [h] Division of Cardiovascular Medicine, Chester County Hospital, West Chester, PA 19380, USA
* Corresponding author. 3400 Civic Center Boulevard, 11th Floor South Tower, Philadelphia, PA 19104.
E-mail address: Brian.Fulton@pennmedicine.upenn.edu

Intervent Cardiol Clin 14 (2025) 225–234
https://doi.org/10.1016/j.iccl.2024.11.008
2211-7458/25/© 2024 Elsevier Inc. All rights reserved, including those for text and data mining, AI training, and similar technologies.

Abbreviations	
AF	atrial fibrillation
CMS	Centers of Medicare and Medicaid Services
CV	cardiovascular
GFR	glomerular filtration rate
HTN	hypertension
ICER	incremental cost-effectiveness ratio
PVI	pulmonary vein isolation
QALY	Quality Adjusted Life Year
RDN	renal denervation
RFA	radiofrequency ablation
RFB	radiofrequency renal denervation of main renal arteries and side branches
RFM	radiofrequency renal denervation of main renal arteries only
rRDN	radiofrequency renal denervation
SBP	systolic blood pressure
SCAI	Society for Cardiovascular Angiography and Interventions
uRDN	ultrasound renal denervation

and renal-specific norepinephrine spillover in blood, decreased plasma renin, and increased renal plasma flow.[5,6]

RDN is poised to offer another modality of treatment for millions of patients with uncontrolled hypertension who are intolerant of medical therapy, unwilling to be on additional medications, or demonstrate resistant hypertension despite maximally tolerated hypertensive therapy (blood pressure >130/80 mm Hg despite being on 3 medications with maximally tolerated doses, including a diuretic). Here, the authors review the existing technologies, procedural details, supporting evidence, and implementation challenges for RDN in the current landscape.

CURRENT DEVICE ITERATIONS

At present, there are 3 methods to perform a successful renal denervation: radiofrequency RDN (rRDN), ultrasound RDN (uRDN), and finally perivascular drug delivery.

Radiofrequency ablation (RFA) RDN is performed by utilizing the Symplicity Spyral catheter (Medtronic, Inc. Dublin, Ireland) and Symplicity G3 radiofrequency generator. This rapid

exchange ablation catheter has 4 radio-opaque electrodes spaced 5 mm apart on a helix-shaped catheter (Fig. 1).[7] The helical shape of the Spyral catheter allows the electrodes to come in contact with the vessel wall while the center of catheter remains nonocclusive in the artery, relying on blood flow to actively cool the vessel walls during an ablation. Main renal arteries, distal branches, as well as accessory renal arteries sized 3 to 8 mm are targets for RFA treatment. During each treatment run, which lasts a total of 60 seconds, radiofrequency waves are emitted from each individual electrode while the generator is actively monitoring impedance and temperature at each electrode site. The generator has built-in algorithms to turn off individual or all the electrodes based upon the impedance/temperature feedback at each electrode site.[8] Each of the 4 electrodes can be turned on or off selectively by the operator to enable more precise treatments or to retreat zones that may have experienced loss of contact.

Ultrasound RDN is performed using the Paradise system (ReCor Medical Inc., Palo Alto, CA, USA) which delivers ultrasound-based energy circumferentially through a piezoelectric crystal transducer that sits inside a balloon (Fig. 2). The system offers 5 different over-the-wire balloons of various sizes which are selected based on the size of the target vessel and sized 1:1. Main renal arteries and accessory arteries (but not the distal branches) sized between 3 and 8 mm are treated. Once satisfactorily placed, the balloon will be connected to the generator that automatically inflates and deflates the balloon. Adequate contact is confirmed with an angiogram showing absent flow of contrast distal to the inflated balloon. This technology relies on a system of sterile water circulation pumped by the generator within the balloon to prevent overheating of the arterial wall during treatment.[8,9] Each treatment run begins with a precooling phase and finally an ultrasound

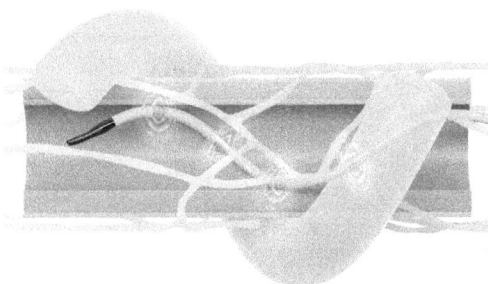

Fig. 1. The Symplicity Spyral radiofrequency renal denervation system. (*Reproduced with permission of Medtronic, Inc.*)

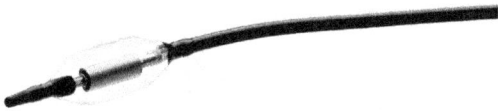

Fig. 2. The Paradise ultrasound renal denervation system. (*With permission from* Recor Medical.)

emission that lasts 7 seconds, and a balloon deflation phase that is controlled by the generator.

Perivascular ethanol ablation is utilized by the Peregrine system (Ablative Solution, Inc., Wakefield, MA, USA). The catheter deploys 3 microneedles spaced 120° apart from one another, into the arterial wall.[10] A potent neurolytic agent, dehydrated alcohol, is injected through the microneedles into the perivascular space.[11] Main renal arteries and accessory arteries are treated but like uRDN, distal branches are not. Unlike the other 2 modalities, this system does not require an external generator. This technology has not yet been approved by the United States Food & Drug Administration (FDA) and is limited to clinical research use only at this time. As such, this document will review and focus on currently FDA-approved devices only.

PROCEDURAL DETAILS
Access & Angiography
Currently, all RDN systems use common femoral artery access, ideally with ultrasound-guided puncture. The Symplicity Spyral (rRDN) is a 6 Fr system while the Paradise (uRDN) and Peregrine systems employ 7 Fr catheters. Aortography and selective renal angiograms are performed to rule out renal artery stenosis, aneurysms, fibromuscular dysplasia, or other renal vascular disease, as well as to assess for the presence and location of accessory renal arteries. Selective renal angiography and subsequent RDN can typically be performed through the following catheter shapes: internal mammary artery, multipurpose, RDN-1, renal double curve or Amplatz catheters. It is important to note that the 55 cm lengths of guiding catheters are most utilized to perform femoral RDN.

Treatment
For rRDN, the targets are main and accessory renal arteries and branches that are between 3 and 8 mm in diameter. The renal arteries targeted for treatment are wired with a 0.014″ nonhydrophilic supportive guidewire. Working in distal to proximal fashion, the Spyral catheter is advanced over the guidewire into the appropriate position, at least 5 mm from major branch points. The wire is retracted back toward the guide allowing the catheter to assume its helical shape and oppose the arterial wall. Prior to delivery of RFA treatment, patients should be given intraarterial nitroglycerin as well as adequate sedation to minimize vasospasm and mitigate pain associated with therapy. After a treatment is delivered, the guidewire can be advanced through the Spyral catheter to be used as a microcatheter to manipulate the guidewire into the remaining target branches. When treating the main renal artery, care is taken to stop ~5 mm from the ostium. A posttreatment selective angiogram is taken to evaluate for potential damage to the artery or the distal renal parenchyma. Treatment is repeated in the contralateral renal artery.

Unlike rRDN, uRDN requires treatment of the main and accessory renal arteries, but not the distal branches. The Paradise system is a balloon-tipped catheter that is advanced over a 0.014″ nonhydrophilic guidewire. Balloon sizes are preselected and range from 3.5 to 8 mm with 1:1 sizing with the renal arterial diameter. Quantitative coronary (vascular) analysis or intravascular ultrasound may be used to assess renal artery diameter. The main and accessory renal arteries are treated from distal to proximal, starting 5 mm from the first branch, and ending 5 mm from the ostium. The balloon has a radiopaque marker in the center. When placement is appropriate, the balloon is inflated and contrast injection from the guide confirms complete apposition to the arterial wall. Intraarterial nitroglycerin and sedation are administered in similar fashion to rRDN. Treatments are then delivered to the desired locations, noting that the catheter must be exchanged for a different balloon size when vessel diameter changes. After completion of uRDN, selective renal angiography is taken, and then attention is turned to the contralateral side.

Post Procedure
Patients are typically discharged later the same day after ensuring no access site or other complications have occurred. Most patients will be seen in follow-up by a member of their hypertension care team (see section on Society Statements below) to ensure no procedure-related issues before transitioning care back to their general cardiologist or primary care physician for ongoing management of their HTN. Follow-up renovascular imaging is not routinely recommended though may be considered in certain clinical scenarios (eg, moderate renal artery atherosclerosis), and laboratory assessment of

renal function should be performed within 3 to 6 months of the procedure.[12]

EVIDENCE FOR RENAL DENERVATION
Clinical Trials

Several contemporary randomized clinical trials have showed consistent benefit of RDN over sham-controlled procedures both for radiofrequency and ultrasound RDN (Table 1). These modalities were initially studied in an off-medication format, in which patients were not taking antihypertensive therapies or medications were temporarily discontinued. The SPYRAL-HTN OFF MED and RADIANCE-HTN SOLO were sham-controlled trials that demonstrated efficacy of rRDN and uRDN, respectively. Patients who underwent rRDN had 24-hour ambulatory systolic blood pressure (SBP) reduction of 4 mm Hg (−6.2 to −1.8) relative to those who received the sham procedure at 3 months.[7] Similarly, patients who underwent uRDN had daytime ambulatory SBP reduction of 6.3 mm Hg (−9.4 to −3.1) relative to the sham-control group at 2 months.[13] This result was duplicated in the larger, pivotal Radiance II trial, where 224 patients were randomized 2:1 to uRDN or sham procedure.[14] There were no significant safety events reported in any of the off med trials with both modalities.

The on-medication trials examined the additive efficacy of RDN on a background of medical therapy. The SPYRAL-HTN ON MED pilot study randomized 80 patients who remained hypertensive (office SBP 150–180 mm Hg and 24-h SBP 140–170 mm Hg) on 1 to 3 antihypertensive medications, on a 1:1 basis to rRDN versus sham procedure. At 6 months follow-up, the rRDN group experienced lowering of 24-h SBP that was 7.4 mm Hg greater than the placebo group.[15] These results were durable in long-term follow-up of 36 months.[16] However, with the addition of an expansion group of an additional 257 patients who were randomized 2:1 to rRDN and placebo procedure, the 24-hour blood pressure lowering was not significantly different between groups at 6 months.[17] Even though the protocol did not allow medication changes unless patients met strict escape criteria, analysis of urine and plasma at baseline and at 6 months showed that among 156 patients enrolled in the United States, medication increases were more common in the control group (37% vs 23%), which could be partly responsible for the lack of difference between groups, in addition to recruitment difficulties during the coronavirus disease 2019 period.[18] Further analysis into medication burdens

between the 2 groups in this study showed that the placebo group was able to achieve similar drops in blood pressure but utilized more medications to do so in comparison to those who underwent RDN.[16]

The safety and efficacy of uRDN in patients taking medications was studied in RADIANCE TRIO trial. One hundred thirty-six patients with resistant hypertension (on ≥3 antihypertensives) were enrolled and switched to a once daily, fixed dose, combination pill of 3 antihypertensives for a run-in period of 4 weeks. Compared to those who received the sham procedure, the uRDN patients experienced a 4.5 mm Hg greater reduction in daytime ambulatory SBP at 6 months follow-up.[19]

Safety outcomes were reported in all sham-controlled trials and established the overall low-risk profile of both procedures. For rRDN and uRDN, procedure-related adverse events were rare and most commonly related to femoral access: 3 patients across different trials had pseudoaneurysm requiring intervention; there was 1 RDN patient in RADIANCE-HTN SOLO who required a renal artery stent (this patient had 40%–50% ostial stenosis at baseline).[13]

It is noteworthy that each of these trials reported slightly different primary outcome measures and at varying time intervals. The SPYRAL studies utilized the 24-hour ambulatory SBP, which was measured at 3 months (OFF-MED) and at 6 months and 36 months (ON-MED). The RADIANCE studies instead used ambulatory daytime SBP, measured at 2 months in both the SOLO and TRIO studies. Thus, the ability to compare the relative efficacy of RDN modalities is limited. RADIOSOUND is the only trial to date comparing uRDN and rRDN, the 2 FDA-approved RDN therapies, head-to head. This trial enrolled 120 patients and randomized 1:1:1 to groups of rRDN main renal artery only (RFM), rRDN of main renal artery and branches (RFB), and uRDN of the main renal artery (US).[20] At 3 month follow-up, the primary-outcome of daytime ambulatory SBP was significantly lower in the US versus RFM group (between group difference, −6.7 mm Hg [−13.2 to −0.2]), while there was no significant difference comparing US to RFB.[20] While results at 6 months showed superiority of uRDN in comparison to both RFM and RFB groups (mean decline in daytime ambulatory SBP −12.1 ± 11.5 mm Hg, compared to −6.0 ± 11 mm Hg for RFM and −4.8 ± 12.1 mm Hg in RFB group), results at 12 months showed there were not significant differences in the modalities of RDN.[21]

Table 1
Randomized trials of renal denervation

Trial	Patients	Medications	Primary Outcome	Follow-up	Systolic Blood Pressure Lowering from Baseline (mm Hg)	Between Group Systolic Blood Pressure Difference (mm Hg)
SPYRAL HTN - OFF MED	166 rRDN, 165 sham	Discontinued	Change in mean 24-h systolic blood pressure (SBP), adjusted for baseline 24-h SBP	3 mo	rRDN −4.7 (−6.4 to −2.9) Sham −0.6 (−2.1-0.9)	−4.0 mm Hg (−6.2 to −1.8, P=.0005)
Spyral HTN - ON MED	38 rRDN, 42 sham	Continued	Change in mean 24-h SBP, adjusted for baseline 24-h SBP	6 mo	rRDN −9.0 (−12.7 to −5.3) Sham −1.6 (−5.2-2.0)	−7.4 mm Hg (−12.5 to −2.3, P=.0051)
Spyral-HTN ON MED Expansion	168 rRDN, 89 sham	Continued	Change in mean 24-h SBP, adjusted for baseline 24-h SBP	6 mo	rRDN −6.5 ± 10 Sham −4.5 ± 10.3	−1.9 mm Hg (−4.4-0.5, P=.12)
Radiance HTN - SOLO	74 uRDN, 72 sham	Discontinued 4 wk before randomization	Change in daytime ambulatory SBP	2 mo	uRDN −8.5 ± 9.3 Sham −2.2 ± 10.0	−6.3 (−9.4 to −3.1, P=.0001)
Radiance II	150 uRDN, 74 sham	Discontinued 4 wk before randomization	Change in daytime ambulatory SBP	2 mo	uRDN −7.9 ± 11.6 Sham −1.8 ± 9.5	−6.3 mm Hg (−9.3 to −3.2, P<.001)
Radiance HTN - TRIO	69 uRDN, 67 sham	Switch to daily, fixed dose, combination pill 4 wk before randomization	Change in daytime ambulatory SBP	2 mo	uRDN −8.0 (−16.4-0.0) Sham −3.0 (−10.3-1.8)	−4.5 mm Hg (−8.5 to −0.3, P=.022)
Radiosound	39 RFM, 39 RFB, 42 uRDN	Continued	Change in daytime ambulatory SBP	3 mo	uRDN −13.2 ± 13.7 RFM -6.5 ± 10.3 RFB -8.3 ± 11.7	uRDN > RFM -6.7 mm Hg (−13.2 to −0.2, P=.043) US ~ RFB (NS)

Abbreviations: NS, non-significant; rRDN, radiofrequency renal denervation; RFM, radiofrequency renal denervation of main renal arteries only; RFB, radiofrequency renal denervation of main renal arteries and side branches; uRDN, ultrasound renal denervation.

Observational Studies

Both rRDN and uRDN continue to be evaluated in post-market, real-world settings through enrollment in global registries. The Global SYMPLICITY registry and its ongoing GSR-DEFINE Study has thus far enrolled over 3300 patients and has demonstrated durable blood pressure-lowering effects of rRDN.[22] Six-month outcomes of over 2200 patients with elevated office SBP despite ≥3 medications showed office SBP decreased by −12.8 ± 26.2 mm Hg and 24-hour ambulatory SBP by −7.2 ± 17.8 mm Hg. At 3 years, blood pressure lowering was even slightly better, with SBP decreases of −16.7 ± 28.6 mm Hg in office and −9.1 ± 20.2 mm Hg in 24-h ambulatory (a result previously seen in 3-year follow-up data from the Symplicity HTN-3 trial, in which the blood pressure-lowering effect of rRDN with the Symplicity Flex catheter became more pronounced over time).[23,24] During this time, the number of medication classes were the same for 46.8% of patients in the registry, while 31.2% decreased, and 22% increased.[23] Decline in estimated glomerular filtration rate (eGFR) was observed but within proportion to that expected for hypertensive populations, including those with chronic kidney disease.[22] Renal complications were rare: 1.6% developed end-stage renal disease and 1.5% had an increase in serum creatinine (sCr) by 50%. Three patients developed renal artery stenosis, including 2 that were successfully treated and one that was medically managed. The Global Paradise Registry is the uRDN registry that aims to enroll 3000 patients with follow-up through 5 years, though no data have yet been reported.[25]

SOCIETY STATEMENTS

The 2021 Society for Cardiovascular Angiography and Interventions (SCAI) and National Kidney Foundation statement underlined principles of patient selection for renal denervation: namely, this treatment is reserved for (1) patients with resistant hypertension (blood pressure >130/80 mm Hg on ≥3 medications with maximally tolerated dose) that is confirmed on ambulatory blood pressure monitoring, particularly those at high risk for cardiovascular events (existing coronary artery disease, diabetes mellitus, stroke, and chronic kidney disease) without secondary causes of hypertension, (2) those who are intolerant of medications, or (3) those unwilling to undergo medication augmentation. Clinical trials excluded patients with GFR less than 40, so the safety of RDN below this threshold has not been established. Shared decision-making between patients and hypertension team is critical.[12,26] In 2023, SCAI published an updated position on RDN reaffirming the prior statement's selection criteria and also outlined standards for physician training and competency and institutional requirements.[12] One of the noteworthy components of this statement is the recommendations for constructing a multidisciplinary team to provide high-quality care for patients considered for RDN.[12] Specifically, it is recommended that patients considered for RDN be evaluated within a dedicated HTN center that employs physicians, advanced practice providers, nursing staff, and ancillary support staff in both invasive and noninvasive specialties to provide a multi-faceted approach to HTN care. This team will serve to streamline referral patterns and facilitate screening, preprocedural testing (eg, exclusion of secondary causes of hypertension), procedural management, and postprocedure care for RDN patients before transitioning care back to their referring providers.[12]

The European Society of Cardiology Council on Hypertension and European Association of Percutaneous Cardiovascular Interventions released a similar statement in 2023.[27] Here, they revised the previous 2018 statement that recommended use of RDN only in clinical trials. Patient selection recommendations are similar to the US statement, including the consideration of global CV risk to prioritize patients most likely to benefit.

IMPLEMENTATION IN THE CURRENT LANDSCAPE

As mentioned earlier, the ReCor Paradise uRDN and Medtronic Spyral rRDN systems are the only 2 devices that have obtained US Food & Drug Administration (FDA) approval in November 2023. Both have similar indications: treatment of uncontrolled hypertension when lifestyle modification and drug therapy fail to achieve adequate blood pressure lowering.

Financial models predict cost effectiveness for both RDN technologies. Cost-effectiveness analysis of uRDN in the UK system resulted in a favorable incremental cost-effectiveness ratio (ICER) with uRDN compared to standard of care was 5600 GBP per Quality Adjusted Life Year (QALY).[28] A similar analysis of SPYRAL HTN-ON MED office SBP lowering predicted similar favorable ICER of 13,899 GBP per QALY (assuming 4.9 mm Hg office SBP lowering).[29] Both these estimates fall below the USD $50,000 per QALY threshold that is viewed as the lower boundary for cost effective health care interventions.[30] A recent analysis of predicted decline in stroke, myocardial infarction, and cardiovascular death in the United States attributable to lowering blood pressure with rRDN showed cost effectiveness of $32,732 per QALY.[31] The omission of clinical events such as arrhythmias and repeat clinical events in these studies makes these models more conservative estimates.

In the United States, while the technology has gained FDA approval, there are no coverage determinations from the Centers of Medicare and Medicaid Services (CMS) yet. Commercial payers currently advise seeking prior authorization. Both the Paradise and Spyral systems are assigned Current Procedural Terminology code category III, which are temporary tracking codes for new and emerging technologies. There is not an associated relative value unit or assigned fees for these codes, which are set by individual Medicare and insurance contractors.[32] This results in difficultly obtaining immediate reimbursement for RDN at this time. This is compounded by the typical delays between FDA approval and designation of an Ambulatory Procedure Code, which determines institutional reimbursement, by CMS. Thus, new RDN programs, particularly those in smaller institutions, will need to rely on temporary transitional pass-through payments from CMS, which serve to subsidize these newer devices and procedures. These are especially important for the uRDN and rRDN systems that require large capital investments (eg, generators) by hospitals. As such, most RDN cases thus far have been performed as a part of postmarketing registry studies rather than commercial use.

FUTURE DIRECTIONS

Long-term follow-up from clinical trials and real-world registries' experience will help clarify where RDN should fit into existing hypertension algorithms. The heterogeneity of results seen in all trials requires further investigation into patient and procedural characteristics that predict success, particularly in patients who are "nonresponders" to RDN treatment, which can affect up to 30% of patients undergoing RDN.[12] This heterogeneity in response is at odds with the broad indication for use that was approved by the FDA, so clinicians should be aware that RDN, while unlikely to cause significant harm, may not be appropriate or successful in all patients. It will also be important to consider how success is measured given that the primary

outcomes used in the trials for uRDN and rRDN are different (24 hour ambulatory SBP vs ambulatory daytime SBP), as were the time points when these were measured. Future trials should aim to standardize clinical endpoints and timepoints to allow for direct comparison and assessment of clinical benefit. Furthermore, as the clinical trials were largely underpowered to study "hard" clinical outcomes, such as cardiovascular morbidity and mortality, we should expect that further data from the larger global registries will shed light on this. In addition, as the adoption of a new technology that carries a high cost evolves, there is a potential to exacerbate health inequity already present in the hypertensive population.[1]

We expect that the indications for RDN will expand beyond the treatment for HTN alone and may extend toward downstream complications of HTN including atrial fibrillation (AF), congestive heart failure, and chronic kidney disease. In fact, several studies have already examined the additive effect of RDN in conjunction with pulmonary vein isolation (PVI) in atrial arrhythmias.[33–35] The Adjunctive Renal Denervation to Modify Hypertension and Sympathetic tone as Upstream Therapy in the Treatment of Atrial Fibrillation (HFIB) pilot studies (HFIB-1 and HFIB-2) randomized a total of 80 patients with AF between the 2 studies to PVI or PVI + RDN. Neither study demonstrated a significant difference in AF recurrence between groups, noting that the RDN devices utilized in those studies were not the 2 that are currently FDA approved.[35] The more recent SYMPLICITY-AF study randomized 70 patients to receive PVI + RDN with the Symplicity Spyral rRDN device or PVI alone. While the study did not meet its primary efficacy endpoint (freedom from ≥2 minutes of AF recurrence or need for repeat AF ablation), it significantly reduced the burden of atrial arrhythmias and dramatically reduced the reliance on antiarrhythmic therapy to achieve similar efficacy on control of AF.[33] Studies are now underway looking at the effect of uRDN on PVI: ULTRA-HFib (NCT04182620) and ULTRA-HFib Redo (NCT05988411). There also have been preliminary trials looking at diastolic heart failure as well with RDN's ability to reduce left ventricular (LV) mass in patents with hypertensive heart disease.[36]

Following in the footsteps of coronary interventions, we expect to see adaptation of RDN systems for radial access in the future. This would reduce the number of procedural access site complications, the majority of which were related to femoral access in clinical trials, and likely increase same-day discharge rates. The challenge for device engineers will be to adapt the current devices for radial access while minimizing substantial deviation from the current iterations, as this could require further FDA approval.

Lastly, the applications of renal denervation techniques to other vascular beds may be the new frontier for this technology. Sympathetic nervous system overactivity is also a driver of dyslipidemia, diabetes, and the metabolic syndrome.[37] Selective hepatic denervation using a single point ablation catheter is currently under investigation.[37]

SUMMARY

Catheter-based RDN is a new modality of antihypertensive treatment for patients whose blood pressure is not adequately controlled by medications, either because they are intolerant of additional medication or do not wish to be on any or additional medications. Two systems, the radiofrequency Spyral rRDN and the ultrasound Paradise uRDN, received approval from the FDA in November 2023. Both devices have demonstrated safety and there is growing evidence from randomized sham-controlled trials as well as global registries supporting their efficacy. The field of RDN has the potential to be a paradigm shifting technology; however, several obstacles remain, including regulatory coverage decisions affecting financial viability, standardization of operator and institutional practice, as well as long-term effects of RDN on clinical events and cardiovascular mortality.

CLINICS CARE POINTS

- Hypertension is a leading cause of cardiovascular morbidity and mortality in the United States and worldwide.
- Many patients fail to meet their blood pressure goals despite optimally tolerated medical therapy.
- Renal denervation (RDN) is a novel catheter-based technique that serves to modify pathologic sympathetic nervous system signaling implicated in the development of hypertension.
- RDN has been shown to be a safe, efficacious, and durable treatment strategy for patients who remain with uncontrolled hypertension despite optimally tolerated medical therapy, or who are unable or unwilling to take additional medications.

DISCLOSURE

Dr T. Kobayashi has served on advisory boards as well as received research funding to the institution from Medtronic, ReCor Medical and Sonivie Medical. Dr D.L. Cohen has served on advisory boards and as well as received research funding to the institution from Medtronic and Recor Medical. She is also on the DSMB for Metavention. Dr B. Fulton has served as a consultant for Medtronic.

REFERENCES

1. Tsao CW, Aday AW, Almarzooq ZI, et al. Heart disease and stroke statistics—2023 update: a report from the American Heart Association. Circulation 2023;147(8). https://doi.org/10.1161/CIR.0000000000001123.
2. Chang TE, Ritchey MD, Park S, et al. National rates of nonadherence to antihypertensive medications among insured adults with hypertension, 2015. Hypertension 2019;74(6):1324–32.
3. Heuser RR, Schlaich M, Sievert H, editors. Renal denervation: a new approach to treatment of resistant hypertension. London: Springer; 2015. https://doi.org/10.1007/978-1-4471-5223-1.
4. Kiuchi MG, Esler MD, Fink GD, et al. Renal denervation update from the international sympathetic nervous system summit. J Am Coll Cardiol 2019;73(23):3006–17.
5. Schlaich MP, Sobotka PA, Krum H, et al. Renal sympathetic-nerve ablation for uncontrolled hypertension. N Engl J Med 2009;361(9):932–4.
6. Mahfoud F, Townsend RR, Kandzari DE, et al. Changes in plasma renin activity after renal artery sympathetic denervation. J Am Coll Cardiol 2021;77(23):2909–19.
7. Böhm M, Kario K, Kandzari DE, et al. Efficacy of catheter-based renal denervation in the absence of antihypertensive medications (SPYRAL HTN-OFF MED Pivotal): a multicentre, randomised, sham-controlled trial. Lancet 2020;395(10234):1444–51.
8. Fulton B, Giri J, Rader F, et al. Renal denervation for hypertension: the current landscape and future directions. Heart Int 2024;18(1). https://doi.org/10.17925/HI.2024.18.1.2.
9. Sakakura K, Roth A, Ladich E, et al. Controlled circumferential renal sympathetic denervation with preservation of the renal arterial wall using intraluminal ultrasound: a next-generation approach for treating sympathetic overactivity. EuroIntervention 2015;10(11):1230–8.
10. Kandzari DE, Weber MA, Pathak A, et al. Effect of alcohol-mediated renal denervation on blood pressure in the presence of antihypertensive medications: primary results from the TARGET BP I randomized clinical trial. Circulation 2024;149(24):1875–84.

11. Fischell TA, Fischell DR, Ghazarossian VE, et al. Next generation renal denervation: chemical "perivascular" renal denervation with alcohol using a novel drug infusion catheter. Cardiovasc Revascularization Med 2015;16(4):221–7.

12. Swaminathan RV, East CA, Feldman DN, et al. SCAI position statement on renal denervation for hypertension: patient selection, operator competence, training and techniques, and organizational recommendations. J Soc Cardiovasc Angiogr Interv 2023;2(6):101121.

13. Azizi M, Schmieder RE, Mahfoud F, et al. Endovascular ultrasound renal denervation to treat hypertension (RADIANCE-HTN SOLO): a multicentre, international, single-blind, randomised, sham-controlled trial. Lancet 2018;391(10137):2335–45.

14. Azizi M, Saxena M, Wang Y, et al. Endovascular ultrasound renal denervation to treat hypertension: the RADIANCE II Randomized Clinical Trial. JAMA 2023;329(8):651.

15. Kandzari DE, Böhm M, Mahfoud F, et al. Effect of renal denervation on blood pressure in the presence of antihypertensive drugs: 6-month efficacy and safety results from the SPYRAL HTN-ON MED proof-of-concept randomised trial. Lancet 2018;391(10137):2346–55.

16. Mahfoud F, Kandzari DE, Kario K, et al. Long-term efficacy and safety of renal denervation in the presence of antihypertensive drugs (SPYRAL HTN-ON MED): a randomised, sham-controlled trial. Lancet 2022;399(10333):1401–10.

17. Kandzari DE, Townsend RR, Kario K, et al. Safety and efficacy of renal denervation in patients taking antihypertensive medications. J Am Coll Cardiol 2023;82(19):1809–23.

18. Townsend RR, Ferdinand KC, Kandzari DE, et al. Impact of antihypertensive medication changes after renal denervation among different patient groups: SPYRAL HTN-on MED. Hypertension 2024;81(5):1095–105.

19. Azizi M, Sanghvi K, Saxena M, et al. Ultrasound renal denervation for hypertension resistant to a triple medication pill (RADIANCE-HTN TRIO): a randomised, multicentre, single-blind, sham-controlled trial. Lancet 2021;397(10293):2476–86.

20. Fengler K, Rommel KP, Blazek S, et al. A three-arm randomized trial of different renal denervation devices and techniques in patients with resistant hypertension (RADIOSOUND-HTN). Circulation 2019;139(5):590–600.

21. Fengler K, Rommel KP, Kriese W, et al. 6- and 12-month follow-up from a randomized clinical trial of ultrasound vs radiofrequency renal denervation (RADIOSOUND-HTN). JACC Cardiovasc Interv 2023;16(3):367–9.

22. Mahfoud F, Böhm M, Schmieder R, et al. Effects of renal denervation on kidney function and long-term outcomes: 3-year follow-up from the Global SYMPLICITY Registry. Eur Heart J 2019;40(42):3474–82.

23. Mahfoud F, Mancia G, Schmieder RE, et al. Outcomes following radiofrequency renal denervation according to antihypertensive medications: subgroup analysis of the global SYMPLICITY registry DEFINE. Hypertension 2023;80(8):1759–70.

24. Bhatt DL, Vaduganathan M, Kandzari DE, et al. Long-term outcomes after catheter-based renal artery denervation for resistant hypertension: final follow-up of the randomised SYMPLICITY HTN-3 Trial. Lancet 2022;400(10361):1405–16.

25. Mahfoud F, Azizi M, Daemen J, et al. Real-world experience with ultrasound renal denervation utilizing home blood pressure monitoring: the Global Paradise System registry study design. Clin Res Cardiol 2023. https://doi.org/10.1007/s00392-023-02325-x.

26. Kandzari DE, Townsend RR, Bakris G, et al. Renal denervation in hypertension patients: proceedings from an expert consensus roundtable cosponsored by SCAI and NKF. Cathet Cardio Intervent 2021;98(3):416–26.

27. Barbato E, Azizi M, Schmieder RE, et al. Renal denervation in the management of hypertension in adults. A clinical consensus statement of the ESC Council on Hypertension and the European Association of Percutaneous Cardiovascular Interventions (EAPCI). Eur Heart J 2023;44(15):1313–30.

28. Taylor RS, Bentley A, Metcalfe K, et al. Cost effectiveness of endovascular ultrasound renal denervation in patients with resistant hypertension. PharmacoEconomics Open 2024;8(4):525–37.

29. Sharp ASP, Cao KN, Esler MD, et al. Cost-effectiveness of catheter-based radiofrequency renal denervation for the treatment of uncontrolled hypertension: an analysis for the UK based on recent clinical evidence. Eur Heart J - Qual Care Clin Outcomes 2024;qcae001. https://doi.org/10.1093/ehjqcco/qcae001.

30. Neumann PJ, Cohen JT, Weinstein MC. Updating cost-effectiveness — the curious resilience of the $50,000-per-QALY Threshold. N Engl J Med 2014;371(9):796–7.

31. Kandzari DE, Cao KN, Ryschon AM, et al. Catheter-based radiofrequency renal denervation in the United States: a cost-effectiveness analysis based on contemporary evidence. Journal of the Society for Cardiovascular Angiography & Interventions 2024102234. https://doi.org/10.1016/j.jscai.2024.102234.

32. Dotson P. CPT ® codes: what are they, why are they necessary, and how are they developed? Adv Wound Care 2013;2(10):583–7.

33. Chinitz L, Böhm M, Evonich R, et al. Long-term changes in atrial arrhythmia burden after renal denervation combined with pulmonary vein isolation. JACC (J Am Coll Cardiol) 2024. https://doi.org/10.1016/j.jacep.2024.04.035. S2405500X24003839.

34. Steinberg JS, Shabanov V, Ponomarev D, et al. Effect of renal denervation and catheter ablation vs catheter ablation alone on atrial fibrillation recurrence among patients with paroxysmal atrial fibrillation and hypertension: the ERADICATE-AF randomized clinical trial. JAMA 2020;323(3):248.

35. Turagam MK, Whang W, Miller MA, et al. Renal sympathetic denervation as upstream therapy during atrial fibrillation ablation. JACC (J Am Coll Cardiol) 2021; 7(1):109–23.

36. Mahfoud F, Urban D, Teller D, et al. Effect of renal denervation on left ventricular mass and function in patients with resistant hypertension: data from a multi-centre cardiovascular magnetic resonance imaging trial. Eur Heart J 2014;35(33): 2224–31.

37. Kiuchi MG, Carnagarin R, Matthews VB, et al. Multi-organ denervation: a novel approach to combat cardiometabolic disease. Hypertens Res 2023; 46(7):1747–58.

Iliac Arterial Intervention

Jacob Ricci, MS[a], Hillary Johnston-Cox, MD, PhD[b],
Andrew J.P. Klein, MD, FSCAI[c],*

KEYWORDS

- Iliac artery • Endovascular intervention • Aortoiliac intervention • Covered stents

KEY POINTS

- Endovascular intervention to obstructive aortoiliac disease is first-line therapy for patients with symptoms or in whom large bore access is required.
- Stenting is often used to treat aortoiliac disease, but balloon angioplasty with provisional stenting has been shown to be cost effective with similar patency rates.
- In iliac chronic total occlusions, covered stents may be more beneficial.
- Intravascular lithotripsy is now available in iliac vessel sizes and may increase vessel compliance and permit increased luminal gain.

INTRODUCTION

Lower extremity peripheral arterial disease (PAD) affects between 8 and 12 million people in the United States.[1] Aortoiliac occlusive arterial disease (AOID) is common among these millions of patients and may be present in upwards of 50% of them.[2] Fortunately, endovascular intervention to this vascular bed has evolved over the last 5 decades[3–5] such that any endovascular first approach is now favored in many patients (reference is 2016 American College of Cardiology/American Heart Association [ACC AHA] guidelines). Symptoms requiring intervention range from lifestyle-limiting claudication to critical limb-threatening ischemia (CLTI) to more recently the need for aortoiliac intervention to permit large bore access for other interventional procedures (Transcatheter Aortic Valve Replacement [TAVR], mechanical circulatory support).[6]

Medical therapy is the foundation of care with any manifestation of atherosclerotic vascular disease and involves antiplatelets along with aggressive risk factor modification. In addition, supervised exercise therapy (SET) has also been shown to be effective for AIOD. The Claudication: Exercise Versus Endoluminal Revascularization (CLEVER) trial was a randomized clinical trial evaluating endovascular therapy (EVT), SET, and optimal medical therapy (OMT).[7] This trial at 18-month demonstrated an improvement in peak walking distance and quality of life scores for SET and EVT compared with OMT. The Endovascular Revascularization and Supervised Exercise for Peripheral Artery Disease and Intermittent Claudication (ERASE) trial is another RCT demonstrating the benefit of SET.[8] This study randomized patients with both aorto-iliac and femoropopliteal disease to EVT + SET versus SET alone. The greatest improvement in walking distance and quality of life (QOL) was in those patients with EVT + SET. In summary, SET is a valid alternative treatment modality for AIOD and may be appropriate for certain patients. CLEVER and ERASE suggest that the combination of SET plus EVT provides the greatest improvement in walking disease and QOL score underscoring that a combination of EVT and exercise therapy may be the best treatment.

Surgical therapy for AIOD with bypass (either aortobifemoral bypass [AFB], ax-femoral bypass [AxFB], or femoral-femoral bypass [FFB]) was previously the treatment of choice in severely

[a] Division of Cardiovascular Medicine, University of Florida College of Medicine, P.O. Box 100288, Gainesville, FL 32611, USA; [b] Northwell Health, 300 Community Drive, Manhasset, NY 11030, USA; [c] Interventional Cardiology, Vascular and Endovascular Medicine, Piedmont Heart Institute, 275 Collier Road Suite 2065, Atlanta, GA 30309, USA
* Corresponding author.
E-mail address: Andrew.Klein@piedmont.org

Intervent Cardiol Clin 14 (2025) 235–242
https://doi.org/10.1016/j.iccl.2024.11.009
2211-7458/25/© 2025 Elsevier Inc. All rights reserved, including those for text and data mining, AI training, and similar technologies.

Abbreviations	
ABI	ankle-brachial index
AFB	aortobifemoral bypass
AOID	aortoiliac occlusive arterial disease
AxFB	ax-femoral bypass
BES	balloon-expandable stents
CIA	common iliac artery
CLEVER	Claudication: Exercise Versus Endoluminal Revascularization
CLTI	critical limb-threatening ischemia
CTA	computed tomography angiography
DAPT	dual antiplatelet therapy
ED	erectile dysfunction
EIA	external iliac artery
ERASE	Endovascular Revascularization and Supervised Exercise for Peripheral Artery Disease and Intermittent Claudication
EVT	endovascular therapy
FFB	femoral-femoral bypass
IIA	internal iliac artery
IVL	intravascular lithotripsy
MRA	magnetic resonance angiography
OMT	optimal medical therapy
PAD	peripheral arterial disease
SES	self-expanding stent
SET	supervised exercise therapy
TASC	Transatlantic Intersociety Consensus

symptomatic patients. However, with improvements in equipment, technique, and operator experience, an "endovascular first" approach is rapidly being adopted by both surgeons and nonsurgeon interventionalists alike (interventional cardiologists and interventional radiologists). In fact, the recently updated ACC/AHA Peripheral Arterial Disease Guidelines support EVT, with primary or provisional stenting as the first-line therapy for patients with AIOD on the basis of its high success rates and lower morbidity and mortality compared with surgical intervention.[9,10] The goal of invasive therapy is the augmentation of blood flow for resolution of symptoms and/or limb salvage. Careful evaluation of medical therapy, history, risk factor status, and evaluation of other comorbid conditions is helpful in the selection of a proper patient population undergoing intervention. In this article, we will provide a substantive review of endovascular treatment strategies for stenotic and AOID.

NONINVASIVE TESTING

Noninvasive testing is crucial for the evaluation of patients with PAD. Initial evaluation often involves the ankle-brachial index (ABI). In patients with AOID, because of the extensive collateral networks possible, the ABI may actually be normal. In patients with a high clinical suspicion and especially in those with suggestions of common iliac artery (CIA)/internal iliac artery (IIA) disease by symptoms of buttock claudication, exercise-induced ABIs may be appropriate and necessary to elicit symptoms and see a drop in the ABIs (Class IB recommendation[11]). Isolated IIA disease patients will have normal ABIs. After ABIs, arterial duplex ultrasound is the most common noninvasive test ordered to evaluate patients with PAD. Though technically possible, duplex is not an ideal choice for AOID disease given the need for specialized techniques and the high prevalence of obesity which impairs visualization. The most commonly used noninvasive imaging technique for AIOD is computed tomography angiography (CTA). CTA, though limited by the need for contrast administration and radiation, provides operators a 3-dimensional view of the aortoiliac system. It can provide detailed information regarding vessel size, degree of calcification, collateral flow as well as provide critical information regarding access site option. In terms of preprocedural planning CTA has become essential for complex AIOD EVT.

In patients who cannot receive iodine-based contrast secondary to renal function and/or allergy, magnetic resonance angiography (MRA) offers a viable alternative. In addition, MRA allows for the evaluation of anatomic location and degree of arterial stenosis without the drawback of radiation exposure to the patient. However, there is often a necessity of using gadolinium contrast agent which excludes patients with significantly impaired kidney function though the use of Feraheme for imaging these vessels is becoming more common and can be used regardless of glomerular filtration rate. MRA does have a tendency to overestimate the degree of stenosis compared with CTA and will be unable to visualize inside previously placed stents. The need for prolonged imaging inside a small MRI tube can pose challenges in patients with claustrophobia.

ANATOMIC CONSIDERATIONS

Treatment strategy for the iliac arteries is influenced by a number of anatomic factors. The common iliac arteries present a challenge when heavily calcified or tortuous, and include ostial disease, which may require a kissing stent strategy even when only one side is affected. The external iliac arteries (EIAs) are highly tortuous posing challenges in the assessment of lesions. The IIA, though frequently overlooked as nonessential, can be important. Significant buttock claudication and lifestyle limitations vasculogenic erectile dysfunction (ED), and critical sources of collateral flow are factors which must be considered when treating patients with AOID and the importance of the IIA should not be underestimated.

The impact of anatomy upon iliac intervention led to the now outdated Trans-Atlantic Inter-Society Consensus (TASC) II guidelines.[12] TASC A and B lesions, traditionally treated with EVT, are shorter in length and typically involve single vessel and no side-branch disease. In contrast, TASC C and D which were thought to be better treated surgically are longer, occlusive, and involve bifurcation and/or the distal aorta.[12]

Open AFB surgery has traditionally been the gold standard for aortoiliac occlusive disease due to high patency rates, but at the expense of increased perioperative morbidity and mortality. The most recent TASC II guidelines recommend aortofemoral bypass for TASC C and TASC D lesions (Fig. 1), without necessarily accounting for patient comorbidities and challenges associated with complex lesions. Endovascular therapies offer a viable alternative especially in those with high-risk cardiovascular comorbidities. Endovascular recanalization of aortoiliac occlusions achieves excellent patency rates with modern techniques and is associated with shorter hospital stays, less morbidity and mortality, along with lower costs.[13–15]

Many operators now opt for EVT with a primary stenting strategy increasingly adopted for most iliac interventions, even TASC C and TASC D lesions. Surgical options are usually reserved for endovascular failure and recalcitrant disease. This is in line with most major society guideline recommendations.[6,16]

INDICATIONS FOR REVASCULARIZATION THERAPY

In June 2024, the ACC/AHA joint committee on clinical practice guidelines released updated guidelines for the management of PAD. Included in this report are recommendations on the use of SET as well as indications for revascularization therapy. Specifically, the use of revascularization therapy is effective in improving quality of life for patients with aortoiliac disease who have not improved with goal-directed medical therapy alone. In patients with functionally limiting claudication and hemodynamically significant aortoiliac disease with inadequate response to goal-directed medical therapy (GDMT) (including structured exercise), endovascular revascularization is effective to improve walking performance and QOL. EVT is also warranted in patients with AIOD who present with CLTI. Per recent guidelines, this is a Class I level of evidence B (LOE B) recommendation to, surgical, endovascular, or hybrid revascularization techniques are recommended, when feasible, to minimize tissue loss, heal wounds, relieve pain, and preserve a functional limb.

ACCESS/APPROACH

The best access location for revascularization of the iliac arteries depends on several factors. These include the nature (stenosis vs occlusion), complexity (tortuosity and/or calcification), and location of target lesion. The optimal access point is ideally large enough to deliver the appropriately size equipment needed to treat the lesion and also be free of significant disease itself and permit safe closure of the arteriotomy. The angulation of the aortoiliac bifurcation, presence of grafts, and body habitus also play a factor. The most common access for treating AOID is and has been the femoral approach. This approach allows for shorter transit distance to the iliacs, compared with radial or brachial approach, and also allows for larger-bore access. When treating disease located in the proximal CIA, ipsilateral femoral access is generally preferred though contralateral access is possible at the potential expense of coaxial support. With distal common iliac disease or external iliac disease, a contralateral approach may be preferred. If there is extensive disease involving the aortoiliac bifurcation, bilateral femoral access may be required particularly if the operator pursues a bilateral simultaneous stent placement strategy.

While the femoral approach remains the most frequent, as operator experience increases and technology continues to advance, the radial and brachial approaches have begun to increase in frequency. Several device manufacturers have developed and tailored equipment specifically for radial and/or brachial access. A meta-analysis of 19 trials and 638 patients demonstrated a high degree of procedural success,

Type A lesions

- Unilateral or bilateral stenoses of CIA
- Unilateral or bilateral single short (≤3 cm) stenosis of EIA

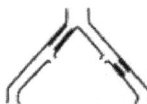

Type B lesions:

- Short (≤3cm) stenosis of infrarenal aorta
- Unilateral CIA occlusion
- Single or multiple stenosis totaling 3–10 cm involving the EIA not extending into the CFA
- Unilateral EIA occlusion not involving the origins of internal iliac or CFA

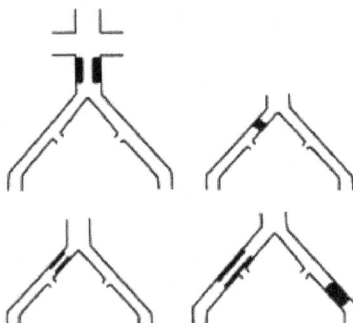

Type C lesions

- Bilateral CIA occlusions
- Bilateral EIA stenoses 3—10 cm long not extending into the CFA
- Unilateral EIA stenosis extending into the CFA
- Unilateral EIA occlusion that involves the origins of internal iliac and/or CFA
- Heavily calcified unilateral EIA occlusion with or without involvement of origins of internal iliac and/or CFA

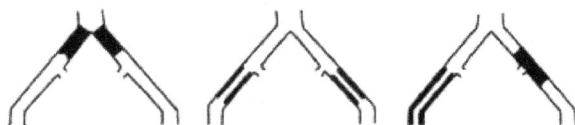

Type D lesions

- Infra-renal aortoiliac occlusion
- Diffuse disease involving the aorta and both iliac arteries requiring treatment
- Diffuse multiple stenoses involving the unilateral CIA, EIA, and CFA
- Unilateral occlusions of both CIA and EIA
- Bilateral occlusions of EIA
- Iliac stenoses in patients with AAA requiring treatment and not amenable to endograft placement or other lesions requiring open aortic or iliac surgery

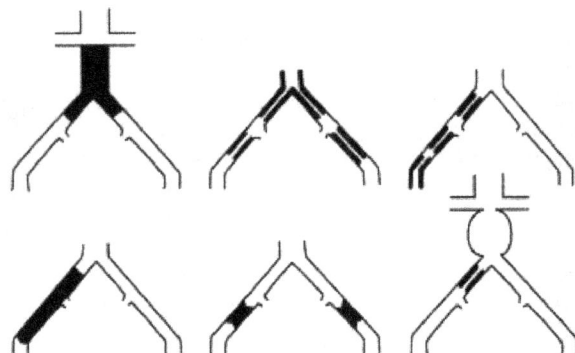

Fig. 1. TASC II anatomic classification of aortoiliac disease. (Norgren L, Hiatt WR, Dormandy JA, et al. Inter-Society Consensus for the Management of Peripheral Arterial Disease (TASC II). J Vasc Surg 2007;45 Suppl S:S5-S67; with permission.)

and safety rates for transradial treatment of aorto-iliac and femoral disease.[17] However, when planning a radial or brachial approach, equipment length must be considered though the armamentarium of longer shaft balloons, stents, drug-coated technologies, etc are rapidly expanding as the R2P (radial to peripheral) movement expands.

Procedural Techniques

While wiring techniques utilized for iliac interventions are generally similar to other interventional procedures, familiarity with devices and their associated wire sizes is imperative. Though 4-F to 6-F systems are available, operators may opt for 7-F to 8-F systems, particularly if there is a concern for vessel perforation as these sizes are required for polytetrafluoroethylene-covered stent delivery and deployment. Given that perforation in the iliac vascular bed can easily be fatal in minutes, operators must constantly be mindful of this potential complication and ensure that the appropriate bailout equipment is available and that the sheath in place is able to deliver the covered stent. Many of the covered stents are restricted to certain size sheaths and/or may only be on a smaller wire (0.018″) platform than may be used.

Typically, lesions are treated with balloon angioplasty followed by stenting given the excellent long-term patency associated with this strategy in these vessels. Vessel preparation for stenting has traditionally been limited to balloon angioplasty only which in heavily calcified lesions can lead to vessel perforation or inadequate vessel preparation which then leads to placement of an under expanded stent which has a high rate of restenosis. Recently, the use of intravascular lithotripsy (IVL) (SHOCKWAVE Medical, Santa Rosa California) has greatly changed the landscape of iliac intervention of heavily calcified lesions. Especially in patients who must undergo iliac intervention for TAVR to permit the large bore sheaths, IVL has been instrumental in facilitating these procedures. In a multicenter observational study, it was noted that the use of IVL increased over the observed years with lesions most often located in the common or external iliac. Though IVL was shown to be an effective addition to TAVI procedures, it should be noted that its use did not reduce periprocedural complication rates seen in patients with severe calcific PAD. While IVL is quickly becoming a clinical mainstay, there remains a gap in controlled investigations of its effectiveness. The largest study looking at IVL is the Disrupt PAD III study which followed 200 patients. They found that IVL is more often used with other balloon devices and was shown to be associated with low residual stenosis and low complication rates.

COMMON ILIAC ARTERY INTERVENTION

Whether an occlusive or stenotic lesion, CIA intervention is frequently associated with substantial improvement in symptoms and resultant mobility. However, given the location of the lesion to be treated, complexity varies.

Focal, or short (<10 cm) stenotic lesions which do not extend into the ostium of the CIA or beyond the iliac bifurcation, a primary stenting strategy is most commonly employed, though provisional stenting has also been shown to be a valid approach (see DUTCH iliac trial) and has yielded excellent clinical results, favoring covered stents.[18–20] Frequently, a unilateral ostial CIA lesion is found, but ultimately requires bilateral stenting to protect the contralateral ostium from plaque shift and compromise of flow.

Stent choice in CIA intervention is mainly dependent on lesion type and location. For lesions which fall into the TASC A or B category, the ICE trial suggested that self-expanding stents (SESs) were more effective than balloon-expandable stents (BESs) as they achieved reduced rates of restenosis and revascularization procedures.[21] However, SES often lack the radial strength needed in these often calcified arteries making many operators choose BES. SES also tend to jump during deployment which makes exact placement challenging. For TASC C and D lesions, the COBEST trial showed that covered stents achieved better patency as compared with bare-metal stents though notably did not affect rates of major limb amputations.[22] This is likely secondary to operators feeling that they can push postdilatation with the safety of a covered stent in place, thereby maximizing luminal gain.

Crossing of aorto-iliac common occlusions (typically TASC C and D lesions), has been aided by the use of the pioneer re-entry catheter (Philips-USA, Cambridge, MA, USA), which is an ultrasound-guided needle reentry device. Other nonimage-guided devices include the Outback (Cordis, Santa Clara, CA, USA), and the Enteer (Medtronic, Minneapolis, MN, USA). Successful reentry rates and high patency rates have been reported with its use and is furthering the prospect of endovascular-first strategies in occlusive disease affecting the infrarenal aorta, unilateral or bilateral iliacs, or aorto-iliac occlusive disease.[23–26]

EXTERNAL ILIAC ARTERY INTERVENTION

One of the main challenges in EIA intervention is the tortuosity of the vessel. This can frequently lead to underestimation of lesion length, and dissection or perforation during balloon angioplasty. Proper initial imaging using a contralateral oblique view can give proper separation of the iliac bifurcation and a better estimation of the lesion length. A marker catheter with 10 mm markers on it can also be beneficial when determining lesion length in highly tortuous vessels. Given the tortuosity associated with the external iliac artery, when stenting, it is best to consider using a self-expanding stent (uncovered or covered), rather than a balloon expandable stent. This is due to the ability of a SES to tolerate movement well and also adjust for discrepancies in vessel size which are often present in the EIA. Noncovered stents are preferred if the lesion extends proximally into the common iliac and involves the bifurcation of the IIA and EIA to preclude IIA occlusion. The IIA often provides collateral flow and should be preserved if possible.

When treating chronically occluded external iliac disease, the approach can be challenging. If treating short lesions, which are favorable to retrograde access and approach, it may be best to use this approach. If the lesion extends distally toward the inguinal ligament, then it is best to consider a contralateral, "up and over" approach. Imaging (intravascular ultrasound [IVUS]) and reentry devices are helpful in this setting when wire-reentry is not easily accomplished. Reentry devices have proven to be safe and effective in improving procedural success.[24]

INTERNAL ILIAC ARTERY INTERVENTION

The IIA is often overlooked as a source of symptoms or limitation. Frequently, buttock claudication and/or vasculogenic ED can be traced to IIA disease. Treatment of IIA stenosis should be along the same lines of treatment of EIA disease, in that tortuosity should be accounted for. SES should be considered, as they are more resistant to movement (similar to use in the EIA). Placement of stents across the origin of the IIA may not result in immediate occlusion, but long-term patency is decreased when the artery is covered. Covering the origin of the IIA should be avoided in order to maintain adequate perfusion of the pelvic viscera.[27] To date, however, there have been no large, multicenter randomized trials evaluating effectiveness of endovascular treatment of IIA disease. To our knowledge, no studies have compared stenting versus angioplasty alone in the IIA. Several smaller series have demonstrated high technical success rates, improvement in symptoms, and safety outcomes, indicating that treatment of IIA disease should be further explored and considered in patients with limiting buttock claudication.[27,28]

COMPLICATIONS OF ILIAC ARTERY INTERVENTION

Though rare, acute perforation of the iliac artery is the most serious potential complication of iliac artery interventions and is mainly due to manipulation of devices within the artery. However, warning signs, particularly patient reports of back pain during balloon inflation should be closely monitored by operators. Given that arterial rupture can lead to rapid exsanguination into the noncontainable retroperitoneal space, operators must always have ready access to covered stents and occlusion balloons as open repair of ruptures is generally not feasible.

POSTENDOVASCULAR THERAPY

The role of extended dual antiplatelet therapy (DAPT) is still unclear; however, common convention is for DAPT for at least 1 to 3 months postintervention. Current ACC/AHA guidelines recommend 1 to 6 months of DAPT post-EVT[11] (reference). In some cases, operators may prefer life-long DAPT, especially in the setting of kissing iliac stents extending into the distal aorta. To date, no randomized trials have examined the results of DAPT versus ASA alone postiliac intervention. In the setting of bare-metal stent usage, generally 1 month of DAPT is acceptable, as endothelialization occurs typically within 2 to 3 weeks of stent implantation. In the setting of covered stent usage, intimal hyperplasia at the edges of the stent can result in stenosis or reocclusion.

Postprocedure follow-up should include ABI (± exercise) in addition to routine clinical follow-up to assess symptomatic improvement and changes in physical examination findings. Most notable on physical examination are the quality and intensity of the CFA pulses as they provide insight into the patents of any upstream stents.

SUMMARY

PAD continues to affect a large patient population prompting continuing evolution of endovascular intervention to affected vascular beds. While medical therapy remains first line, for those patients who fail to see improvement in QOL, an "endovascular first" strategy is becoming a common approach. When electing to perform an endovascular intervention, careful consideration must be taken to identify not only the anatomic location of the target lesion but also tortuosity of the vascular bed itself. This characterization can be accomplished through the use of noninvasive testing modalities such as CTA, duplex ultrasound, or MRA. Generally, procedural technique is similar to other endovascular approaches. However, the location of the target lesion (CIA vs EIA vs IIA) can present unique challenges that operators must be prepared for. Overall, these procedures are safe and effective with low complication rates though there remains a risk of acute perforation. Generally, patients tolerate these procedures well. The role and duration of DAPT remains not well defined poststenting. Regardless, adequate follow-up should include ankle brachial index as well as thorough assessment of symptomatic improvement and other physical examination changes.

CLINICS CARE POINTS

- Aortoiliac occlusive disease (AOID) is common and can result in lifestyle limiting claudication as well as critical limb threatening ischemia.
- Many patients with AOID can be treated with minimally invasive endovascular techiques in an outpatient setting.
- Though stenting is often performed, for TASC A and B lesions, angioplasty alone is a cost-effective and provides similar long term patency at 5 years as was shown in the Dutch iliac stent trial.
- Covered stents may offer an advantage over non-covered stents when treating iliac occlusions, perhaps due to the ability to further expand them without the fear of vessel perforation/rupture.
- Iliac perforation/rupture can be lethal and operators must be constantly vigilant for this complication and insure that appropriate bail-out equipment (covered stents, aortic occlusion balloons) are on standby and available.

DISCLOSURE

The authors have nothing to disclose.

REFERENCES

1. Hirsch AT, Criqui MH, Treat-Jacobson D, et al. Peripheral arterial disease detection, awareness, and treatment in primary care. JAMA 2001;286(11):1317–24.
2. Aboyans V, Desormais I, Lacroix P, et al. The general prognosis of patients with peripheral arterial disease differs according to the disease localization. J Am Coll Cardiol 2010;55(9):898–903.
3. Dotter CT, Judkins MP. Description of a new technic and a prelimina report of its application. Circulation 1964;904–20.
4. Gruntzig A, Hopff H. [Percutaneous recanalization after chronic arterial occlusion with a new dilator-catheter (modification of the Dotter technique) (author's transl)]. Dtsch Med Wochenschr 1974;99(49):2502–10, 2511.
5. Palmaz JC, Sibbitt RR, Reuter SR, et al. Expandable intraluminal graft: a preliminary study. Work in progress. Radiology 1985;156(1):73–7.
6. Klein AJ, Jaff MR, Gray BH, et al. SCAI appropriate use criteria for peripheral arterial interventions: an update. Cathet Cardiovasc Interv 2017;90(4):E90–110.
7. Reynolds RM, Apruzzese P, Galper BZ, et al. Cost-effectiveness of supervised exercise, stenting, and optimal medical care for claudication: results from the claudication: exercise versus endoluminal revascularization (CLEVER) Trial. J Am Heart Assoc 2014;3(6):e001233.
8. Fakhry F, Spronk S, van der Laan L, et al. Endovascular revascularization and supervised exercise for peripheral artery disease and intermittent claudication. JAMA 2015;314(18):1936.
9. Ruggiero JN, Jaff RM. The current management of aortic, common iliac, and external iliac artery disease: basic data underlying clinical decision making. Ann Vasc Surg 2011;25(7):990–1003.
10. Correction to: 2016 AHA/ACC guideline on the management of patients with lower extremity peripheral artery disease: a report of the American College of Cardiology/American Heart association Task Force on clinical practice guidelines. Circulation 2017;135(12):e791–2.
11. Gornik LH, Gornik HL, Aronow HD, et al. 2024 ACC/AHA/AACVPR/APMA/ABC/SCAI/SVM/SVN/SVS/SIR/VESS guideline for the management of lower extremity peripheral artery disease. J Am Coll Cardiol 2024;83(24):2497–604.
12. Norgren L, Hiatt WR, Dormandy JA, et al. Inter-society consensus for the management of peripheral arterial disease (TASC II). J Vasc Surg 2007;45(Suppl S):S5–67.
13. Tang L, Paravastu SCV, Thomas SD, et al. Cost analysis of initial treatment with endovascular revascularization, open surgery, or primary major amputation in patients with peripheral artery disease. J Endovasc Ther 2018;25(4):504–11.
14. Fanari Z, Weintraub WS. Cost-effectiveness of medical, endovascular and surgical management of peripheral vascular disease. Cardiovasc Revasc Med 2015;16(7):421–5.
15. Doshi R, Changal KH, Gupta R, et al. Comparison of outcomes and cost of endovascular management versus surgical bypass for the management of lower extremities peripheral arterial disease. Am J Cardiol 2018;122(10):1790–6.
16. Conte MS, Pomposelli FB. Society for vascular surgery practice guidelines for atherosclerotic occlusive disease of the lower extremities management of asymptomatic disease and claudication. Introduction. J Vasc Surg 2015;61(3 Suppl):1S.
17. Meertens MM, Ng E, Loh SEK, et al. Transradial approach for aortoiliac and femoropopliteal interventions: a systematic review and meta-analysis. J Endovasc Ther 2018;25(5):599–607.
18. Mwipatayi BP, Thomas S, Wong J, et al. A comparison of covered vs bare expandable

stents for the treatment of aortoiliac occlusive disease. J Vasc Surg 2011;54(6):1561–70.

19. Bekken JA, Vos JA, Aarts RA, et al. DISCOVER: Dutch Iliac Stent trial: COVERed balloon-expandable versus uncovered balloon-expandable stents in the common iliac artery: study protocol for a randomized controlled trial. Trials 2012;13:215.

20. Laird JR, Loja M, Zeller T, et al. iCAST balloon-expandable covered stent for iliac artery lesions: 3-year results from the iCARUS Multicenter Study. J Vasc Intervent Radiol 2019;30(6):822–829 e4.

21. Krankenberg H, Zeller T, Ingwersen M, et al. Self-expanding versus balloon-expandable stents for iliac artery occlusive disease. JACC Cardiovasc Interv 2017;10(16):1694–704.

22. Mwipatayi PB, Sharma S, Daneshmand A, et al. Durability of the balloon-expandable covered versus bare-metal stents in the Covered versus Balloon Expandable Stent Trial (COBEST) for the treatment of aortoiliac occlusive disease. J Vasc Surg 2016;64(1):83–94.e1.

23. Jacobs DL, Cox DE, Motaganahalli R. Crossing chronic total occlusions of the iliac and femoral-popliteal vessels and the use of true lumen reentry

devices. Perspect Vasc Surg Endovasc Ther 2006; 18(1):31–7.

24. Krishnamurthy VN, Eliason JL, Henke PK, et al. Intravascular ultrasound-guided true lumen reentry device for recanalization of unilateral chronic total occlusion of iliac arteries: technique and follow-up. Ann Vasc Surg 2010;24(4):487–97.

25. Minko P, Katoh M, Opitz A, et al. Subintimal revascularization of chronic iliac artery occlusions using a reentry-catheter. Röfo 2011;183(6):549–53.

26. Tetteroo E, van der Graaf Y, Bosch JL, et al. Randomised comparison of primary stent placement versus primary angioplasty followed by selective stent placement in patients with iliac-artery occlusive disease. Dutch Iliac Stent Trial Study Group. Lancet 1998;351(9110):1153–9.

27. Vinogradova M, Lee HJ, Armstrong EJ, et al. Patency of the internal iliac artery after placement of common and external iliac artery stents. Ann Vasc Surg 2017;38:184–9.

28. Prince FJ, Smits MLJ, van Herwaarden JA, et al. Endovascular treatment of internal iliac artery stenosis in patients with buttock claudication. PLoS One 2013;8(8):e73331.

Femoropopliteal Interventions for Peripheral Artery Disease

A Review of Current Evidence and Future Directions

Adam P. Johnson, MD, MPH[a,b,*], Rajesh V. Swaminathan, MD[b,c,d], Samantha D. Minc, MD, MPH[a,e], Jorge Antonio Gutierrez, MD, MHS[b,c]

- Femoropopliteal • Peripheral artery disease • Pndovascular

- Peripheral artery disease (PAD) affects millions globally, with the femoropopliteal segment being a common site for occlusive disease. Isolated disease of this segment most often presents as claudication of varying severity.
- Diagnosis involves noninvasive tests like ankle brachial index (ABI) and imaging techniques such as duplex ultrasonography, Computed Tomography Angiography (CTA), or Magnetic Resonance Angiography (MRA). Anatomic classification systems include the Trans-Atlantic Inter-Society Consensus (TASC-II) and the more recently described Global Limb Anatomic Staging System (GLASS).
- Treatment options include medical management, smoking cessation, and supervised exercise therapy for all patients. Those with severe symptomatic disease and who have failed medical treatment may benefit from endovascular interventions (eg, angioplasty, stenting, atherectomy) or surgical revascularization.
- Endovascular treatments have evolved with technologies like drug-coated balloons (DCBs), drug-eluting stents (DES), and atherectomy devices. These interventions aim to improve patency rates and reduce the need for reintervention, though long term outcomes and durability remain areas of ongoing research.
- New technologies and techniques, such as intravascular ultrasound, intravascular lithotripsy, mimetic stents, and bioabsorbable stents, are being adopted to improve long-term outcomes. Future research should focus on diverse patient populations and aim for patient-centered outcomes, including functional independence and quality of life.

---

[a] Department of Surgery, Division of Vascular and Endovascular Surgery, Duke University Health System, Durham, NC, USA; [b] Durham Veterans Administration Medical Center, Durham, NC, USA; [c] Department of Medicine, Division of Cardiology, Duke University Health System, 508 Fulton Street, Durham, NC 27705, USA; [d] Duke Clinical Research Institute, Durham, NC, USA; [e] Department of Surgery, Division of Vascular Surgery, West Virginia University School of Medicine, Morgantown, WV, USA
* Corresponding author. Department of Surgery, Duke University Medical Center, DUMC Box 3538, Durham, NC 27710.
E-mail address: adam.johnson@duke.edu

Intervent Cardiol Clin 14 (2025) 243–256
https://doi.org/10.1016/j.iccl.2024.11.010
2211-7458/25/Published by Elsevier Inc.

Abbreviations	
ABI	ankle brachial index
BMS	bare metal stents
CLTI	chronic limb-threatening ischemia
CTA	computed tomography angiography
CTO	chronic total occlusion
DCB	drug-coated balloon
DES	drug-eluting stent
ELA	excimer laser atherectomy
FDA	Food and Drug Administration
GLASS	Global Limb Anatomic Staging System
ISR	in-stent restenosis
IVL	intravascular lithotripsy
IVUS	intravascular ultrasound
MALE	major adverse limb events
MRA	magnetic resonance angiography
PAD	peripheral artery disease
PTA	percutaneous transluminal angioplasty
SET	supervised exercise therapy
SFA	superficial femoral artery
TASC-II	Trans-Atlantic Inter-Society Consensus
TLR	target lesion revascularization
VOYAGER PAD	vascular outcomes study of ASA along with rivaroxaban in endovascular or surgical limb revascularization for PAD

INTRODUCTION

Peripheral artery disease (PAD) affects approximately 40 million people in the US and Europe and 230 million worldwide.[1,2] The femoropopliteal arterial segment is the most common cause of claudication in patients with lower extremity atherosclerotic disease.[3] It is less frequently associated with tissue loss and subsequent amputation, especially when it is the only level of disease involved.[4] Consequently, isolated femoropopliteal disease is often treated to improve quality of life. In contrast, treating femoropopliteal disease in a multilevel disease setting may be necessary for limb salvage.

Due to its location, the femoropopliteal segment is particularly amenable to endovascular treatment solutions. However, direct comparisons of new technologies through randomized controlled trials are limited. In addition, although procedural and short term outcomes are favorable for many newer technologies, longer-term durability still needs to be discovered. Recent evidence argues that early intervention in the femoropopliteal segment for asymptomatic or minimally symptomatic disease may increase the need for reintervention and worsen long term outcomes.[5,6] We aim to summarize the current evidence for diagnosing, classifying, and treating symptomatic PAD in this segment, focusing on approaches that maximize long term outcomes.

DIAGNOSIS AND CLASSIFICATION

The initial decision to pursue revascularization of the femoropopliteal segment depends on the patient's presenting symptoms and the results of noninvasive perfusion pressures. PAD symptoms can often overlap with neurologic, musculoskeletal, and venous disorders of the lower extremity. Therefore, a close review of patient symptoms' severity, character, and timing and whether this aligns with noninvasive perfusion testing is critical. Rutherford's classification is most commonly used to characterize presenting symptoms from PAD, but this has been reclassified based on the most recent 2024 American Heart Association (AHA) guidelines (Table 1).[7,8] Isolated PAD of the femoropopliteal segment should be reflected in a diminished but measurable ankle brachial index (ABI). An exercise treadmill ABI may be helpful in special circumstances, as ABIs may be normal at rest but decrease between 1 and 5 minutes after exercise. Noncompressible or unmeasurable ABI may suggest severe calcification or tibial disease.

Due to its easily accessible anatomic location, the femoropopliteal segment can also be evaluated with duplex ultrasonography. A triphasic waveform with normal velocities in the common femoral artery suggests adequate inflow. Elevated velocities with degradation of waveforms distally suggest hemodynamically significant stenosis. Many interventions of the isolated femoropopliteal segment can be planned entirely by duplex ultrasonography. Computed tomography angiography (CTA) or magnetic resonance angiography (MRA) may be helpful if inflow disease is suspected, in settings where the patient has a large body habitus, making ultrasound unfeasible, or if the patient has bilateral disease that needs to be characterized expeditiously. Guidelines recommend against anatomic imaging in patients whose symptoms or perfusion measurements do not warrant revascularization.[8]

Table 1
Symptoms of peripheral artery disease

Rutherford category	Presenting symptom	2024 American Heart Association clinical subset
0	Asymptomatic	Asymptomatic PAD
1	Mild claudication	Chronic symptomatic PAD
2	Moderate claudication	
3	Severe claudication	
4	Ischemic rest pain	Chronic limb-threatening ischemia
5	Minor tissue loss – focal ulcer isolated to the toes	
6	Major tissue loss – extending proximal to the transmetatarsal region	

Definitive anatomic classification is performed through catheter-based peripheral angiography with contrast media. Carbon dioxide angiography can provide adequate resolution in this vascular territory and has been associated with reduced postcontrast acute kidney injury (3.9% vs 4.8%, $P = .03$) in patients with chronic kidney disease.[9] Historically, the disease burden in the femoropopliteal segment has been classified according to the Trans-Atlantic Inter-Society Consensus (TASC-II) document on management of PAD (Fig. 1).[10] The Global guidelines for managing chronic limb-threatening ischemia (CLTI) have also outlined a classification system termed the Global Limb Anatomic Staging System (GLASS), which is focused on defining the severity of disease in the femoropopliteal segment with greater attention to the full extent of the patient's disease. GLASS separates the staging of inflow and outflow and grades severity into 4 categories (Fig. 2). Generally, the less severe anatomic classes (TASC A/B or GLASS 1/2) have high technical success rates with endovascular interventions. The more severe anatomic classes (TASC D and GLASS 4) with chronic total occlusion (CTO) have high failure rates and may be candidates for early surgical revascularization. Finally, the intermediate severity (TASC C or GLASS 3) has a high failure rate for endovascular therapy but may be appropriate in patients who are too high-risk for surgery.

TREATMENT
Medical Management and Behavior Modification

The medical management of PAD is discussed in depth in an earlier article. Here, we focus on the management strategies that should (1) be attempted and failed first in patients with mild/ moderate symptoms before intervention, and (2) ensure optimal longevity of interventions once pursued. Regardless of symptomatology, primary prevention for patients with atherosclerotic disease of any vascular bed is recommended with a single antiplatelet agent, usually a low-dose aspirin (81 mg), and high-intensity statin therapy. A subanalysis of the Cardiovascular Outcomes for People Using Anticoagulation Strategies trial in patients with symptomatic PAD found a 4.2% (95% CI, 1.9%–6.2%) absolute risk reduction for adverse cardiac or limb events at 30 months with the addition of rivaroxaban 2.5 mg twice daily. It is important to note that this clinical benefit decreased to 3.2% (95% CI, 0.6%–5.3%) once fatal or critical bleeding was considered. No data surrounding symptom improvement was captured.[12]

Smoking cessation is a vital component of primary and secondary prevention in PAD, although it is poorly utilized.[13] Ongoing periprocedural smoking increases the risk of morbidity and mortality.[14] Guideline-directed best practice in smoking cessation often includes a pharmacologic agent with or without nicotine replacement and referral to a smoking cessation program. It is usually recommended that pharmacologic agents are started before the anticipated quit date so that the patient is medically preconditioned before any behavioral intervention.[15] In a randomized controlled trial, patients with PAD were 3 times more likely to quit when enrolled in an intensive smoking cessation counseling program supplemented by pharmacologic agents.[16] At a minimum, clinicians should adopt the Ask-Advice-Connect framework with every clinical visit, where they (1) ask directly about the use of tobacco products, (2) provide advice on the impact of quitting on their health status, and (3) connect to cessation programs.

Type A lesions

- Single stenosis ≤10 cm in length
- Single occlusion ≤5 cm in length

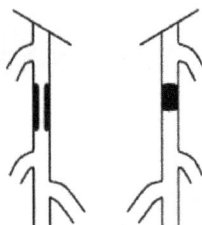

Type B lesions:

- Multiple lesions (stenoses or occlusions), each ≤5 cm
- Single stenosis or occlusion ≤15 cm not involving the infrageniculate popliteal artery
- Single or multiple lesions in the absence of continuous tibial vessels to improve inflow for a distal bypass
- Heavily calcified occlusion ≤5 cm in length
- Single popliteal stenosis

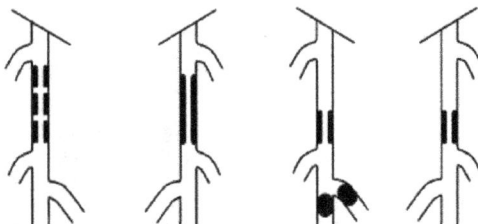

Type C lesions

- Multiple stenoses or occlusions totaling >15 cm with or without heavy calcification
- Recurrent stenoses or occlusions that need treatment after two endovascular interventions

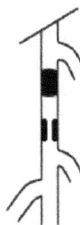

Type D lesions

- Chronic total occlusions of CFA or SFA (>20 cm, involving the popliteal artery)
- Chronic total occlusion of popliteal artery and proximal trifurcation vessels

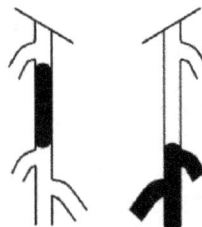

Fig. 1. TASC classification of femoral popliteal lesions.[10] CFA, common femoral artery; SFA, superficial femoral artery. (Figure is reproduced with permission from the publisher.)

The risk of poor periprocedural outcomes can be a helpful way to frame the message to support smoking cessation in this particularly high risk patient population.[17]

Several medications have demonstrated improvements in symptoms and quality of life in patients with intermittent claudication without revascularization. A Cochrane review demonstrated increased pain-free walking distance (mean difference of 26.49 m higher; 95% confidence interval [CI] 18.93–34.05) and total walking distance (mean difference of 39.57 m higher; 95% CI 21.80–57.33) after 3 to 6 months of cilostazol use compared with placebo. However, patients reported an increased incidence of headaches, diarrhea, palpitations, and dizziness, and there was no difference in mortality,

amputation, or major adverse limb events (MALE).[18] We recommend initiating patients on 50 mg twice daily for the first 2 weeks before increasing to a full dose of 100 mg twice daily to help mitigate side effects.

Supervised exercise therapy (SET) increases walking distance and quality of life in patients with intermittent claudication. This has been demonstrated through randomized trials for patients with and without revascularization. For example, a meta-analysis of 25 randomized trials found SET alone to be associated with an improvement of 180 m (95% CI, 130–238) in peak walking time and 128 m (95% CI, 92–195) in claudication onset time among patients with PAD.[19] Furthermore, the most improved effects on walking performance occurred when SET was

0	Mild or no significant (<50%) disease	
1	• Total length SFA disease <1/3 (<10 cm) • May include single focal CTO (< 5 cm) as long as not flush occlusion • Popliteal artery with mild or no significant disease	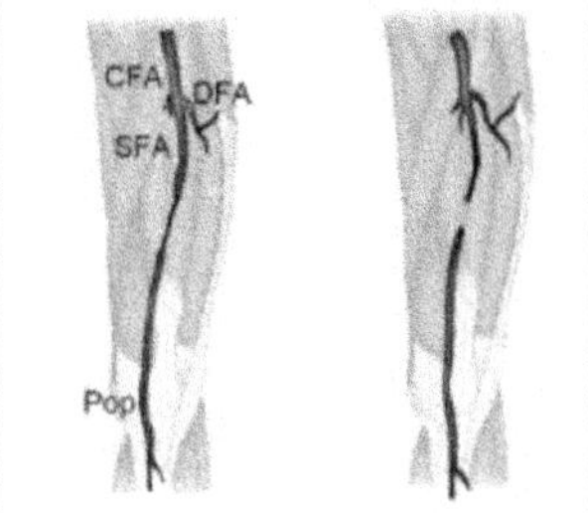
2	• Total length SFA disease 1/3–2/3 (10-20 cm) • May include CTO totaling < 1/3 (10 cm) but not flush occlusion • Focal popliteal artery stenosis <2 cm, not involving trifurcation	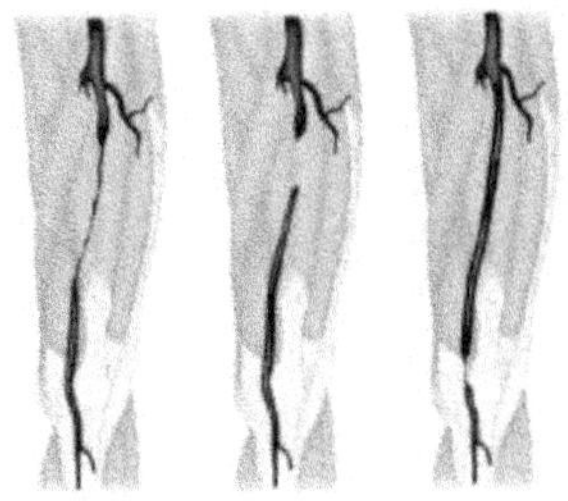
3	• Total length SFA disease >2/3 (>20 cm) length • May include any flush occlusion <20 cm or non-flush CTO 10–20 cm long • Short popliteal stenosis 2–5 cm, not involving trifurcation	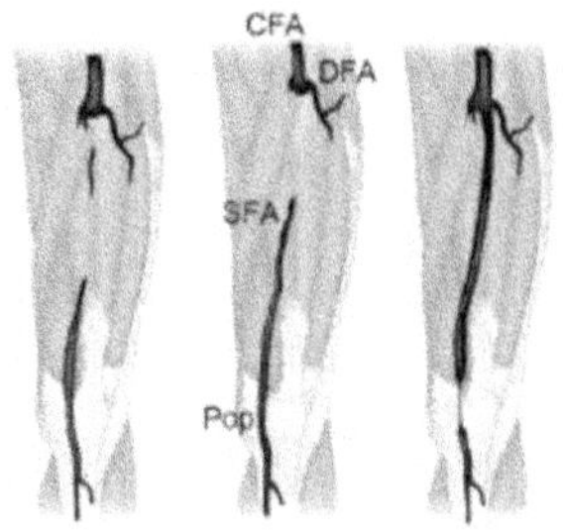
4	• Total length SFA occlusion > 20 cm • Popliteal disease >5 cm or extending into trifurcation • Any popliteal CTO	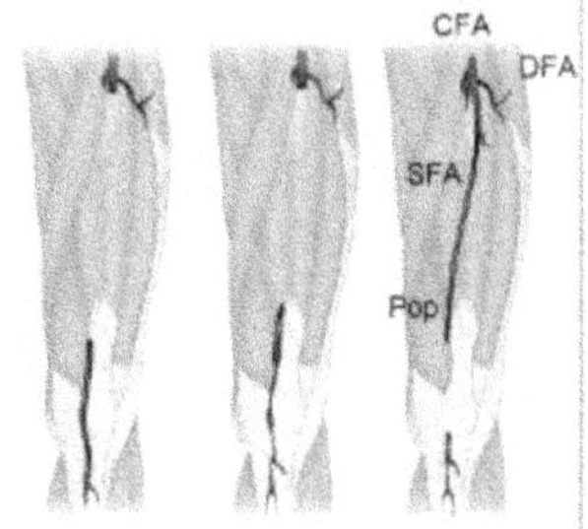

Fig. 2. Femoropopliteal GLASS.[11] Trifurcation is defined as the termination of the popliteal artery at the confluence of the anterior tibial (AT) artery and tibioperoneal trunk. CFA, Common femoral artery; CTO, chronic total occlusion; DFA, deep femoral artery; Pop, popliteal; SFA, superficial femoral artery. (The figure is reproduced with permission from the publisher.)

combined with revascularization.[20] As such, we recommend that all patients should be enrolled in a SET program regardless of the decision to revascularize.[21–23]

Guidelines recommend initiating medical therapy before offering any intervention to patients with claudication as the gold standard of care. However, reviews of periprocedural patients often show that only one quarter to one half of patients are on optimal medical therapy before their intervention.[24,25] Poor reimbursement or access to medical treatment, smoking cessation, and exercise therapy are likely contributing to poor adherence before endovascular intervention.[26] Further research is needed to understand the barriers compromising the implementation of this guideline. Regardless of a decision to revascularize, patients benefit from optimal medical treatment, smoking cessation, and SET.[21–23]

Anatomic Decision Making

The specific anatomic constraints of each femoro-popliteal segment drive therapeutic success and are essential to understand when considering a treatment plan. The common femoral artery undergoes significant angulation with hip flexion and is relatively superficial and easily accessible by surgical approach, even under local anesthesia. Isolated common femoral disease, even with concomitant profunda or proximal superficial femoral artery (SFA) disease, is primarily still treated with surgical endarterectomy. The flexion forces and proximity to the profunda bifurcation pose a significant risk for failure of endovascular therapies or sacrificing the profunda artery when treating through to the SFA. Most patients with isolated disease in this area will tolerate surgical therapy, and endovascular treatment should be pursued only in high-risk patients.[27]

The SFA is a long, straight segment of the artery that passes through the medial compartment of the thigh. It is often discussed in segments (see Figs. 1 and 2). The ostium is the most proximal segment. When involved with disease, this is usually addressed surgically with the common femoral artery. Endovascular treatment of the ostium is complex as it risks embolization, dissection, or coverage of the ostium of the profunda artery. Proximal and mid segments are relatively straight segments with minimal torsion forces from hip or knee flexion. However, there are often many collaterals in this segment. Therefore, this segment is usually treated with angioplasty and noncovered stents. The distal SFA segment is proximal to Hunter's canal; however, it can experience significant torsion forces and may be prone to stent restenosis and fracture.[28,29] Therefore, antiproliferative drug delivery and novel mimetic stents have been developed to address these mechanical challenges.

The popliteal artery is also divided into 3 segments. The P1 segment is the most proximal and extends from Hunter's canal to behind the knee. This segment carries significant flexion forces, like the distal SFA. As such, the primary endovascular treatment modality is angioplasty rather than stenting if possible. P1 is also a common site of arterial inflow or outflow for surgical bypass and should be preserved, if possible, during endovascular interventions. The P2 segment is behind the knee and has significant flexion forces, making traditional stents prone to fracture in this region. Debulking with atherectomy and drug delivery may be used as adjuncts to angioplasty in this region. New mimetic stents may hold promise to avoid

fractures in these patients. The P3 segment is below the knee and proximal to the anterior tibial (AT) bifurcation. This is best treated by angioplasty, and drug delivery should be considered as an adjunct to avoid stenting. P3 is also an important site for outflow for bypasses of the femoropopliteal segment. All efforts should be made to preserve this site when attempting to treat complex or occlusive lesions of the femoropopliteal segment.

Many patients have multilevel disease (ie, arterial beds above and below the femoropopliteal are impacted). This is particularly the case in patients presenting with more advanced PAD, such as CLTI/chronic wounds and rest pain. When intervening in these patients, it's essential to understand that the successful patency of a single segment is highly dependent on patent inflow and outflow segments. Therefore, if all diseased segments cannot be successfully treated endovascularly to restore in-line flow, an alternative strategy may be warranted, such as a hybrid (endovascular and surgery) or open repair.

Endovascular Interventions

Historically, angioplasty has been the mainstay of endovascular interventions. Initial evaluation of balloon angioplasty alone in the femoropopliteal segment demonstrated an excellent safety profile but poor long-term patency.[30] Advances in adjunctive therapies, such as stenting, drug delivery, and debulking, have aimed to extend angioplasty's durability. However, it is essential to understand that most efficacy studies have focused on data related to patency and the need for target lesion revascularization (TLR), which is not necessarily translatable to limb preservation outcomes. Studies must focus on clinically relevant outcomes such as wound healing, MALE, amputation, mortality, and patient-reported outcomes such as functional independence and freedom from pain.[11] Practitioners who treat the femoropopliteal segment should be keenly aware of the failure modes for each novel endovascular therapy so that they can be applied most effectively to the appropriate lesions and patient populations.

Access Considerations

Most endovascular femoropopliteal interventions are performed via a contralateral retrograde femoral access. This allows imaging of the entire femoropopliteal system and larger bore access for device delivery. However, contralateral access requires the crossover technique up and over the aortic bifurcation with longer catheters. This should be avoided in patients with severe iliac tortuosity, aortobiiliac endovascular, or open surgical grafts.[31] Isolated distal femoral and popliteal disease can be treated from an antegrade ipsilateral approach, which provides additional support for crossing complex, calcified, and chronically occluded lesions. Antegrade access directly into the most proximal SFA, followed by manual compression, is safe and optimizes successful SFA cannulation.[32]

Retrograde ipsilateral pedal approaches reduce the complications related to common femoral access and allow the crossing of CTOs that are inaccessible from the antegrade approach due to plaque morphology. However, the sheath size is smaller, limiting the delivery of devices.[33,34] Due to these limitations, pedal access is often performed only for lesion crossing. The wire is then externalized proximally through femoral access, allowing for larger bore device delivery, such as stents or debulking devices often needed in the femoropopliteal segment. This technique of subintimal arterial flossing with antegrade-retrograde interventions overcomes the barrier of pedal access size while maximizing options for device delivery via the antegrade approach.[31,35]

Transradial approaches have gained popularity and have become the gold standard for coronary angiography because they have shown significant reductions in access complications when compared to transfemoral access.[36] Treatment of the femoropopliteal segment from transradial access is complicated due to the distance to intervention and limitations of sheath size. New long sheaths and device delivery systems are available for transradial approaches but have not been widely adopted.[37]

Balloon Angioplasty

Percutaneous transluminal angioplasty (PTA) or plain balloon angioplasty works through plaque compression and arterial lumen expansion. In the Bypass versus Angioplasty in Severe Ischemia of the Leg (BASIL) trial, a balloon angioplasty-first strategy demonstrated similar 6-month amputation-free survival compared with a bypass surgery-first strategy, fostering widespread adoption due to reduced periprocedural complications.[38] This was found to be particularly true for patients who might require a prosthetic conduit. However, BASIL also demonstrated that bypass surgery after an attempt at endovascular therapy had worse outcomes. Concerning balloon choice, using PTA

to treat femoropopliteal disease was traditionally the preferred treatment option and is still a common practice. To further improve patency and reduce the need for reintervention, several adjuncts to angioplasty have been developed. These include drug delivery, stenting, and debulking.

Drug-Coated Balloons

Drug-coated balloons (DCB) deliver antimetabolite medication to the angioplasty site, most commonly paclitaxel, to prevent neo-intimal hyperplasia during remodeling. Specific formulations of paclitaxel dosing (2 $\mu g/mm^2$–3.5 $\mu g/mm^2$) and how it is bonded to the balloon excipient to enhance delivery vary widely across manufacturers. The US Food and Drug Administration (FDA) has approved the following 4 DCBs for femoropopliteal disease: IN.PACT (Medtronic Vascular, Santa Rose, California), Lutonix (Bard Lutonix, New Hope Minnesota), Ranger (Boston Scientific, Marlborough, MA, USA), and Stellarex (Royal Philips, Amsterdam, The Netherlands). Meta-analyses of paclitaxel-coated devices versus PTA have demonstrated superior primary patency and freedom from TLR at 2 years with DCB.[39,40] For example, in a meta-analysis of 44 studies between 2010 to 2021 in which 5282 limbs were treated, DCB demonstrated the highest patency rate, 0.83 (95% CI: 0.78–0.88), at 1 year for lesions longer than 15 cm compared to other endovascular techniques.[41] In terms of studies comparing outcomes by low versus high paclitaxel doses (specifically, Ranger 2 $\mu g/mm^2$ vs IN.PACT Admiral 3.5 $\mu g/mm^2$), randomized trials have demonstrated comparable primary patency rates, clinically driven TLR, and all-cause mortality at 2 years.[42] It is important to note that residual stenosis of greater than 30%, smaller reference vessel diameter, and higher severity of disease on presentation have been associated with a heightened risk of subsequent loss of patency loss.[43,44]

In 2018, a meta-analysis raised concerns about increased long-term mortality risk associated with paclitaxel-coated devices.[45] Furthermore, this risk was considered to be dose-related. These findings were criticized since most of the trials analyzed in the study centered on short term patency outcomes rather than long-term mortality. In response to these findings, a subsequent patient-level pooled analysis of 10 trials representing 2666 patients with a median follow up of 4.9 years found no significant increased risk of death among patients treated with paclitaxel-coated devices.[46] Furthermore, after an intense review of contemporary paclitaxel trials with long-term follow up (Swedish drug elution trial in peripheral arterial disease and vascular outcomes study of ASA along with rivaroxaban in endovascular or surgical limb revascularization for PAD [VOYAGER PAD]), American and European real-world databases (Medicare, the US Veterans Health Administration, and the German Barmer health insurance), the FDA found no risk of late mortality associated with paclitaxel-coated devices.[47–52]

Stenting

Stents used to treat femoropopliteal disease are self-expanding and constructed of the nickel-titanium alloy, nitinol (an essential consideration if a patient has a known nickel allergy). Due to the dynamic forces exerted on the SFA, bare metal stents are limited by delayed healing, stent fracture, in-stent restenosis (ISR), and stent thrombosis. To better handle the physiologic stress of daily activities, bare metal stents (BMS) such as the Supera were developed with interwoven wires to increase flexibility without sacrificing radial strength. Interwoven BMS have yet to be compared to traditional stents in prospective comparative studies.

To overcome ISR and stent thrombosis, drug-eluting stents (DES) with antiproliferative properties were developed for use in the peripheral space. The FDA has approved two paclitaxel-based devices, Zilver PTX and Eluvia. The former has paclitaxel-coated directly onto the nitinol stent. The landmark Zilver PTX randomized controlled trial evaluated the Zilver PTX stent versus PTA in 474 patients with femoropopliteal disease. Zilver PTX had superior patency rates at 2 years versus angioplasty alone, 75% versus 27%, $P = .01$.[53] The Zilver PTX stent was also compared to paclitaxel-coated DCBs in the REAL PTX trial. Primary patency rates at 12 months were similar, 79% versus 80% ($P = .96$), respectively. Patency at 36 months was 54% for Zilver PTX compared to 38% for DCB. However, this did not meet statistical significance as the study was not powered to evaluate patency beyond the first year ($P = .17$).[54] The Eluvia DES differs from Zilver PTX in 2 ways. First, the paclitaxel dose is lower, 0.167 µg/mm^2 versus 3.0 µg/mm^2, respectively. Second, whereas the Zilver PTX releases 95% of paclitaxel within 24 hours of deployment, Eluvia utilizes a polymer to release 90% of paclitaxel over 1 year.[55] The Eluvia DES was assessed in the trial comparing Eluvia versus BMS in treatment of superficial femoral and/or proximal

popliteal artery (IMINENT) trial, where it was found to have a superior primary patency rate at 1 year (83% vs 74% for BMS, $P<.01$).[56] The randomized trial comparing the ELUVIA DES versus Zilver PTX stent for treatment of superficial femoral and/or proximal popliteal arteries (IMPERIAL) trial was the first study to compare these 2 devices. Eluvia had a primary patency rate of 87% at 1 year versus 82% with Zilver PTX, $P<.0001$.[57]

There are 2 common strategies for using stenting in femoropopliteal disease—the first advocates for primary stenting in lesions with significant length, severity, and calcification. The second supports the use of provisional stenting only in the setting of failed angioplasty, which can occur in more severe lesions. Provisional stenting is recommended in flow-limiting dissection, recoil stenosis greater than 50%, or persistent translesion gradient greater than 10 mm Hg, which is found to occur in 25% to 40% of long or calcified lesions.[58] A recent small pragmatic multicenter trial (BEST-SFA) investigated a drug-coated stent-preferred (N = 60) or stent-avoidant strategy (N = 59) for candidate SFA lesions and found no difference in 12-month primary patency (78.6% vs 78.2%, $P = 1.00$) or freedom from major adverse events (94.9% vs 93.1%, $P = .717$).[59] However, a meta-analysis including 10 randomized trials inclusive of 1631 patients/lesions that compared primary with provisional bare metal stenting showed that primary stenting may demonstrate improved short term (<1 year, odds ratio [OR] 2.24, CI 1.08–4.66) and medium term (1–2 years, OR 1.38, CI 1.01–1.89) patency over provisional stenting; however, no difference in long-term outcomes was seen (> 2 years, OR 1.33, CI 0.82–2.16).[40] This same trend was seen for TLR. Selective focal or "spot" stenting has been shown to have improved patency (HR 2.04, CI: 1.25–3.32) and TLR (HR 13.06, CI: 10.69–15.86) over long stenting in the femoropopliteal region.[60]

The FDA has also approved using covered stents (Viabahn, W.L. Gore & Associations, Flagstaff, AZ) for treating SFA disease. With a helical nitinol stent on the surface of a polytetrafluoroethylene graft, covered stents are believed to be more flexible and adept at withstanding the physiologic forces of the SFA. This is likely the etiology of the low stent fracture rates, 2.6%, at 3 years seen in the VIBRANT study, which found no statistically significant difference in primary patency rates between Viabahn-covered stents versus BMS at 3 years (24 vs 26%, $P = .39$).[61] However, it should be noted that covered stenting in the SFA occludes many collateral vessels with a risk of distal embolization and more severe ischemia in the setting of in-stent thrombosis.

Adjunct Therapies

The utilization of debulking techniques has nearly doubled in the past 10 years.[62] Atherectomy is often implemented to allow delivery of therapies (balloons and stents), facilitate adequate expansion of devices, and enhance endothelial contact with antiproliferative agents. Debulking devices include directional atherectomy, rotational atherectomy, and orbital atherectomy. A recent Cochrane review and meta-analysis found debulking atherectomy devices associated with reduced dissection and bailout stenting.[63,64] However, the same review conceded that evidence was of very low certainty due to a high risk of bias, imprecision, and inconsistency in the available literature. Atherectomy also carries a risk of perforation, dissection, and distal embolization. These rates have not been found to differ from balloon angioplasty alone in recent meta-analyses of randomized trials; however, conclusions regarding the severity of these complications were not assessed.[63,65] Overall, atherectomy remains a controversial topic, and detractors argue that it poses a significant cost burden without a durable outcome to support its value.[66] Larger studies focused on clinically relevant outcomes are critical to determine whether atherectomy should continue to be routinely used in this disease space. Finally, excimer laser atherectomy (ELA) is an alternative plaque modification therapy. ELA has demonstrated improved 1-year freedom from TLR among patients undergoing PTA alone (OR = 0.11, 95% CI 0.02–0.56).[65] ELA has also been found to be a reasonable and beneficial therapy for ISR.[44]

Additional specialty balloons include intravascular lithotripsy (IVL), scoring, cutting, and semicompliant balloons. Intravascular lithotripsy implements acoustic energy to fracture calcium and improve vessel compliance, allowing for the delivery of equipment.[67] This therapy is ideal in severely calcified focal femoropopliteal lesions that may be resistant to balloon angioplasty alone or in locations that may not be amenable to stent placement, such as the distal SFA or popliteal segments.[68] This aligns with current evidence as a significant benefit of IVL demonstrated in randomized trials and meta-analysis is freedom from provisional stent placement, reduced postangioplasty dissection, and reduced residual stenosis. For example, a meta-analysis of nine studies, including 681 patients, found post-IVL diameter stenosis reduction to be 59.3% (95% CI

53.30%–65.31%) with only a 1.24% rate (95% CI 0.60%–2.61%) of flow-limiting dissection.[69,70] Lithotripsy can also be used to optimize postprocedural luminal gain before stenting in particularly resistant stenoses.

Intravascular Imaging

Intravascular ultrasound (IVUS) to guide percutaneous coronary intervention has long been associated with improved outcomes. Observational and randomized evidence suggests that this benefit may extend into the peripheral space. Analysis of the Japanese Diagnosis Procedure Combination database found 59.5% of peripheral interventions, 59,925 patients, to have undergone IVUS-guided peripheral vascular interventions. Using propensity score matching, the IVUS was associated with a 20% decrease in 12-month amputation risk. More recently, a single-center trial of 150 patients undergoing femoropopliteal intervention randomized patients to angiography alone versus angiography plus IVUS. The 12-month rate of freedom from binary restenosis, defined as $\geq 50\%$ stenosis on duplex ultrasound, was significantly higher in the IVUS cohort (72.4% vs 55.4%; $P=$ .008).[71] A multidisciplinary consensus from 6 major US vascular societies has graded IVUS as appropriate for all femoropopliteal artery intraprocedural and postintervention optimization scenarios.[72]

Surgical Therapy

Surgical targets for bypass include the common femoral artery for inflow and above-knee popliteal, below-knee popliteal arteries, and tibial vessels for outflow. Stenting in these segments can severely compromise subsequent open surgical attempts at revascularization; therefore, these should be preserved whenever possible. Multidisciplinary collaboration with patients with advanced peripheral artery disease requires medical, endovascular, and open surgical management expertise. In patients who have failed endovascular therapy or in patients with severe femoropopliteal disease at high risk for complication and failure of endovascular treatment, such as GLASS stage 4 or TASC C/D therapy, the BEST-CLI trial has shown a reduction in MALE (42.6% vs 57.4%, $P<.001$) over a follow up of 2.7 years for femoropopliteal bypass with single segment great saphenous vein if available.[73] However, there was no difference in above-the-ankle amputation rates, death, and bypass with alternative conduits over those patients able to be treated with endovascular therapies.[73,74]

Postprocedural Management and Surveillance

Following femoropopliteal intervention, antiplatelet and antithrombotic therapies are the cornerstone of therapy to mitigate the risk of subsequent MALE and major adverse cardiac events. Guidelines recommend both antiplatelet and antithrombotic therapy, low-dose aspirin, and low-dose rivaroxaban (2.5 mg twice daily).[8] The VOYAGER PAD trial demonstrated aspirin and rivaroxaban to be superior to aspirin alone in preventing subsequent acute limb ischemia (HR 0.67 95% CI 0.55–0.82) and unplanned index-limb revascularization for recurrent limb ischemia (HR 0.88 95% CI 0.79–0.99).[75] Dual antiplatelet therapy of low-dose aspirin and a P2Y12 inhibitor may also be considered for 1 to 6 months.[8]

The optimal surveillance frequency following femoropopliteal intervention is still being determined. The primary goal of surveillance postrevascularization is the early identification of intervention sites with new severe restenosis despite the absence of new symptoms. Performing an ABI and arterial duplex ultrasound within 1 to 3 months post procedure, then at 6 and 12 months, and then yearly is reasonable. A reduction in ABI of greater than 0.15 from the prior value is proposed to identify the failure of revascularization; however, it is recommended this be used in conjunction with duplex ultrasound.[8]

Emerging Technologies

Endovascular technology is evolving to minimize the body's reaction to foreign body material. One strategy is described as mimetic stents, or stents that mimic the biophysical properties of the artery. These are often accomplished through woven nitinol struts that have increased resistance to stretch and torsion forces. The theory is these will have better patency in the highly flexible popliteal arterial segments behind the knee.[76] The current evidence demonstrates adequate periprocedural safety and comparable mid-term outcomes, with a 1-year patency of 81% and a 5-year patency of 63%.[77] These adjuncts may be helpful for patients at high risk for surgical bypass, particularly in CLTI.[77,78] However, this technology may not be as beneficial as DES or DCBs.[79] A second technology to reduce the long-term effects of implanted stents is bioabsorbable stents, particularly in the below-knee popliteal artery. Early studies have shown promise with this technology, but it remains largely experimental.[80]

Finally, percutaneous transmural bypass, the PQ Bypass DETOUR system, utilizes a needle to cross between the common femoral or proximal SFA into the femoral vein and then reenter into a healthy distal popliteal artery and deploys a covered stent through the femoral vein between inflow and outflow targets. In the DETOUR2 study, a prospective, single-arm trial of 202 patients with complex femoropopliteal disease, the 1-year primary patency was found to be 72.1%.[81]

CONCLUSIONS AND FUTURE DIRECTIONS

The femoropopliteal segment is one of the most affected anatomic segments in symptomatic lower extremity atherosclerotic disease. Disease of the femoropopliteal segment most often presents with claudication but can also present as rest pain and tissue loss. In the setting of functionally limiting claudication with an inadequate response to guideline-directed medical therapy and in cases of acute or chronic limb-threatening ischemia, endovascular revascularization is a crucial therapy. Understanding this vascular bed's failure mechanisms and anatomic constraints is essential in selecting an endovascular approach that optimizes technical success and long-term durability while minimizing periprocedural complications. There are still many limitations on the data related to treating femoropopliteal disease. Trials have historically enrolled fewer women and racially/ethnically diverse patients and often focus on patients with intermittent claudication rather than patients with more severe disease.[82] Future trials should focus on enrolling diverse, representative patient populations that are particularly understudied and be powered for patient-centered, limb-related, and mortality outcomes, both short and long term, in their design.[39]

DISCLOSURE

APJ and SDM have no relevant disclosures. Relevant disclosures for RVS include ACIST Medical (research support), Philips (Advisory board/consulting), Boston Scientific (Speakers bureau/consulting). Relevant disclosures for J Antonio Gutierrez include Veterans Health Administration (research support).

REFERENCES

1. Mensah GA, Fuster V, Murray CJL, et al. Global burden of cardiovascular diseases and risks, 1990-2022. J Am Coll Cardiol 2023;82(25):2350–473.
2. Aday AW, Matsushita K. Epidemiology of peripheral artery disease and polyvascular disease. Circ Res 2021;128(12):1818–32.

3.. White C. Clinical practice. Intermittent claudication. N Engl J Med 2007;356(12):1241–50.

4. Abry L. Peripheral artery disease leading to major amputation: trends in revascularization and mortality over 18 years. Ann Vasc Surg 2022;78.

5. Golledge J, Moxon JV, Rowbotham S, et al. Risk of major amputation in patients with intermittent claudication undergoing early revascularization. Br J Surg 2018;105(6):699–708.

6. Madabhushi V, Davenport D, Jones S, et al. Revascularization of intermittent claudicants leads to more chronic limb-threatening ischemia and higher amputation rates. J Vasc Surg 2021;74(3):771–9.

7. Rutherford RB, Baker JD, Ernst C, et al. Recommended standards for reports dealing with lower extremity ischemia: Revised version. J Vasc Surg 1997;26(3):517–38.

8. Gornik HL, Aronow HD, Goodney PP, et al. ACC/AHA/AACVPR/APMA/ABC/SCAI/SVM/SVN/SVS/SIR/VESS guideline for the management of lower extremity peripheral artery disease: a report of the American College of Cardiology/American Heart association Joint Committee on clinical practice guidelines. Circulation 2024;149(24).

9. Lee SR, Ali S, Cardella J, et al. Carbon dioxide angiography during peripheral vascular interventions is associated with decreased cardiac and renal complications in patients with chronic kidney disease. J Vasc Surg 2023;78(1):201–8.

10. Norgren L, Hiatt WR, Dormandy JA, et al. Inter-society consensus for the management of peripheral arterial disease (TASC II). Eur J Vasc Endovasc Surg 2007;33(1):S1–75.

11. Conte MS, Bradbury AW, Kolh P, et al. Global vascular guidelines on the management of chronic limb-threatening ischemia. J Vasc Surg 2019;69(6):3S–125S.e40.

12. Kaplovitch E, Eikelboom JW, Dyal L, et al. Rivaroxaban and aspirin in patients with symptomatic lower extremity peripheral artery disease: a subanalysis of the COMPASS randomized clinical trial. JAMA Cardiol 2020. https://doi.org/10.1001/jamacardio.2020.4390.

13. Patel KK, Jones PG, Ellerbeck EF, et al. Underutilization of evidence-based smoking cessation support strategies despite high smoking addiction burden in peripheral artery disease specialty care: insights from the international PORTRAIT registry. J Am Heart Assoc 2018;7(20):e010076.

14. Reitz KM, Althouse AD, Meyer J, et al. Association of smoking with postprocedural complications following open and endovascular interventions for intermittent claudication. JAMA Cardiol 2022;7(1):45.

15. Barua RS, Rigotti NA, Benowitz NL, et al. ACC expert consensus decision pathway on tobacco cessation treatment. J Am Coll Cardiol 2018; 72(25):3332–65.

16. Hennrikus D, Joseph AM, Lando HA, et al. Effectiveness of a smoking cessation program for peripheral artery disease patients. J Am Coll Cardiol 2010;56(25):2105–12.

17. Creager MA, Hamburg NM. Smoking cessation improves outcomes in patients with peripheral artery disease. JAMA Cardiol 2022;7(1):15.

18. Brown T, Forster RB, Cleanthis M, et al. Cilostazol for intermittent claudication. In: Vascular Group Cochrane, editor. Cochrane Database Syst Rev 2021;2021(6).

19. Fakhry F, Van De Luijtgaarden KM, Bax L, et al. Supervised walking therapy in patients with intermittent claudication. J Vasc Surg 2012;56(4):1132–42.

20. Treat-Jacobson D, McDermott MM, Bronas UG, et al. Optimal exercise programs for patients with peripheral artery disease: a scientific statement from the American Heart Association. Circulation 2019;139(4).

21. Fakhry F, Fokkenrood HJ, Spronk S, et al. Endovascular revascularisation versus conservative management for intermittent claudication. Cochrane Vascular Group. Cochrane Database Syst Rev 2018;2018(3).

22. Pandey A, Banerjee S, Ngo C, et al. Comparative efficacy of endovascular revascularization versus supervised exercise training in patients with intermittent claudication. JACC Cardiovasc Interv 2017; 10(7):712–24.

23. Malgor RD, Alalahdab F, Elraiyah TA, et al. A systematic review of treatment of intermittent claudication in the lower extremities. J Vasc Surg 2015;61(3):54S–73S.

24. Levin SR, Farber A, Cheng TW, et al. Patients undergoing interventions for claudication experience low perioperative morbidity but are at risk for worsening functional status and limb loss. J Vasc Surg 2020;72(1):241–9.

25. Jones DW, Goodney PP, Eldrup-Jorgensen J, et al. Active smoking in claudicants undergoing lower extremity bypass predicts decreased graft patency and worse overall survival. J Vasc Surg 2018;68(3):796–806.e1.

26. McDermott MM. Erasing disability in peripheral artery disease: the role of endovascular procedures and supervised exercise. JAMA 2015; 314(18):1921.

27. Shammas NW, Abi Doumet A, Karia R, et al. An overview of the treatment of symptomatic common femoral artery lesions with a focus on endovascular therapy. Vasc Health Risk Manag 2020;16:67–73.

28. Scheinert D, Scheinert S, Sax J, et al. Prevalence and clinical impact of stent fractures after femoropopliteal stenting. J Am Coll Cardiol 2005;45(2):312–5.

29. Cheng CP, Wilson NM, Hallett RL, et al. In Vivo MR angiographic quantification of axial and twisting deformations of the superficial femoral artery

resulting from maximum hip and knee flexion. J Vasc Intervent Radiol 2006;17(6):979–87.

30. Bradbury AW, Adam DJ, Bell J, et al. Bypass versus angioplasty in severe ischaemia of the Leg (BASIL) trial: an intention-to-treat analysis of amputation-free and overall survival in patients randomized to a bypass surgery-first or a balloon angioplasty-first revascularization strategy. J Vasc Surg 2010; 51(5 SUPPL):5S–17S.

31. Dubosq M, Raux M, Nasr B, et al. Algorithm of femoropopliteal endovascular treatment. Medicina (Mex) 2022;58(9):1293.

32. Nasr B, Hauguel A, Yven C, et al. Antegrade superficial femoral artery approach using manual compression and 4-f delivery system for infrainguinal occlusive disease. Ann Vasc Surg 2022;78:1–8.

33. Martin G, Covani M, Saab F, et al. A systematic review of the ipsilateral retrograde approach to the treatment of femoropopliteal arterial lesions. J Vasc Surg 2021;74(4):1394–405.e4.

34. Giannopoulos S, Palena LM, Armstrong EJ. Technical success and complication rates of retrograde arterial access for endovascular therapy for critical limb ischaemia: a systematic review and meta-analysis. Eur J Vasc Endovasc Surg 2021;61(2):270–9.

35. Solimeno G, Salcuni M, Capparelli G, et al. Technical perspectives in the management of complex infrainguinal arterial chronic total occlusions. J Vasc Surg 2022;75(2):732–9.

36. Mason PJ, Shah B, Tamis-Holland JE, et al. An update on radial artery access and best practices for transradial coronary angiography and intervention in acute coronary syndrome: a scientific statement from the American Heart Association. Circ Cardiovasc Interv 2018;11(9):e000035.

37. Sher A, Posham R, Vouyouka A, et al. Safety and feasibility of transradial infrainguinal peripheral arterial disease interventions. J Vasc Surg 2020;72(4):1237–46.e1.

38. Bradbury AW, Adam DJ, Beard JD, et al. Bypass versus angioplasty in severe ischaemia of the leg (BASIL): multicentre, randomised controlled trial. Lancet 2005;366(9501):1925–34.

39. D'Oria M, Mastrorilli D, Secemsky E, et al. Robustness of longitudinal safety and efficacy after paclitaxel-based endovascular therapy for treatment of femoro-popliteal artery occlusive disease: an updated systematic review and meta-analysis of randomized controlled trials. Ann Vasc Surg 2024;101:164–78.

40. Koeckerling D, Raguindin PF, Kastrati L, et al. Endovascular revascularization strategies for aortoiliac and femoropopliteal artery disease: a meta-analysis. Eur Heart J 2023;44(11):935–50.

41. Dubosq-Lebaz M, Fels A, Chatellier G, et al. Systematic review and meta-analysis of clinical outcomes after endovascular treatment in patients with femoropopliteal lesions greater than 150

mm. J Endovasc Ther 202315266028231202709. https://doi.org/10.1177/15266028231202709.

42. Steiner S, Schmidt A, Zeller T, et al. COMPARE: prospective, randomized, non-inferiority trial of high- vs. low-dose paclitaxel drug-coated balloons for femoropopliteal interventions. Eur Heart J 2020;41(27):2541–52.

43. Krishnan P, Farhan S, Schneider P, et al. Determinants of drug-coated balloon failure in patients undergoing femoropopliteal arterial intervention. J Am Coll Cardiol 2022;80(13):1241–50.

44. Feldman DN, Armstrong EJ, Aronow HD, et al. SCAI consensus guidelines for device selection in femoral-popliteal arterial interventions. Cathet Cardiovasc Interv 2018;92(1):124–40.

45. Katsanos K, Spiliopoulos S, Kitrou P, et al. Risk of death following application of paclitaxel-coated balloons and stents in the femoropopliteal artery of the leg: a systematic review and meta-analysis of randomized controlled trials. J Am Heart Assoc 2018;7(24).

46. Parikh SA, Schneider PA, Mullin CM, et al. Mortality in randomised controlled trials using paclitaxel-coated devices for femoropopliteal interventional procedures: an updated patient-level meta-analysis. Lancet 2023;402(10415):1848–56.

47. Gutierrez JA, Rao SV, Jones WS, et al. Survival and causes of death among veterans with lower extremity revascularization with paclitaxel-coated devices: insights from the veterans health administration. J Am Heart Assoc 2021;10(4):e018149.

48. Nordanstig J, James S, Andersson M, et al. Mortality with paclitaxel-coated devices in peripheral artery disease. N Engl J Med 2020;383(26):2538–46.

49. Secemsky EA, Shen C, Schermerhorn M, et al. Longitudinal assessment of safety of femoropopliteal endovascular treatment with paclitaxel-coated devices among medicare beneficiaries: the SAFE-PAD Study. JAMA Intern Med 2021;181(8):1071.

50. Hess CN, Patel MR, Bauersachs RM, et al. Safety and effectiveness of paclitaxel drug-coated devices in peripheral artery revascularization. J Am Coll Cardiol 2021;78(18):1768–78.

51. Freisinger E, Koeppe J, Gerss J, et al. Mortality after use of paclitaxel-based devices in peripheral arteries: a real-world safety analysis. Eur Heart J 2020; 41(38):3732–9.

52. Schneider PA, Laird JR, Doros G, et al. Mortality not correlated with paclitaxel exposure. J Am Coll Cardiol 2019;73(20):2550–63.

53. Dake MD, Ansel GM, Jaff MR, et al. Sustained safety and effectiveness of paclitaxel-eluting stents for femoropopliteal lesions. J Am Coll Cardiol 2013;61(24):2417–27.

54. Bausback Y, Wittig T, Schmidt A, et al. Drug-eluting stent versus drug-coated balloon revascularization in patients with femoropopliteal arterial disease. J Am Coll Cardiol 2019;73(6):667–79.

55. Gasior P, Cheng Y, Valencia AF, et al. Impact of fluoropolymer-based paclitaxel delivery on neointimal proliferation and vascular healing: a comparative peripheral drug-eluting stent study in the familial hypercholesterolemic swine model of femoral restenosis. Circ Cardiovasc Interv 2017;10(5):e004450.

56. Gouëffic Y, Torsello G, Zeller T, et al. Efficacy of a drug-eluting stent versus bare metal stents for symptomatic femoropopliteal peripheral artery disease: primary results of the EMINENT randomized trial. Circulation 2022;146(21):1564–76.

57. Müller-Hülsbeck S, Benko A, Soga Y, et al. Two-year efficacy and safety results from the imperial randomized study of the eluvia polymer-coated drug-eluting stent and the zilver PTX Polymer-free Drug-Coated Stent. Cardiovasc Intervent Radiol 2021;44(3):368–75.

58. Thieme M, Von Bilderling P, Paetzel C, et al. The 24-month results of the Lutonix global SFA registry. JACC Cardiovasc Interv 2017;10(16):1682–90.

59. Wittig T, Schmidt A, Fuß T, et al. Randomized trial comparing a stent-avoiding with a stent-preferred strategy in complex femoropopliteal lesions. JACC Cardiovasc Interv 2024;17(9):1134–44.

60. Bontinis A, Bontinis V, Koutsoumpelis A, et al. A systematic review aggregated data and individual participant data meta-analysis of spot stenting in the treatment of lower extremity peripheral arterial disease. Ann Vasc Surg 2022;85:424–32.

61. Geraghty PJ, Mewissen MW, Jaff MR, et al. Three-year results of the VIBRANT trial of VIABAHN endoprosthesis versus bare nitinol stent implantation for complex superficial femoral artery occlusive disease. J Vasc Surg 2013;58(2):386–95.e4.

62. Mohan S, Flahive JM, Arous EJ, et al. Peripheral atherectomy practice patterns in the United States from the vascular quality initiative. J Vasc Surg 2018;68(6):1806–16.

63. Wardle BG, Ambler GK, Radwan RW, et al. Atherectomy for peripheral arterial disease. Cochrane Vascular Group. Cochrane Database Syst Rev 2020;2020(9).

64. Wu Z, Huang Q, Pu H, et al. Atherectomy combined with balloon angioplasty versus balloon angioplasty alone for de novo femoropopliteal arterial diseases: a systematic review and meta-analysis of randomised controlled trials. Eur J Vasc Endovasc Surg 2021;62(1):65–73.

65. Pan D, Guo J, Su Z, et al. Efficacy and safety of atherectomy combined with balloon angioplasty vs balloon angioplasty alone in patients with femoro-popliteal lesions: a systematic review and meta-analysis of randomized controlled trials. J Endovasc Ther 202315266028231215354. https://doi.org/10.1177/15266028231215354.

66. Gupta R, Siada S, Lai S, et al. Critical appraisal of the contemporary use of atherectomy to treat femoropopliteal atherosclerotic disease. J Vasc Surg 2022;75(2):697–708.e9.

67. Shammas NW, Mangalmurti S, Bernardo NL, et al. Intravascular lithotripsy for treatment of severely calcified common femoral artery disease: results from the disrupt PAD III observational study. J Endovasc Ther 202415266028241255622. https://doi.org/10.1177/15266028241255622.

68. Stavroulakis K, Bisdas T, Torsello G, et al. Intravascular lithotripsy and drug-coated balloon angioplasty for severely calcified femoropopliteal arterial disease. J Endovasc Ther 2023;30(1):106–13.

69. Tepe G, Brodmann M, Werner M, et al. Intravascular lithotripsy for peripheral artery calcification. JACC Cardiovasc Interv 2021;14(12):1352–61.

70. Wong CP, Chan LP, Au DM, et al. Efficacy and safety of intravascular lithotripsy in lower extremity peripheral artery disease: a systematic review and meta-analysis. Eur J Vasc Endovasc Surg 2022;63(3):446–56.

71. Allan RB, Puckridge PJ, Spark JI, et al. The impact of intravascular ultrasound on femoropopliteal artery endovascular interventions. JACC Cardiovasc Interv 2022;15(5):536–46.

72. Secemsky EA, Mosarla RC, Rosenfield K, et al. Appropriate use of intravascular ultrasound during arterial and venous lower extremity interventions. JACC Cardiovasc Interv 2022;15(15):1558–68.

73. Farber A, Menard MT, Conte MS, et al. Surgery or endovascular therapy for chronic limb-threatening ischemia. N Engl J Med 2022;13.

74. Bradbury AW, Moakes CA, Popplewell M, et al. A vein bypass first versus a best endovascular treatment first revascularisation strategy for patients with chronic limb threatening ischaemia who required an infra-popliteal, with or without an additional more proximal infra-inguinal revascularisation procedure to restore limb perfusion (BASIL-2): an open-label, randomised, multicentre, phase 3 trial. Lancet 2023. https://doi.org/10.1016/S0140-6736(23)00462-2. S0140673623004622.

75. Bonaca MP, Bauersachs RM, Anand SS, et al. Rivaroxaban in peripheral artery disease after revascularization. N Engl J Med 2020;382(21):1994–2004.

76. Peker A, Balendran B, Paraskevopoulos I, et al. Demystifying the use of self-expandable interwoven nitinol stents in femoropopliteal peripheral arterial disease. Ann Vasc Surg 2019;59:285–92.

77. Chan YC, Cheng SW, Cheung GC. A midterm analysis of patients who received femoropopliteal helical interwoven nitinol stents. J Vasc Surg 2020;71(6):2048–55.

78. Okuno S, Iida O, Iida T, et al. Comparison of clinical outcomes between endovascular therapy with self-expandable nitinol stent and femoral–popliteal bypass for trans-atlantic inter-society consensus II C and D femoropopliteal lesions. Ann Vasc Surg 2019;57:137–43.

79. Haine A, Schmid MJ, Schindewolf M, et al. Comparison between interwoven nitinol and drug eluting stents for endovascular treatment of femoropopliteal artery disease. Eur J Vasc Endovasc Surg 2019;58(6):865–73.

80. Varcoe RL, DeRubertis BG, Kolluri R, et al. Drug-eluting resorbable scaffold versus angioplasty for infrapopliteal artery disease. N Engl J Med 2023. https://doi.org/10.1056/NEJMoa2305637. NEJMoa2305637.

81. Lyden SP, Soukas PA, De A, et al. DETOUR2 trial outcomes demonstrate clinical utility of percutaneous transmural bypass for the treatment of long segment, complex femoropopliteal disease. J Vasc Surg 2024;79(6):1420–7.e2.

82. Michos ED, Reddy TK, Gulati M, et al. Improving the enrollment of women and racially/ethnically diverse populations in cardiovascular clinical trials: an ASPC practice statement. Am J Prev Cardiol 2021;8:100250.

Chronic Limb-Threatening Ischemia
A Comprehensive Review Paper

Ghassan Daher, MD[a], Satawart Upadhyay, MD[b],
Jun Li, MD, FSCAI[a,c,d,*]

KEYWORDS

- Chronic limb-threatening ischemia (CLTI) • Peripheral artery disease (PAD)
- Endovascular interventions • Socioeconomic disparities • No-option CLTI

KEY POINTS

- CLTI is a highly prevalent, underdiagnosed, and limb-threatening disease with significant burden of cardiovascular morbidity and mortality.
- Timely and appropriate diagnosis and treatment is of the utmost importance for limb salvage, while medical optimization helps prevent further deterioration from both a life and limb perspective.
- CLTI is a multifaceted disorder, requiring multiple health care providers for interdisciplinary collaboration to optimize outcomes.
- Disparities in PAD management have historically been underrecognized, but equity in care delivery is emerging as a foremost goal of the endovascular community's efforts for improvement.

INTRODUCTION

Lower extremity peripheral artery disease (PAD) is estimated to affect 10 to 12 million individuals over the age of 40 in the United States alone. Worldwide, the prevalence of PAD is estimated to be between 113 and 236 million individuals. Chronic limb-threatening ischemia (CLTI), the end-stage manifestation of the disease state, affects 11% to 20% of patients with known PAD.[1–3] CLTI is defined by >2-week duration of a non-healing wound or the presence of ischemic rest pain attributable to arterial occlusive disease. Unfortunately, despite significant advancements in therapeutic strategies and guideline-directed medical therapy (GDMT), CLTI continues to cause significant morbidity and mortality, with major amputation rates of up to 30% and mortality rates ranging 25% to 35% within a year.[1,4,5] This article provides a comprehensive overview of CLTI, including diagnostic assessment, treatment options, and the ongoing challenges in its management.

HISTORICAL PERSPECTIVE

By the early twentieth century, the relationship of arteriosclerosis and its role in limb ischemia was becoming more evident. The term "intermittent claudication" was used to describe exercise-induced pain due to poor blood flow. The mainstay of therapy during that time was purely surgical as the primary contributors of atherosclerosis were yet to be elucidated. In the mid-twentieth century, the term "critical limb ischemia" emerged to describe the most

[a] Harrington Heart and Vascular Institute, University Hospitals Cleveland Medical Center, 11100 Euclid Avenue, Cleveland, OH 44106, USA; [b] Department of Medicine, University Hospitals, Lakeside Building, Suite 3500, 11100 Euclid Avenue, Cleveland, OH 44106, USA; [c] Vascular Center, Pulmonary Embolism Response Team, University Hospitals Harrington Heart & Vascular Institute; [d] Case Western Reserve University School of Medicine, 6525 Powers Boulevard, MAC III, Suite 301, Parma, OH 44129, USA
* Corresponding author. University Hospitals Harrington Heart and Vascular Institute, 6525 Powers Boulevard, MAC III, Suite 301, Parma, OH 44129.
E-mail address: Jun.Li@UHhospitals.org

Intervent Cardiol Clin 14 (2025) 257–272
https://doi.org/10.1016/j.iccl.2024.11.011
2211-7458/25/© 2025 Elsevier Inc. All rights reserved, including those for text and data mining, AI training, and similar technologies.

Abbreviations	
ABI	ankle-brachial index
ASCVD	atherosclerotic cardiovascular disease
AT	anterior tibial
BASIL	Bypass versus Angioplasty in Severe Ischemia of the Leg
BTK	below-the-knee
CKD	chronic kidney disease
CLTI	chronic limb-threatening ischemia
CTA	computed tomography angiography
CTO	chronic total occlusion
DAPT	dual antiplatelet therapy
DPI	dual pathway inhibition
DRS	drug-eluting resorbable scaffold
DSA	digital subtraction angiography
ECM	extracellular matrix
GDMT	guideline-directed medical therapy
LDL	low-density lipoprotein
MACE	major adverse cardiac event
MALE	major adverse limb event
MRA	magnetic resonance angiography
NOP-CLTI	no-option CLTI
PAD	peripheral artery disease
PTA	percutaneous transluminal angioplasty
PVR	pulse volume recordings
SCB	sirolimus-coated balloons
SPP	skin perfusion pressure
TADV	transcatheter arterialization of the deep veins
TBI	toe-brachial index

severe form of PAD, characterized by rest pain, nonhealing ulcers, and gangrene. The mid-twentieth to late-twentieth century was marked by the beginnings of medical therapy, heralded by the introduction of aspirin and statins. Concurrently, early developments in endovascular interventions emerged, with Dr Charles Dotter performing the first angioplasty of a stenotic superficial femoral artery in 1964, thereby revolutionizing the management of PAD.

In 2017, the European Society of Vascular Surgery proposed the term "chronic limb-threatening ischemia" to replace critical limb

ischemia, to address several issues.[6] CLTI implies chronicity to the disease state, as many patients survive with a threatened limb for extended periods of time. Additionally, aside from arterial disease, other factors affecting a threatened limb (including diabetes, neuropathy, and infection) contribute to the risk of major amputation.

CLASSIFICATION SYSTEMS

Multiple classification schemas exist for PAD and CLTI (Table 1), varying based on clinical and objective characteristics. The first classification system by Fontaine and colleagues emerged from the European Society of Cardiovascular Surgery in the 1950s and was solely based on clinical symptoms, without other diagnostic tests.[7] The symptomatic classification was adapted by Rutherford and colleagues to delineate PAD into acute and chronic limb ischemia, emphasizing differences in treatment algorithms required for each. The Rutherford classification also associates clinical symptoms with objective findings, including ankle pressure and pulse volume recordings.[8]

Bollinger and colleagues proposed an angiographic methodology for classification based on smaller segments of the lower extremity arteries. This method uses the occlusive pattern (plaque vs stenosis vs complete occlusion) along with the number of lesions visualized on an angiogram to provide an additive score.[9] Although Bollinger methods of classification were used in the Bypass versus Angioplasty in Severe Ischemia of the Leg (BASIL) trial, this system is not used in clinical settings.

In 1987, Taylor and Palmer introduced the angiosome concept, dividing the human body into 3-dimensional blocks of tissue, each supplied by specific arterial and venous sources known as angiosomes.[10] These angiosomes are interconnected by collateral or choke vessels, which can provide indirect flow to a vascular territory when direct flow is absent. Under this concept, the goal of revascularization is to restore blood flow to the affected ischemic angiosomes. The infrapopliteal territory is served by 3 main arteries (Fig. 1): the anterior tibial, posterior tibial, and peroneal. Together, these arteries supply 6 angiosomes: the anterior tibial artery supplies the anterior shin and dorsum of the foot, the posterior tibial artery supplies the medial heel and the medial and lateral plantar angiosomes, and the peroneal artery supplies the lateral aspect of the heel and the lateral border of the foot.[11] A meta-analysis showed a 60% relative risk reduction in

Table 1
Classification schemas for defining stages of peripheral artery disease and chronic limb-threatening ischemia

Classification	Symptom Based	Anatomic	Direct Treatment	Apply to Acute Limb Ischemia	Specifically for Diabetes	Pros	Cons
Fontaine	Yes	No	Yes	Not classically	No	Historically proven; easy to apply to patient	No objective criteria
Rutherford	Yes	No	Yes	Yes	No	Historically proven, quickly apply to patient, objective	Classically should not be applied in diabetes, no consideration for wounds
Bollinger	No	Yes	No	No	No	Categorical variable can be used in research, allows for documentation of change in follow-up	No basis on symptoms, applied poorly to diabetes
Graziani	No	Yes	No	No	Yes	Application in diabetes	Does not address aortoileal disease, does not direct therapy
Wifi	Yes	No	Yes	No	Yes	Robust to account for several factors in PAD	New and not validated in many research studies
TASC II	No	Yes	Yes	Yes	No	Defined disease process, used in several research studies	Treatment recommendations not widely accepted and may need updating
Angiosome	No	Yes	Yes	Not described	No	May help optimize revascularization strategy	Needs further validation
AMA	Yes	No	No	Yes	No	Good for use in disability, reflects state of the patients global health	Not intended to direct treatment, mixed arterial and venous categories

Abbreviations: AMA, American Medical Association; PAD, peripheral artery disease; TASC II, Trans-Atlantic Inter-Society Consensus Document; WIfI, wound, Ischemia, foot Infection.
Adapted from Hardman RL, Jazaeri O, Yi J, et al. Overview of classification systems in peripheral artery disease. Semin Intervent Radiol 2014;31(4):378–88. https://doi.org/10.1055/s-0034-1393976. PMID: 25435665; PMCID: PMC4232437.

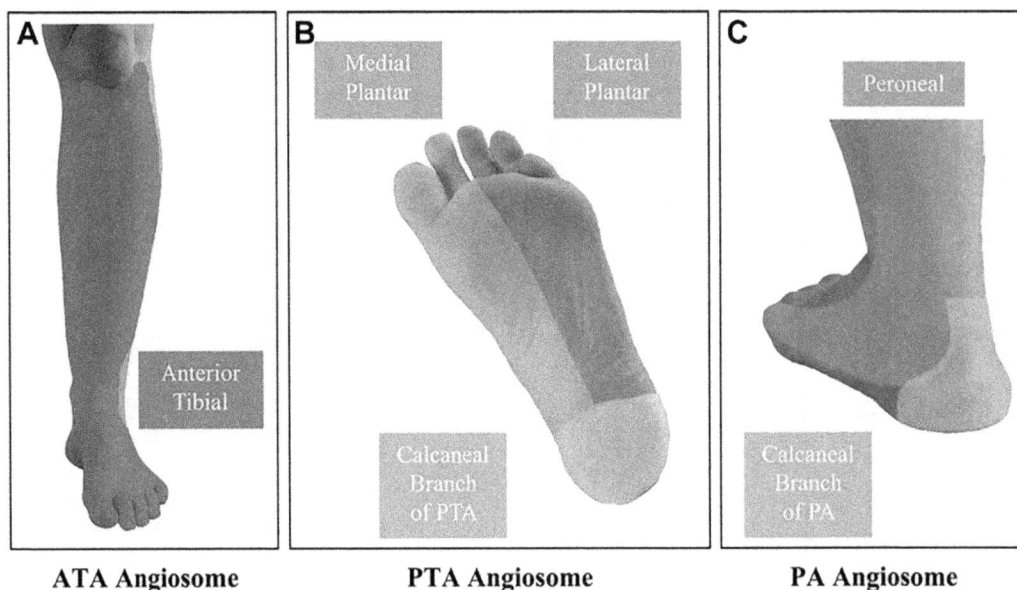

ATA Angiosome   **PTA Angiosome**   **PA Angiosome**

Fig. 1. Below-the-knee angiosomes, based on supply of artery into the target territory of wound. The anterior tibial artery (ATA) supplies the dorsal aspect of the foot (A), while the posterior tibial artery (PTA) supplies the heel and plantar territories (B). A complete pedal arch will allow crossover from ATA to PTA, and vice versa. The peroneal artery (PA) provides lateral distribution perfusion to the ankle and heel (C). (Osamu Iida et al., Long-term results of direct and indirect endovascular revascularization based on the angiosome concept in patients with critical limb ischemia presenting with isolated below-the-knee lesions, Journal of Vascular Surgery, 55 (2), 2012, 363-370.e5, https://doi.org/10.1016/j.jvs.2011.08.014.)

major amputations with angiosome-guided direct revascularization versus indirect revascularization, though high heterogeneity exists amongst these retrospective and observational studies.[12] Wound blush has been proposed by some operators to be reasonable surrogates for successful wound healing,[13] regardless of direct or indirect revascularization, but this is a difficult to quantify endpoint and can vary based on contrast injection techniques.

To provide insight into interplay of wound, perfusion, and infection in overall limb salvage success, the Society of Vascular Surgery proposed the Wound, Ischemia, and foot Infection (WIfI) classification system.[14,15] A separate grade is given to the wound (based on location and depth of ulcer), ischemia (based on ankle or toe perfusion), and infection, which combine to provide an overall assessment of major amputation risk and potential for benefit derived from revascularization.[14,16]

PATHOPHYSIOLOGY

Atherosclerosis is a multifaceted process involving various biological pathways, including lipid metabolism, inflammation, and vascular cell biology.[17,18] The initiation of atherosclerosis stems from endothelial dysfunction, which is characterized by impaired nitric oxide bioavailability and altered hemodynamic responses. This facilitates low-density lipoprotein (LDL) retention in the arterial intima, where it undergoes oxidative modifications, creating proinflammatory particles crucial to disease progression.[17,18] Oxidized LDLs and other proinflammatory cytokines lead to sustained endothelial activation and upregulation of adhesion molecules and chemokines which lead to monocyte recruitment and foam cell activation. Eventual apoptosis of these cells leads to formation of a necrotic core, which is covered by recruited vascular smooth muscle cells and extracellular matrix (ECM), providing structural integrity to the plaque. ECM vesicles released by these dying cells eventually lead to plaque calcification through a mechanism known as cellular trans-differentiation where they start to express osteoblast-like phenotypes.[19,20]

DIAGNOSTIC ASSESSMENT

Hemodynamic and anatomic assessments are critical for diagnosing CLTI. In patients with suspected CLTI, initial hemodynamic assessment with resting ankle-brachial index (ABI) with or without pulse volume recordings (PVR) and/or Doppler waveforms is a class I indication for establishing diagnosis.[1] Nonetheless, ABI and

PVR have limitations in CLTI diagnosis, particularly in patients with noncompressible vessels. Multiple analyses have shown toe-brachial index (TBI) to be more sensitive than ABI and PVR for diagnosis of CLTI in patients with infrapopliteal disease.[21–23] Generally, ABI conveys information on above-the-knee or inflow hemodynamics, but TBI provides an end-organ perfusion assessment with conglomerate evaluation of below-the-knee (BTK) and inframalleolar flow. For this reason, the authors favor obtaining screening TBI in addition to ABI in patients suspected of CLTI (Fig. 2). Typically, TBI of ≤0.70 suggests evidence of disease, while absolute toe pressures <30 mm Hg are associated with worst clinical outcomes.[1] Supplemental tests with transcutaneous oxygen pressure (TcPO$_2$) and skin perfusion pressure (SPP) may be helpful, though utility remains low in clinical practice.

Additional imaging may assist endovascular interventionists and surgeons in identification of optimal vascular access, locating the culprit lesion(s), and determining the feasibility and modality of revascularization. Anatomic assessment with duplex ultrasound, computed tomography angiography (CTA), magnetic resonance angiography (MRA), or digital subtraction angiography (DSA) is an option. Duplex ultrasound is commonly used but is limited in obese patients and in those with significantly calcified arteries, as shadowing prohibits proper insonation of velocities. CTA provides detailed information but involves exposure to radiation and contrast agents, which is limited in patients with kidney disease, and can result in overexaggeration of calcium. MRA is limited by long acquisition times, patient motion, and the inability to visualize distal tibial and inframalleolar arteries. DSA can be performed at same time as an intervention, but is an invasive procedure. Emerging technologies like indocyanine green angiography and vascular optical tomographic imaging show promise for future diagnostic improvements but are yet to be adopted in clinical practice.[24–27]

SURGICAL VERSUS ENDOVASCULAR REVASCULARIZATION

Revascularization therapy has received a Class 1 recommendation by all professional guidelines and has become the primary treatment for CLTI(1). By 1 year, up to 40% of CLTI patients will need a lower limb amputation in the absence of revascularization.[1] In addition, there is an increased risk of ipsilateral leg ulcers or death (mortality of 19.2%, 48.7%, and 61.3% at 1, 3,

and 5 years, respectively, after major amputation), and a significant increase of contralateral lower limb amputation (5.7% at 1 year to 11.5% at 5 years) following a primary amputation.[28,29] Therefore, every effort should be made to provide patients with CLTI the most timely, effective, safe, and cost-efficient revascularization.

Depending on patient comorbidities, lesion location, and vessel characteristics, multiple revascularization options exist, including endovascular, surgical, or hybrid. The BASIL trial was a multicenter randomized control trial published in 2005 comparing bypass surgery versus balloon angioplasty in 452 patients among 27 United Kingdom hospitals, with follow-up to 5.5 years.[30] The study showed similar outcomes at final follow-up between both treatment modalities in amputation-free survival and mortality rates. The decade following BASIL saw a substantial increase in endovascular revascularization, coinciding with reduced rates of major amputation, though this does not imply a causative relationship.[29,31] Given advancements in the endovascular armamentarium, and associated increased length of stay and cost with open surgical revascularization, some practitioners have favored the "endovascular first" approach.[32]

More recently, 2 randomized controlled trials have reintroduced the question of whether a surgical or endovascular approach should be used as the initial revascularization strategy for CLTI. The Best Endovascular versus Best Surgical Therapy in Patients with critical limb ischemia (CLI) or BEST-CLI trial included patients with infrainguinal disease who are deemed candidates for either revascularization strategy.[33] Matriculation rate was slow in the trial, drawing criticisms on its applicability in a real-world CLTI population. Furthermore, 15% of the endovascular cohort (in those with native vein conduits present) underwent unsuccessful revascularization necessitating crossover in treatment arm to surgery, raising questions of whether true clinical equipoise was present based on anatomy in preprocedural assessment. Nonetheless, the authors concluded major adverse limb event (MALE) or all-cause death was statistically higher in the endovascular population.[34] Conversely, the subsequently published BASIL-2 trial, evaluating bypass surgery compared to best endovascular therapy in patients with infrapopliteal disease (with or without additional proximal lesion), showed that the primary outcome of amputation free-survival was more favorable in the endovascular group.[33]

The opposing findings in these 2 contemporary trials highlight the importance of individualizing

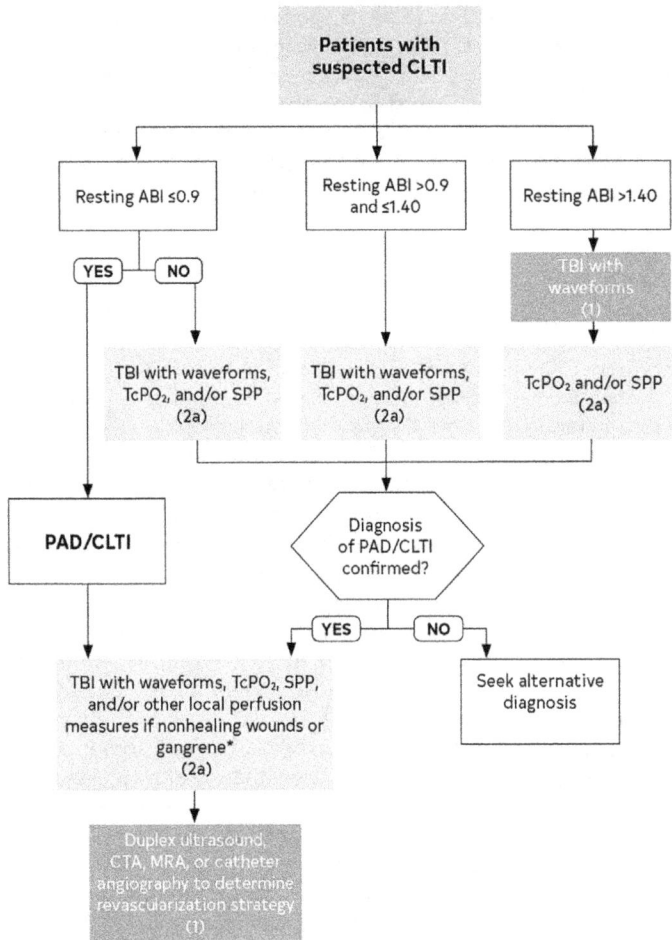

Fig. 2. Algorithm for diagnostic testing in patients for suspected CLTI, adapted from the 2024 multi-societal PAD guidelines. *If not already performed. ABI, ankle-brachial index; Class 1, strong recommendation (benefit >>> risk); Class 2a, moderate strength recommendation (benefit >> risk); CLTI, chronic limb-threatening ischemia; CTA, computed tomography angiography; MRA, magnetic resonance angiography; PAD, peripheral artery disease; SPP, skin perfusion pressure; TBI, toe-brachial index; TcPO$_2$, transcutaneous oxygen pressure. (*Adapted from* Gornik HL, Aronow HD, Goodney PP, et al. 2024 ACC/AHA/AACVPR/APMA/ABC/SCAI/SVM/SVN/SVS/SIR/VESS Guideline for the Management of Lower Extremity Peripheral Artery Disease: A Report of the American College of Cardiology/American Heart Association Joint Committee on Clinical Practice Guidelines. Circulation 2024;149(24):e1313-e1410. https://doi.org/10.1161/CIR.0000000000001251. Epub 2024 May 14. PMID: 38743805.)

ABI Interpretation	
Normal	1.00-1.40
Borderline	0.91-0.99
Abnormal	≤0.90
Noncompressible	>1.40

TBI Interpretation	
Normal	>0.70
Abnormal	≤0.70

treatment strategies based on multiple considerations: (1) patient-related clinical factors such as age, medical comorbidities, life expectancy, compliance, and anesthesia risk; (2) anatomic factors, including presence of a venous conduit, calcification, lesion length, distal target and perfusion, and prior history of previous procedures; and (3) the skillset and comfort level of the regional operators with the proposed revascularization strategy. Shishehbor and colleagues demonstrated the efficacy of real-time multidisciplinary discussions to offer the best available revascularization technique to the patients destined for major amputation, with an improvement in amputation-free survival.[35]

To this end, multi-societal consensus guidelines and experts advocate for an interdisciplinary approach in treating patients with CLTI (1, 35). Ideally, a multimodality treatment approach encompassing wound care specialists (podiatry and/or vascular medicine), vascular specialist (both vascular surgery and endovascular specialist), infectious disease specialist, endocrinologist if applicable, and other supportive personnel (eg, care coordinator, nursing, pharmacy, and social work) would work toward the overall care of patients with CLTI (Fig. 3). A structured, synchronized approach with focus on timely restoration of blood flow and optimization to promote wound closure is imperative, and open communication amongst practitioners is vital to the success of healing.

ENDOVASCULAR REVASCULARIZATION TECHNIQUES

For the purposes of this article, current best-practices in endovascular revascularization techniques will be described. The objectives of revascularization for rest pain, or Rutherford class 4 symptoms, differ from wound healing for Rutherford class 5 to 6 symptom patients. For the former, typically restoration of inflow vessels is sufficient, regardless of the presence or absence of in-line flow in the tibial arteries. Management and revascularization techniques for inflow disease, including aortoiliac and femoropopliteal segments, are described in detail in the previous articles in this issue. On the other hand, in the presence of wounds, optimization of preferably in-line flow into the target territory will help expedite wound healing. Nonetheless, for patients with no in-line options, indirect revascularization of a nontarget tibial artery can still augment wound healing in the presence of collaterals to the target territory, as described earlier.

Lesion Crossing

Access can be obtained via a contralateral crossover or antegrade approach directly into the ipsilateral limb. In patients with known patent inflow vessels, particularly in those with challenging BTK occlusions, direct antegrade access into the ipsilateral common femoral artery is advised. Detailed knowledge of typical anatomic findings as outlined in Fig. 4,[36] as well as common variants, is an integral aspect of an endovascular CLTI operator. Depending on the lesion and cap morphology, a combination of antegrade and retrograde approach may be indicated to cross areas of occlusion (Fig. 5).[36]

Preparation of the affected leg with antiseptic solution prior to draping of the patient will allow for rapid transition into retrograde approach and improve procedural efficiency. Ultrasound

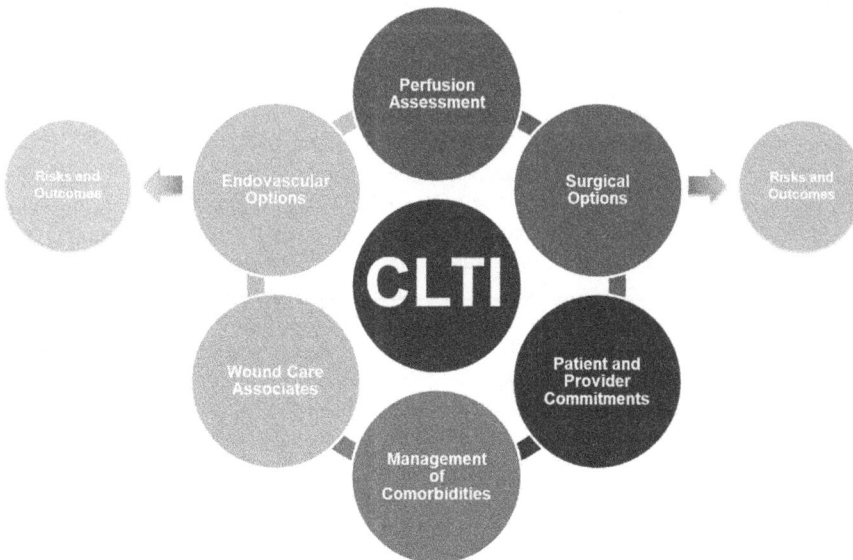

Fig. 3. A network of care providers necessary to help traverse care management for patients with CLTI. An integral aspect to ensure success in management is patient engagement and involvement to ensure adherence with follow-up and medical optimization. CLTI, chronic limb-threatening ischemia.

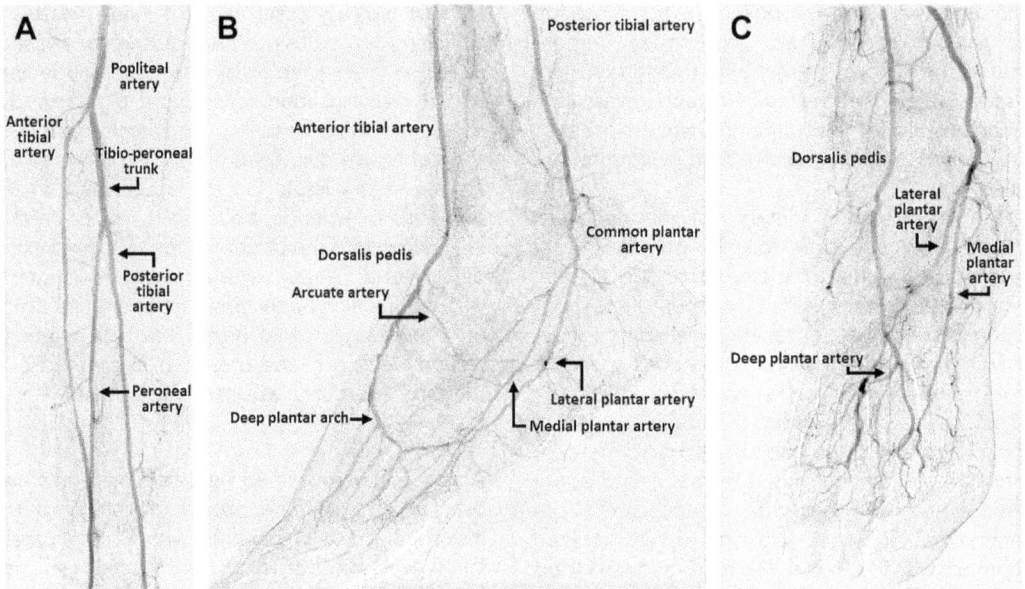

Fig. 4. (A–C) Angiographic appearance of a normal variant of pedal flow. (*Adapted from* Li J, Varcoe R, Manzi M, et al. Below-the-Knee Endovascular Revascularization: A Position Statement. JACC Cardiovasc Interv 2024;17(5):589-607. https://doi.org/10.1016/j.jcin.2023.11.040. Epub 2024 Jan 17. PMID: 38244007.)

guidance is feasible for the majority of alternative access points, although distal peroneal and proximal anterior tibial (AT) artery may be difficult to visualize depending on body habitus. Typically, retrograde access points are utilized for crossing only and do not warrant sheath placement. Hemostasis can be achieved easily with manual compression with or without balloon tamponade for sheathless access. In certain patients requiring additional maneuvers to rendezvous the antegrade and retrograde systems, double or parallel balloon may be needed; in these situations, a short (7 cm) 4 French sheath may be utilized to help with winged balloon transition for removal from the body. For patients with sheath access retrograde, external compression with a blood pressure cuff whilst applying internal balloon tamponade can help secure hemostasis intraprocedurally. Patients with sheath access in the distal AT or distal posterior tibial artery could achieve hemostasis post procedurally using a TR band (Trans-Radial band, Terumo, Tokyo, Japan) with the rounded support plate removed. However, in CLTI patients, it is more desirable to ascertain hemostasis on the table and ensure adequate distal perfusion (especially if single runoff only) to the wound prior to leaving the angiography suite.

Wire selection will be dependent on lesion length, composition, and presence of an occlusion.[36] Generally, a hydrophilic wire with lower tip load is sufficient to traverse short segment occlusions. Those with moderate tip load can be utilized in more fibrotic lesions to penetrate difficult caps. Wires designed to cross heavily calcific or hard fibrotic caps have heavier, 30-g tips. Wires should be shaped in a fashion to optimize engagement into chronic total occlusion (CTO) cap, with 30° to 45° bend at 1 mm from the tip. Hydrophilic wires are designed to "knuckle" into a J tip to traverse through dissection planes easily. A combination of 0.014″ and 0.018″ wires is typically utilized in BTK CTO crossing, with microcatheters or over-the-wire balloons for support.

Treatment Options

Percutaneous transluminal angioplasty (PTA) remains the primary treatment modality for BTK disease, though midterm patency rates remain abysmal.[37] To date, atherectomy and lithotripsy trials have been heterogeneous in design, with only 2 randomized controlled trials.[38] Incongruent designs and results limit interpretation of atherectomy benefits over PTA. Antiproliferative therapy with paclitaxel-coated balloons have yielded mixed results as seen in the Lutonix BTK investigational device exemption (IDE) Study. Single-armed trials[39,40] to evaluate the use of sirolimus-coated balloons (SCB) BTK have been promising, though randomized controlled trials evaluating SCB to PTA (SELUTION4BTK [NCT05055297] and MAGICAL BTK [NCT06182397]) are ongoing. To date,

Flowchart (Fig. 5):

Occlusion → No / Yes

No → Antegrade → Light-bodied, hydrophilic wire → • Pilot 200 • Command ES • Gladius • Regalia

Yes → Occlusion length → Short / Long

Short → Antegrade → Intimal tracking → Limited subintimal dissection and re-entry → Intermediate-bodied, hydrophilic wire → • Command ES/ST • Gladius • V18 • Gaia PV • Glidewire Gold

Long → Heavy calcium → Yes / No

Heavy calcium Yes → Antegrade dissection and re-entry → Hydrophilic wire for crossing → • Glidewire Gold • Command ES/ST • Gladius • V18 → ± CTO wire for re-entry → • Connect 250T • Astato 30 • Astato XS 40 • Winn 200T • Approach CTO • Confianza Pro 12

Heavy calcium No → Antegrade intimal tracking → Intermediate- to heavy-bodied wire → • Pilot 200 • Gaia PV • Treasure 12 • Winn 200T • Approach CTO • Connect 250T

No → Limited subintimal dissection and re-entry → Intermediate-bodied, hydrophilic wire → • Command ES/ST • Gladius • V18 • Glidewire Gold • Gaia PV

Failed antegrade → Retrograde → Intermediate-bodied, hydrophilic wire* → • Glidewire Gold • Command ES/ST • V18

Retrograde → Successful rendezvous → Yes / No

Yes → Externalize wire → Consider wire exchange over long microcatheter → Intervention and hemostasis

No → Interrogate different subintimal planes → Reverse CART / CART / Double balloon

Pedal artery treatment† → Yes / No

Yes → Soft-tipped, hydrophilic wire → • Regalia • Fielder XT • Pilot 200

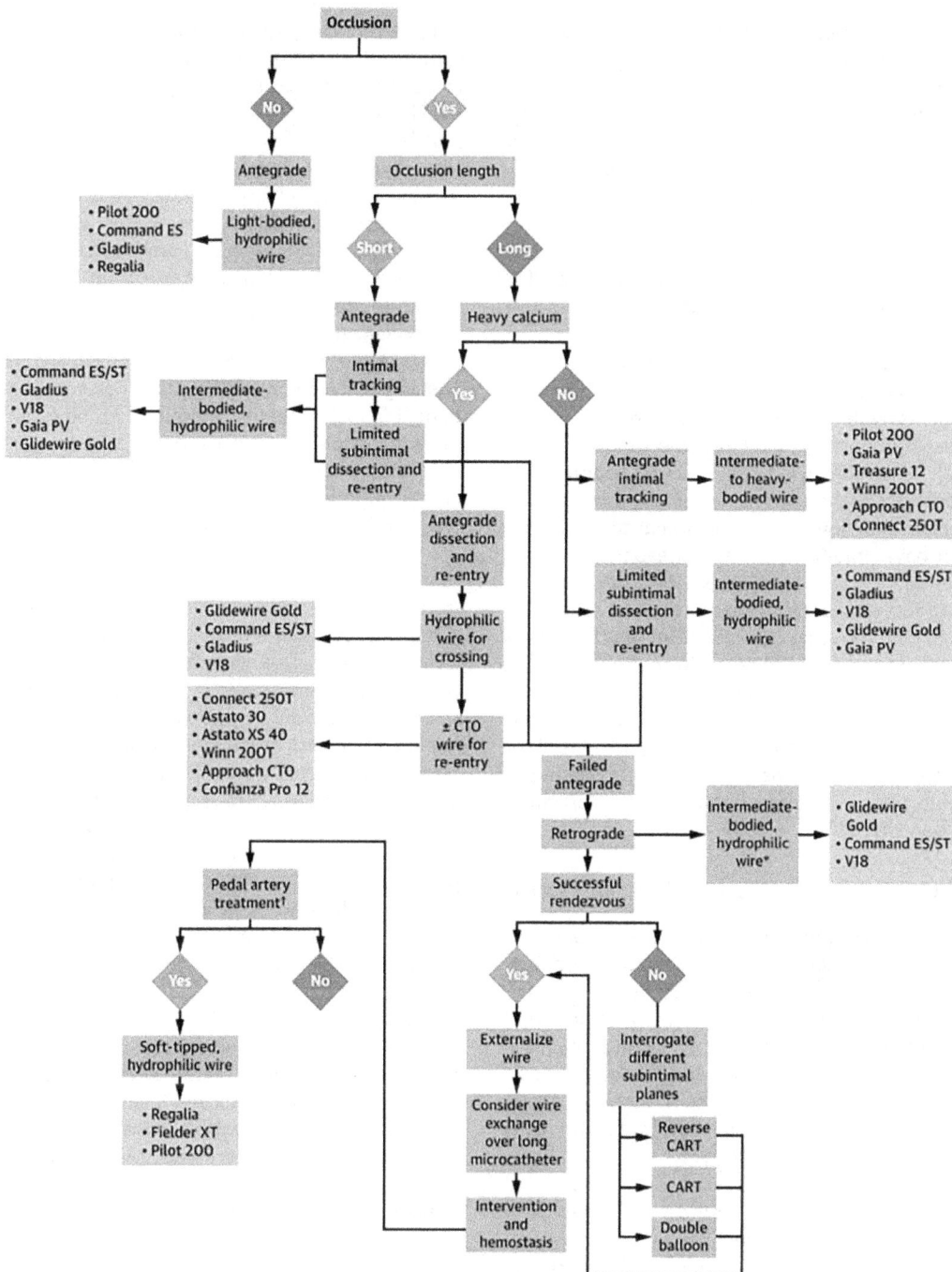

Fig. 5. A proposed algorithm for approach and wire escalation technique for below-the-knee interventions. *Wire escalation may be necessary based on lesion characteristics. †Decision to treat pedal artery depends on patency of loop and targeted angiosome. CART, controlled antegrade and retrograde tracking; CTO, chronic total occlusion. (*Adapted from* Li J, Varcoe R, Manzi M, et al. Below-the-Knee Endovascular Revascularization: A Position Statement. JACC Cardiovasc Interv 2024;17(5):589-607. https://doi.org/10.1016/j.jcin.2023.11.040. Epub 2024 Jan 17. PMID: 38244007.)

drug-coated balloons have not been approved for use in BTK lesions in the United States.

Inherent in the method of PTA is the creation of dissection planes to generate luminal gain. However, acute elastic recoil resulting in early lumen loss as well as flow-limiting dissection oftentimes warrant consideration of scaffold use. Drug-eluting stents have been shown to reduce target lesion revascularization and amputation compared to PTA and bare-metal stents,[41] though still at the cost of leaving a permanent implant. More recently, drug-eluting resorbable scaffold (DRS) has been shown to have improved outcomes compared to PTA, with outcomes being driven primarily by freedom from binary restenosis of target lesion and clinically driven target lesion revascularization at 1 year.[42] DRS is currently approved for use for BTK disease in patients with CLTI.

No-Option Chronic Limb-Threatening Ischemia Patients

Patients with "desert foot" or the lack of any meaningful arterial flow into the foot fall within the no-option CLTI (NOP-CLTI) population. Noninvasive therapies such as hyperbaric oxygen, arterial flow pump, and spinal cord stimulation have traditionally been the only therapies offered.[36,43] However, recent data have shown favorable amputation-free survival rates of 66% at 6 months using transcatheter arterialization of the deep veins (TADV) in these critically ill patients compared to amputation-free survival rates of 42% prior to emergence of TADV. TADV with the LimFlow device (Inari Medical, Irvine, California) is now approved for use in patients with no other suitable revascularization options for CLTI.[43]

GUIDELINE-DIRECTED MEDICAL THERAPY

While revascularization is the primary treatment for CLTI, medical therapy plays a crucial supportive role in preventing cardiovascular events, progression of limb-threatening ischemia and symptoms, and promoting wound healing. Optimal medical therapy in PAD has previously been introduced in this issue, though several important considerations specific to the CLTI population will be highlighted.

Antiplatelet and Antithrombotic Therapies

Following lower extremity revascularization, antiplatelet therapy has traditionally been recommended, although placebo-controlled trials are limited. Dual antiplatelet therapy (DAPT) is often employed after endovascular revascularization, a practice extrapolated from coronary intervention protocols and supported by observational studies suggesting potential benefits. For long-term management strategy, previous trials have suggested that P2Y12 inhibition with clopidogrel or ticagrelor monotherapy may be more effective than aspirin in prevention of secondary cardiovascular events.[44,45]

More recently, dual pathway inhibition (DPI) with low-dose antithrombotic therapy along with low-dose aspirin has been suggested to be effective in reducing major adverse cardiac events (MACE) and MALE compared to low-dose aspirin alone, with the latter primarily secondary to reduction in acute limb ischemia.[46,47] To date, no randomized controlled trial exists evaluating DAPT versus DPI in post revascularization for PAD or CLTI. Recommendations from the most recent multisocietal guidelines regarding post-revascularization antiplatelet and antithrombotic strategies are outlined in Fig. 6. Importantly, full-intensity oral anticoagulation alone has not shown benefit in PAD patients without other indications for anticoagulation and increases bleeding risk. This underscores the importance of tailoring antithrombotic strategies to individual patient characteristics and risk factors.[1]

Management of Comoribidities

Aggressive atherosclerotic risk factor modification is vital in patients with CLTI, independent of revascularization status, to minimize cardiovascular outcomes. Key components of GDMT include smoking cessation, high-dose statins, diabetes management, and anti-hypertensive medications. High-intensity statins are a class 1 indication with a goal of achieving >50% reduction in LDL levels.[1] Recent American College of Cardiology expert consensus guidelines recommend an even tighter goal of LDL goal of <55 mg/dL for patients with known stable atherosclerotic cardiovascular disease (ASCVD) at very high risk of future recurrent events.[48] High-risk conditions include age ≥65 years old, history of cardiac revascularization outside of the major ASCVD event, diabetes mellitus, hypertension, chronic kidney disease (CKD), congestive heart failure, heterozygous familial hypercholesterolemia, current smoking, and elevated LDL ≥100 mg/dL despite maximally tolerated statin and ezetimibe. Management of other comorbidities such as hypertension, diabetes mellitus, and smoking are addressed elsewhere in this issue.

Microvascular Circulation

Patients with concomitant CKD and long-standing diabetes mellitus are more likely to develop significant microvascular disease, resulting in poor outflow to territory of wound.[49] In the absence of TADV revascularization, vasodilatory medications to augment nitric oxide release,[50] coupled with additional noninvasive strategies outlined earlier for NOP-CLTI, may expedite wound healing. It is imperative for all CLTI patients, particularly those with poor

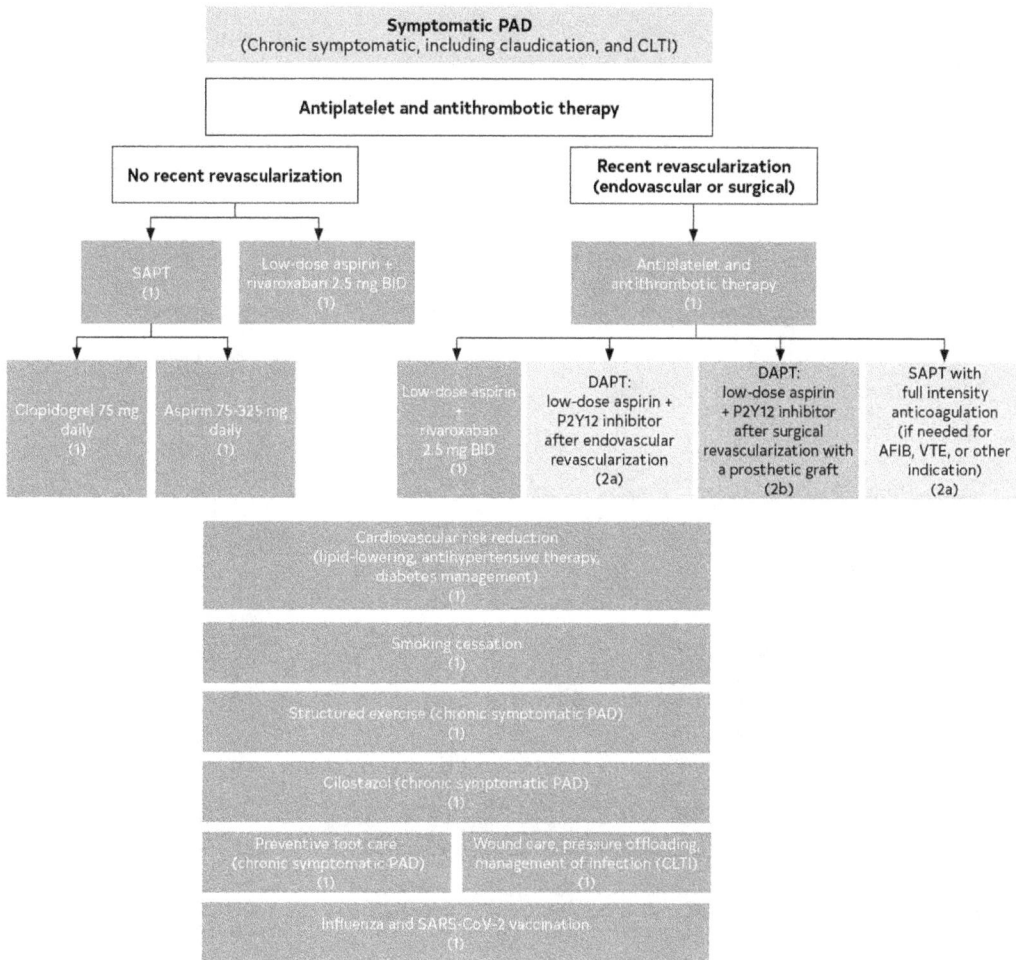

Fig. 6. Recommended medical therapy and foot care for patients with symptomatic PAD. AFIB, atrial fibrillation; BID, twice daily; CLTI, chronic limb-threatening ischemia; DAPT, dual antiplatelet therapy; PAD, peripheral artery disease; SAPT, single antiplatelet therapy; SARS-CoV-2, severe acute respiratory syndrome coronavirus 2; VTE, venous thromboembolism. (*Adapted from* Gornik HL, Aronow HD, Goodney PP, et al. 2024 ACC/AHA/AACVPR/APMA/ABC/SCAI/SVM/SVN/SVS/SIR/VESS Guideline for the Management of Lower Extremity Peripheral Artery Disease: A Report of the American College of Cardiology/American Heart Association Joint Committee on Clinical Practice Guidelines. Circulation 2024;149(24):e1313-e1410. https://doi.org/10.1161/CIR.0000000000001251. Epub 2024 May 14. PMID: 38743805.)

outflow, to have meticulous and consistent follow-ups in cardiovascular clinic, and optimal wound care management is crucial in preventing morbidity and mortality.

DISPARITIES IN VASCULAR CARE

All patients with PAD are at an elevated risk of MACE and MALE, but additional factors have been identified that further amplify this risk and lead to poorer outcomes.[51–53] Chronic comorbidities such as diabetes, hypertension, CKD (particularly end-stage renal disease), and ongoing smoking are well-known risk factors for development of PAD and association with

MACE and MALE. Furthermore, patients with microvascular diseases such as retinopathy, neuropathy, and nephropathy are at an increased risk of MALE among patients with PAD. Lastly, depression has been identified as a prevalent comorbidity among patients with PAD and leads to higher rates of MACE and MALE outcomes in this cohort of patients.

Although disparities in detection, management, and outcomes of PAD have long been evident in the United States, certain patient demographics and health disparities related to social determinants of health have also been associated with disproportionately greater risk of MACE and MALE among patients with

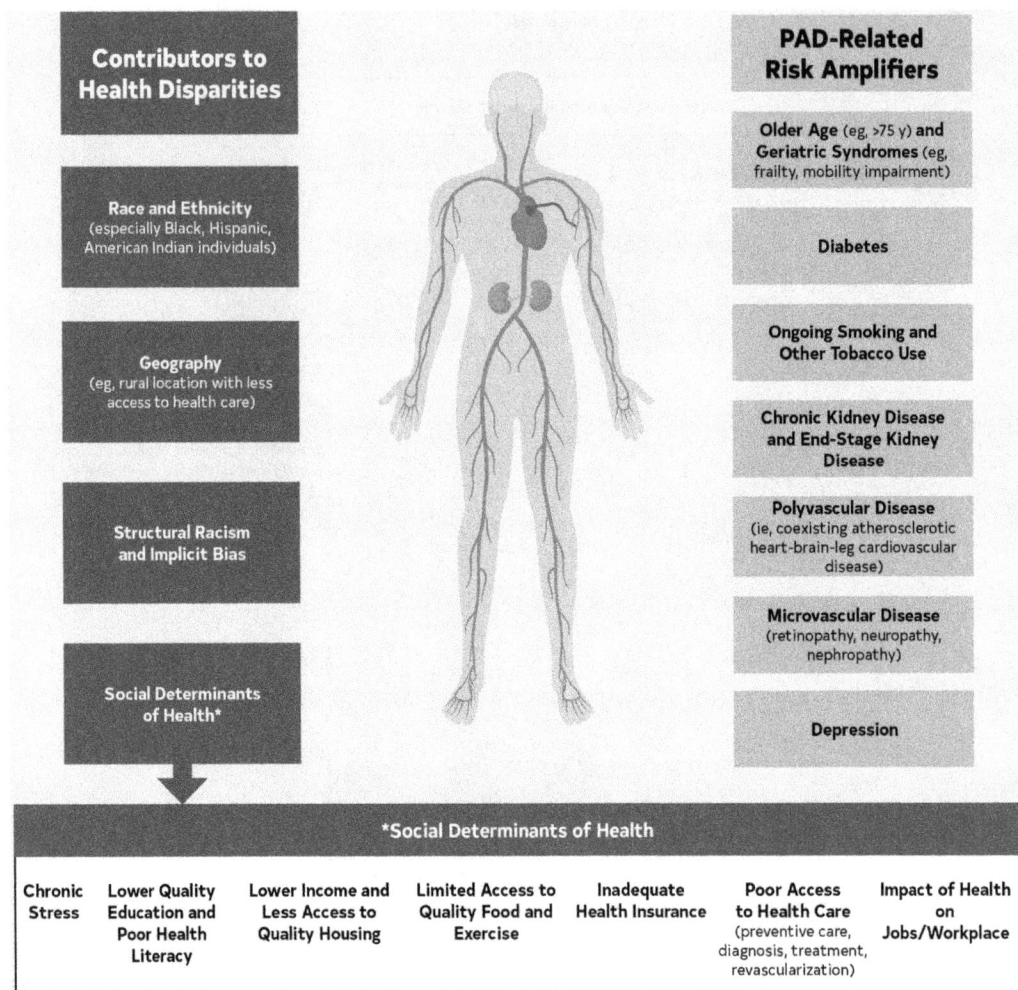

Fig. 7. The breadth of contributors to ongoing disparities in care delivery, along with traditional risk amplifiers of PAD. PAD, peripheral artery disease. (*Adapted from* Gornik HL, Aronow HD, Goodney PP, et al. 2024 ACC/AHA/AACVPR/APMA/ABC/SCAI/SVM/SVN/SVS/SIR/VESS Guideline for the Management of Lower Extremity Peripheral Artery Disease: A Report of the American College of Cardiology/American Heart Association Joint Committee on Clinical Practice Guidelines. Circulation 2024;149(24):e1313-e1410. https://doi.org/10.1161/CIR.0000000000001251. Epub 2024 May 14. PMID: 38743805.)

PAD.[51,52,54] These disparities cannot be fully accounted for by the presence of greater burden of risk-amplifying comorbidities alone (Fig. 7). Housing insecurity, access to health care, education attainment, income inequity, and generational wealth are only some of the social issues that limit equitable access to social and economic resources. Unfortunately, structural racism has perpetuated these inequities for generations. Disenfranchised communities are more likely to have lower wages, lower quality school system, poorer health literacy, and limited access to consistent primary and specialty care. In the United States, a combination of these factors leads to almost a 4-fold higher rate of major amputation, 30% higher rate of cardiovascular mortality, and 45% higher rate of stroke among Black Americans compared with non-Hispanic White Americans.[55]

Differences between sexes also exist. Studies have shown that women with PAD usually tend to present 10 to 20 years later than men, attributed to changes in sex hormones during menopause, and they tend to have more atypical symptoms and poor functional status when compared to men with PAD at similar ABI values.[56–58] Differences in management also exist, with women being at a greater risk of undergoing above-knee versus below-knee amputation and increased periprocedural mortality irrespective of the procedure performed.[56] Unfortunately, despite the prevalence of PAD in women with poorer limb outcomes, women continue to be underdiagnosed, undertreated, and underrepresented in clinical trials.

Racial, ethnic, and sex disparities remain on the forefront of the endovascular community's goal for improvement in care delivery. Multiple societal statements have been published proposing various strategies to address the contributing factors,[59,60] though these efforts remain nascent. Interventions are necessary at every level, including national policies and regulations, professional societies to help increase awareness and education, regional incentives to promote recruitment of providers to underserved areas, health care system-based patient screening and quality improvement, education of the communities at risk, and self-awareness of the provider to examine his or her own practice and commitment to improving equity of care.[60]

SUMMARY

CLTI is a severe and complex manifestation of PAD that demands a comprehensive approach to diagnosis, treatment, and follow-up care. Despite significant progress in revascularization techniques and medical therapies, ensuring timely and equitable care for all patients remains a challenge. Ongoing research and interdisciplinary collaboration are crucial to improving outcomes and reducing the burden of CLTI. By implementing comprehensive management strategies that incorporate appropriate diagnostic tools, advanced revascularization techniques, and adjunctive therapies, health care providers can more effectively address the needs of the patients with CLTI and enhance their quality of life. This multifaceted approach holds promise for better long-term outcomes in this challenging patient population.

CLINICS CARE POINTS

- Chronic Limb-Threatening Ischemia often represents the advanced stage of peripheral artery disease. Early recognition through history (non-healing wounds or rest pain >2 weeks) and diagnostic tools like ABI and TBI is crucial for optimizing outcomes.

- Hemodynamic assessments (ABI, TBI, TcPO2, or SPP) and concurrent anatomic assessments -using imaging modalities such as CTA, MRA, or DSA, should be made as soon as CLTI is suspected to provide a comprehensive evaluation.

- A multidisciplinary approach involving vascular specialists, wound care experts, endocrinologists, and others is critical in optimizing patient outcomes, focusing on both revascularization and wound healing.

- Revascularization is the cornerstone of CLTI management, reducing the risk of major amputation and mortality. An individualized approach (endovascular vs. surgical vs. hybrid strategy) is favored based on patient anatomy, comorbidities, and operator expertise.

- Comprehensive medical management, including antiplatelet therapy, lipid-lowering agents, and tight glycemic control, is essential in reducing the risks of major adverse cardiovascular events (MACE) and limb events (MALE).

- Recognizing socioeconomic and racial disparities in care is vital to ensuring equitable access to timely diagnosis and treatment for the vulnerable populations.

DISCLOSURES

Dr J. Li receives research funding from Abbott Vascular, United States and Inari Medical, United States. She is on the advisory board for Boston Scientific, Inari Medical, and Medtronic. The remainder of authors have no disclosures.

REFERENCES

1. Gornik HL, Aronow HD, Goodney PP, et al. 2024 ACC/AHA/AACVPR/APMA/ABC/SCAI/SVM/SVN/SVS/SIR/VESS guideline for the management of lower extremity peripheral artery disease: a Report of the American College of Cardiology/American heart association Joint committee on clinical practice guidelines. Circulation 2024;149(24):e1313–410.

2. Song P, Rudan D, Zhu Y, et al. Global, regional, and national prevalence and risk factors for peripheral artery disease in 2015: an updated systematic review and analysis. Lancet Glob Health 2019;7(8):e1020–30.

3. Eid MA, Mehta K, Barnes JA, et al. The global burden of peripheral artery disease. J Vasc Surg 2023;77(4):1119–11126.e1.

4. Norgren L, Hiatt WR, Dormandy JA, et al. Inter-society consensus for the management of peripheral arterial disease (TASC II). Eur J Vasc Endovasc Surg 2007;33(Suppl 1):S1–75.

5. Wübbeke LF, Kremers B, Daemen JHC, et al. Mortality in octogenarians with chronic limb threatening ischaemia after revascularisation or conservative

therapy alone. Eur J Vasc Endovasc Surg 2021;61(2):350–1.

6. Aboyans V, Ricco JB, Bartelink MEL, et al. 2017 ESC guidelines on the diagnosis and treatment of peripheral arterial diseases, in collaboration with the European society for vascular surgery (ESVS): document covering atherosclerotic disease of extracranial carotid and vertebral, mesenteric, renal, upper and lower extremity arteriesEndorsed by: the European stroke organization (ESO)the task force for the diagnosis and treatment of peripheral arterial diseases of the European society of Cardiology (ESC) and of the European society for vascular surgery (ESVS). Eur Heart J 2018;39(9):763–816.

7. Fontaine R, Kim M, Kieny R. [Surgical treatment of peripheral circulation disorders]. Helv Chir Acta 1954;21(5–6):499–533.

8. Rutherford RB, Baker JD, Ernst C, et al. Recommended standards for reports dealing with lower extremity ischemia: revised version. J Vasc Surg 1997;26(3):517–38.

9. Bollinger A, Breddin K, Hess H, et al. Semiquantitative assessment of lower limb atherosclerosis from routine angiographic images. Atherosclerosis 1981;38(3–4):339–46.

10. Taylor GI, Palmer JH. The vascular territories (angiosomes) of the body: experimental study and clinical applications. Br J Plast Surg 1987;40(2):113–41.

11. Shishehbor MH, White CJ, Gray BH, et al. Critical limb ischemia: an expert statement. J Am Coll Cardiol 2016;68(18):2002–15.

12. Bosanquet DC, Glasbey JC, Williams IM, et al. Systematic review and meta-analysis of direct versus indirect angiosomal revascularisation of infrapopliteal arteries. Eur J Vasc Endovasc Surg 2014;48(1):88–97.

13. Utsunomiya M, Takahara M, Iida O, et al. Wound blush obtainment is the most important angiographic endpoint for wound healing. JACC Cardiovasc Interv 2017;10(2):188–94.

14. Mills JL, Sr, Conte MS, Armstrong DG, et al. The society for vascular surgery lower extremity threatened limb classification system: risk stratification based on wound, ischemia, and foot infection (WIfI). J Vasc Surg 2014;59(1):220–34.e1-2.

15. Hardman RL, Jazaeri O, Yi J, et al. Overview of classification systems in peripheral artery disease. Semin Intervent Radiol 2014;31(4):378–88.

16. Darling JD, McCallum JC, Soden PA, et al. Predictive ability of the Society for Vascular Surgery Wound, Ischemia, and foot Infection (WIfI) classification system following infrapopliteal endovascular interventions for critical limb ischemia. J Vasc Surg 2016;64(3):616–22.

17. Jebari-Benslaiman S, Galicia-García U, Larrea-Sebal A, et al. Pathophysiology of atherosclerosis. Int J Mol Sci 2022;23(6).

18. Favero G, Paganelli C, Buffoli B, et al. Endothelium and its alterations in cardiovascular diseases: life style intervention. BioMed Res Int 2014;2014:801896.

19. Libby P. Inflammation in atherosclerosis. Nature 2002;420(6917):868–74.

20. Badimon L, Padró T, Vilahur G. Atherosclerosis, platelets and thrombosis in acute ischaemic heart disease. Eur Heart J Acute Cardiovasc Care 2012;1(1):60–74.

21. Shishehbor MH, Hammad TA, Zeller T, et al. An analysis of IN.PACT DEEP randomized trial on the limitations of the societal guidelines-recommended hemodynamic parameters to diagnose critical limb ischemia. J Vasc Surg 2016;63(5):1311–7.

22. Randhawa MS, Reed GW, Grafmiller K, et al. Prevalence of tibial artery and pedal arch patency by angiography in patients with critical limb ischemia and noncompressible ankle brachial index. Circ Cardiovasc Interv 2017;10(5):e004605.

23. Sukul D, Grey SF, Henke PK, et al. Heterogeneity of ankle-brachial indices in patients undergoing revascularization for critical limb ischemia. JACC Cardiovasc Interv 2017;10(22):2307–16.

24. Met R, Bipat S, Legemate DA, et al. Diagnostic performance of computed tomography angiography in peripheral arterial disease: a systematic review and meta-analysis. JAMA 2009;301(4):415–24.

25. Menke J, Larsen J. Meta-analysis: accuracy of contrast-enhanced magnetic resonance angiography for assessing steno-occlusions in peripheral arterial disease. Ann Intern Med 2010;153(5):325–34.

26. de Vries SO, Hunink MG, Polak JF. Summary receiver operating characteristic curves as a technique for meta-analysis of the diagnostic performance of duplex ultrasonography in peripheral arterial disease. Acad Radiol 1996;3(4):361–9.

27. Khalil MA, Kim HK, Hoi JW, et al. Detection of peripheral arterial disease within the foot using vascular optical tomographic imaging: a clinical pilot study. Eur J Vasc Endovasc Surg 2015;49(1):83–9.

28. Glaser JD, Bensley RP, Hurks R, et al. Fate of the contralateral limb after lower extremity amputation. J Vasc Surg 2013;58(6):1571–1577 e1.

29. Rowe VL, Lee W, Weaver FA, et al. Patterns of treatment for peripheral arterial disease in the United States: 1996-2005. J Vasc Surg 2009;49(4):910–7.

30. Adam DJ, Beard JD, Cleveland T, et al. Bypass versus angioplasty in severe ischaemia of the leg (BASIL): multicentre, randomised controlled trial. Lancet 2005;366(9501):1925–34.

31. Agarwal S, Sud K, Shishehbor MH. Nationwide trends of hospital admission and outcomes among critical limb ischemia patients: from 2003-2011. J Am Coll Cardiol 2016;67(16):1901–13.

32. Jaff MR, White CJ, Hiatt WR, et al. An update on methods for revascularization and expansion of

the TASC lesion classification to include below-the-knee arteries: a supplement to the inter-society consensus for the management of peripheral arterial disease (TASC II). Vasc Med 2015;20(5):465–78.

33. Bradbury AW, Moakes CA, Popplewell M, et al. A vein bypass first versus a best endovascular treatment first revascularisation strategy for patients with chronic limb threatening ischaemia who required an infra-popliteal, with or without an additional more proximal infra-inguinal revascularisation procedure to restore limb perfusion (BASIL-2): an open-label, randomised, multicentre, phase 3 trial. Lancet 2023;401(10390):1798–809.

34. Menard MT, Farber A. The BEST-CLI trial: a multidisciplinary effort to assess whether surgical or endovascular therapy is better for patients with critical limb ischemia. Semin Vasc Surg 2014;27(1):82–4.

35. Shishehbor MH, Hammad TA, Rhone TJ, et al. Impact of interdisciplinary system-wide limb salvage advisory council on lower extremity major amputation. Circ Cardiovasc Interv 2022;15(1):e011306.

36. Li J, Varcoe R, Manzi M, et al. Below-the-Knee endovascular revascularization: a position statement. JACC Cardiovasc Interv 2024;17(5):589–607.

37. Schmidt A, Ulrich M, Winkler B, et al. Angiographic patency and clinical outcome after balloon-angioplasty for extensive infrapopliteal arterial disease. Catheter Cardiovasc Interv 2010;76(7):1047–54.

38. Benfor B, Sinha K, Lumsden AB, et al. Scoping review of atherectomy and intravascular lithotripsy with or without balloon angioplasty in below-the-knee lesions. J Vasc Surg Cases Innov Tech 2023;9(2):101185.

39. Choke E, Tang TY, Peh E, et al. MagicTouch PTA sirolimus coated balloon for femoropopliteal and below the knee disease: results from XTOSI pilot study up to 12 months. J Endovasc Ther 2022;29(5):780–9.

40. Tang TY, Yap CJQ, Soon SXY, et al. 12-Months results from the PRESTIGE study using sirolimus drug-eluting balloons in the treatment of complex BTK tibial atherosclerotic lesions in CLTI patients. Cardiovasc Revasc Med 2022;43:143–6.

41. Fusaro M, Cassese S, Ndrepepa G, et al. Drug-eluting stents for revascularization of infrapopliteal arteries: updated meta-analysis of randomized trials. JACC Cardiovasc Interv 2013;6(12):1284–93.

42. Varcoe RL, DeRubertis BG, Kolluri R, et al. Drug-eluting resorbable scaffold versus angioplasty for infrapopliteal artery disease. N Engl J Med 2024;390(1):9–19.

43. Shishehbor MH, Powell RJ, Montero-Baker MF, et al. Transcatheter arterialization of deep veins in chronic limb-threatening ischemia. N Engl J Med 2023;388(13):1171–80.

44. Committee CS. A randomised, blinded, trial of clopidogrel versus aspirin in patients at risk of ischaemic events (CAPRIE). CAPRIE Steering Committee. Lancet 1996;348(9038):1329–39.

45. Berger JS, Abramson BL, Lopes RD, et al. Ticagrelor versus clopidogrel in patients with symptomatic peripheral artery disease and prior coronary artery disease: insights from the EUCLID trial. Vasc Med 2018;23(6):523–30.

46. Eikelboom JW, Connolly SJ, Bosch J, et al. Rivaroxaban with or without aspirin in stable cardiovascular disease. N Engl J Med 2017;377(14):1319–30.

47. Bonaca MP, Bauersachs RM, Anand SS, et al. Rivaroxaban in peripheral artery disease after revascularization. N Engl J Med 2020;382(21):1994–2004.

48. Lloyd-Jones DM, Morris PB, Ballantyne CM, et al. 2022 ACC expert consensus decision pathway on the role of nonstatin therapies for LDL-cholesterol lowering in the management of atherosclerotic cardiovascular disease risk: a Report of the American College of Cardiology solution set oversight committee. J Am Coll Cardiol 2022;80(14):1366–418.

49. Ferraresi R, Mauri G, Losurdo F, et al. BAD transmission and SAD distribution: a new scenario for critical limb ischemia. J Cardiovasc Surg 2018;59(5):655–64.

50. Ahmed R, Augustine R, Chaudhry M, et al. Nitric oxide-releasing biomaterials for promoting wound healing in impaired diabetic wounds: state of the art and recent trends. Biomed Pharmacother 2022;149:112707.

51. Arya S, Binney Z, Khakharia A, et al. Race and socioeconomic status independently affect risk of major amputation in peripheral artery disease. J Am Heart Assoc 2018;7(2):e007425.

52. Mustapha JA, Fisher BT Sr, Rizzo JA, et al. Explaining racial disparities in amputation rates for the treatment of peripheral artery disease (PAD) using decomposition methods. J Racial Ethn Health Disparities 2017;4(5):784–95.

53. Carnethon MR, Pu J, Howard G, et al. Cardiovascular health in african Americans: a scientific statement from the American heart association. Circulation 2017;136(21):e393–423.

54. Minc SD, Hendricks B, Misra R, et al. Geographic variation in amputation rates among patients with diabetes and/or peripheral arterial disease in the rural state of West Virginia identifies areas for improved care. J Vasc Surg 2020;71(5):1708–17017 e5.

55. Creager MA, Matsushita K, Arya S, et al. Reducing nontraumatic lower-extremity amputations by 20% by 2030: time to get to our feet: a policy statement from the American heart association. Circulation 2021;143(17):e875–91.

56. Hirsch AT, Allison MA, Gomes AS, et al. A call to action: women and peripheral artery disease: a

scientific statement from the American Heart Association. Circulation 2012;125(11):1449–72.

57. McDermott MM, Greenland P, Liu K, et al. Sex differences in peripheral arterial disease: leg symptoms and physical functioning. J Am Geriatr Soc 2003; 51(2):222–8.

58. Pabon M, Cheng S, Altin SE, et al. Sex differences in peripheral artery disease. Circ Res 2022;130(4):496–511.

59. Allison MA, Armstrong DG, Goodney PP, et al. Health disparities in peripheral artery disease: a scientific statement from the American heart association. Circulation 2023;148(3):286–96.

60. Grines CL, Klein AJ, Bauser-Heaton H, et al. Racial and ethnic disparities in coronary, vascular, structural, and congenital heart disease. Catheter Cardiovasc Interv 2021;98(2):277–94.

Acute Limb Ischemia Interventions

Asmaa Ahmed, MD[a], Nauman Naeem, MD[a], Aakriti Jain, MD[a], Sahej Arora, MD[a], Islam Y. Elgendy, MD, FACC, FAHA, FSCAI, FSVM, FESC[b],*

KEYWORDS

- Acute limb ischemia • Catheter-directed thrombolysis • Endovascular
- Surgical revascularization

KEY POINTS

- Incidence of acute limb ischemia (ALI) has been stable worldwide ~ 1 to 1.5 cases per 10,000 annually, with higher rates in the lower limbs than the upper limbs.
- Patients typically present with sudden-onset pain, pallor, pulse deficit, paralysis, paresthesia, and poikilothermia.
- Diagnosis is mainly based on clinical evaluation and can be supported by imaging when needed; however, imaging should not delay treatment in cases of suspected ALI.
- Treatment options include anticoagulation, catheter-directed thrombolysis, mechanical thrombectomy, and surgical revascularization. The Rutherford Classification helps guide therapeutic interventions.
- Timely diagnosis and intervention can significantly impact limb salvage rates, with delayed or inadequate treatment often leading to irreversible damage and amputation.

BACKGROUND

Acute limb ischemia (ALI) is defined as a sudden reduction in limb perfusion threatening the viability of the limb, requiring urgent evaluation and management.[1] ALI is a treatable, but potentially devastating form of peripheral arterial disease. Different etiologies are implicated in ALI including arterial embolism, arterial thrombosis due to plaque progression or rupture, graft thrombosis, arterial trauma, aortic dissection, or iatrogenic complications related to endovascular procedures.[1,2] Almost half of the cases are attributed to a cardioembolic source such as atrial fibrillation, prosthetic heart valves not receiving appropriate anticoagulation, left ventricular thrombus, or paradoxical embolism.[3] The most common site of embolism is usually the femoral artery bifurcation (~35%–50% of the cases).[1,4,5] Acute thrombosis is most likely to occur at the site of an atherosclerotic plaque but may also occur in arterial aneurysms (especially the popliteal artery).[1] In autogenous vein bypass graft, thrombosis tends to occur at the site of anastomoses, the site of retained valves, and kinks.[1] While in prosthetic bypass grafts, thrombosis can occur anywhere in the graft (Fig. 1).[1]

EPIDEMIOLOGY

The incidence of ALI is estimated to be 1 to 1.5 cases per 10,000 individuals annually. Most patients are older (>75 years), with no sex predilection.[1,6] The incidence of acute lower limb ischemia is comparatively higher than upper limb ischemia, with 9 to 16 cases versus 1 to 3 cases per 100,000 individuals. Patients with

[a] Department of Internal Medicine, Rochester General Hospital, 1425 Portland Avenue, Rochester, NY 14621, USA; [b] Division of Cardiovascular Medicine, Gill Heart and Vascular Institute, University of Kentucky, 900 South Limestone Street, Suite CTW 320, Lexington, KY 40536, USA
* Corresponding author.
E-mail address: iyelgendy@gmail.com
Twitter: @islamelgendy83 (I.Y.E.)

Intervent Cardiol Clin 14 (2025) 273–282
https://doi.org/10.1016/j.iccl.2024.11.012
2211-7458/25/Published by Elsevier Inc.

Abbreviations	
ALI	acute limb ischemia
CDT	catheter-directed thrombolysis
CTA	computed tomography angiography
DUS	duplex ultrasound
MRA	magnetic resonance angiography
PMT	percutaneous mechanical thrombectomy

DIAGNOSIS

Clinical Presentation

The clinical features of ALI are described by the mnemonic "6 Ps"—pain, pallor, pulse deficit, paralysis, paresthesia, and poikilothermia.[11] Patients often present with new or worsening claudication, or sudden onset of severe limb pain which is out of proportion to the physical examination findings. Additionally, sensory or motor deficits may develop depending on the severity. The presence of edema may further worsen tissue perfusion due to compression of the arterial supply.[12] Patients with ALI usually present within 14 days of symptom onset and should be differentiated from those with chronic limb ischemia for whom symptoms develop over a longer duration.[1]

Differentiating thrombotic and embolic causes of ALI may be challenging but is crucial for selecting treatment strategies. The presence of atherosclerotic risk factors (smoking, diabetes, dyslipidemia, and hypertension), peripheral arterial disease, coronary artery disease, stroke, or history of claudication may indicate a thrombotic cause.[13] Pre-existing atherosclerosis leads to formation of collateral vessels in the affected limb and may mask overt symptoms of ischemia.[14] By contrast, embolic events present

acute lower limb ischemia tend to be slightly younger compared with those with upper limb ischemia.[7,8] In the United States, the incidence of ALI is 15 to 26 cases per 100,000 each year, with acute lower limb ischemia incidence about 20 times higher than in the upper extremity.[9] The incidence of ALI has remained nearly the same over the years and in different regions worldwide. For example, one national registry in the United Kingdom showed that the incidence of ALI was 14.3 per 100,000 individuals annually,[10] and another national registry in Sweden showed that the incidence rate was 12.2 per 100,000 individuals annually.[10]

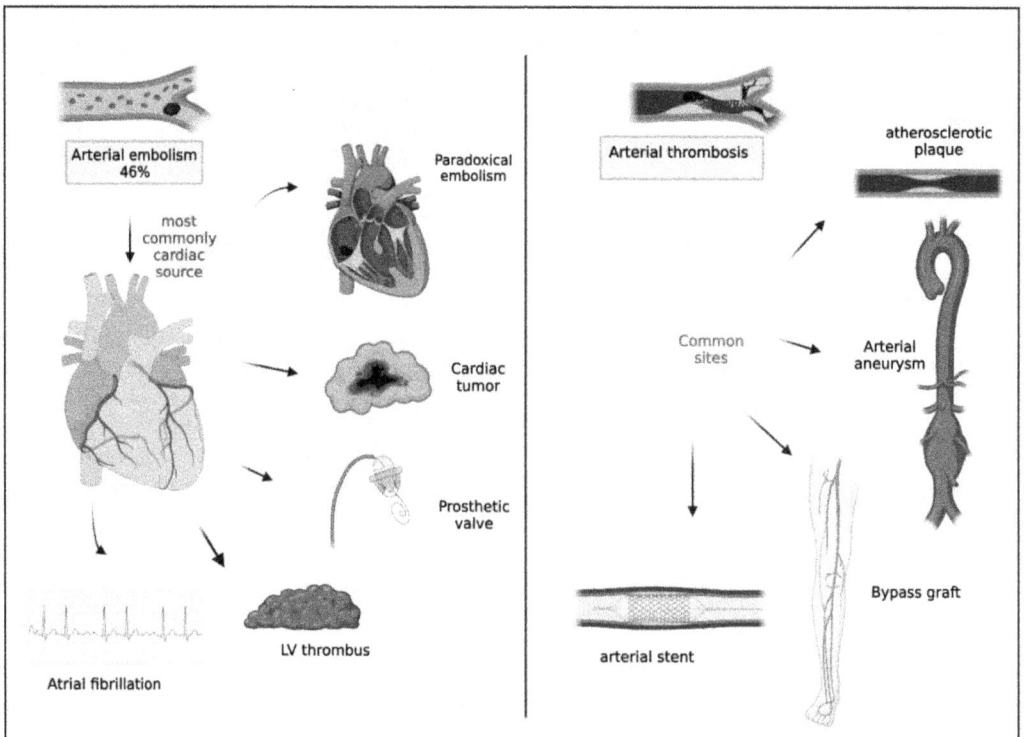

Fig. 1. Pathogenesis and etiologies of ALI.

more acutely with a clear onset of symptoms. The affected limb appears "marble" like and may subsequently appear mottled after reperfusion with deoxygenated blood.[15] Patients might have a known source of emboli, a history of embolic event, or arrhythmia, and often do not have a history of claudication.[16–18]

Assessment

The physical examination should include checking the pulses bilaterally which may indicate the site of occlusion or presence of arrhythmia. Capillary refill and assessment of pulses with hand-held continuous arterial and venous Doppler should be performed next.[4,13] The absence of a palpable pulse on one side suggests embolism, whereas bilaterally absent pulses indicates underlying atherosclerotic disease. A neurologic examination should also be performed at regular intervals to assess for motor or sensory deficits.[13] The severity of symptoms can range from mild discomfort to profound ischemia threatening limb viability, depending on the extent and location of vascular occlusion. Rutherford and colleagues classified ALI into viable and threatened categories based on the clinical findings and associated prognosis (Table 1).[19]

Imaging

The diagnosis of ALI is mainly clinical and requires a comprehensive approach integrating clinical evaluation and diagnostic imaging.[13] Urgent evaluation of patients with suspected ALI by experienced clinicians to assess limb viability and potential for limb salvage is recommended.

If the clinical findings are highly suggestive of ALI, imaging should be deferred and anticoagulation should be promptly initiated. Imaging should only be reserved for patients with a complicated history of revascularization procedures.[20,21] Imaging modalities confirm the diagnosis and delineate vascular anatomy, the extent of arterial occlusion, and tissue viability. These modalities include duplex ultrasound (DUS), computed tomography angiography (CTA), and magnetic resonance angiography (MRA). DUS is often the initial imaging modality of choice, offering real-time assessment of blood flow, detecting arterial occlusions, and evaluating collateral circulation. It is easily accessible and does not require contrast agents. However, it has lower sensitivity and specificity than CTA and MRA and is also limited by its inability to visualize iliac vessels, very distal arteries, collaterals, and has lower spatial resolution.[11] CTA and MRA provide detailed visualization of the arterial tree, allowing for precise localization of occlusions and assessment of collateral perfusion to aid intervention planning. The results from CTA and MRA are usually comparable. The use of individual modalities depends on availability, cost, and operator expertise.[2] Conventional catheter angiography is considered the "gold standard" for ALI diagnosis. Due to its invasive nature and associated risk of complications, it should not replace noninvasive imaging as the diagnostic modality and should only be performed if an intervention is planned.[2] These imaging modalities are very helpful in guiding treatment decisions to restore blood flow and prevent irreversible tissue damage. A

Table 1
Rutherford classification of stages of acute limb ischemia

| Stage | Description/Prognosis | Findings | | Doppler Signal | |
		Sensory Loss	Motor Weakness	Arterial	Venous
I Viable	Not immediately threatened	None	None	Audible	Audible
II Threatened					
a Marginally	Salvageable if promptly treated	Minimal (toes)	None	Often inaudible	Audible
b Immediately	Salvageable with immediate revascularization	More than toes, pain at rest	Mild or moderate	Inaudible	Audible
III Irreversible	Major tissue loss or permanent nerve damage inevitable	Profound, anesthetic	Paralysis (rigor)	Inaudible	Inaudible

stage III (irreversibly damaged) limb should not be considered for imaging or revascularization.[13]

MANAGEMENT

Patients with suspected ALI should be preferably managed at centers with full-time access to vascular services given the intricacies in diagnosis and management. With the possibility of amputation as well as other complications, interventional or surgical team involvement is necessary. ALI management is usually guided by Rutherford Classification. Patients with class 1/viable limb are usually managed with systemic anticoagulation, and further evaluation of the underlying etiology and severity through pertinent imaging.[1,9,22] Patients with class IIa also have time for noninvasive imaging but require more urgent revascularization while those in class IIb need an emergent revascularization procedure (either endovascular or surgical) as discussed further.[1,9,22] Patients with class III symptoms have irreversible ischemia and often require amputation[1,9,22] (Fig. 2).

Systemic Anticoagulation

Unfractionated heparin, unless contraindicated, should be initiated for any patients with suspected ALI (irrespective of the etiology), to prevent further clot propagation and preserve distal circulation.[23] Heparin is administered as a bolus of 70 to 100 IU/kg, followed by infusion at the rate of 12 to 18 units/kg/h monitored by activated clotting time or activated partial thromboplastin time. In patients with suspected or confirmed heparin-induced thrombocytopenia, bivalirudin or argatroban are available options.[20]

Catheter-Directed Thrombolysis

Catheter-directed thrombolysis (CDT) is a minimally invasive procedure in which a multisided hole catheter is percutaneously placed across the thrombus to deliver a localized infusion of a thrombolytic agent at low doses among patients who have no absolute contraindications to thrombolytic therapy (Box 1).[21] Infusion of thrombolytics is coupled with peripheral administration of intravenous (IV) heparin, aiming for an activated partial thromboplastin time of less than 60 seconds. Thrombolysis is typically administered over 24 to 48 hours while the patient is monitored in the intensive care unit. A relook angiography is subsequently performed, often followed by definitive revascularization procedures such as angioplasty or stenting. This technique is the preferred treatment for

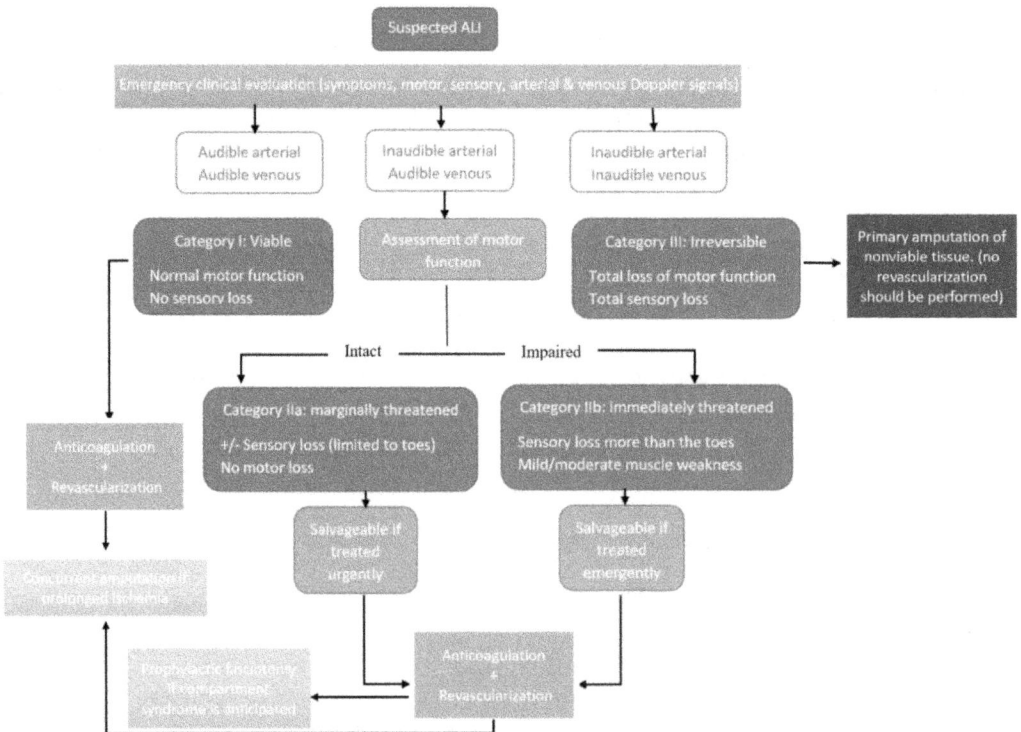

Fig. 2. Diagnosis and management of ALI.

Box 1
Contraindications to thrombolytic therapy

Absolute contraindications:

1. Established cerebrovascular event (including transient ischemic attacks) within last 2 months

2. Active bleeding diathesis

3. Recent gastrointestinal bleeding (<10 days)

4. Neurosurgery (intracranial, spinal) within the last 3 months

5. Intracranial trauma within the last 3 months

Relative major contraindications:

1. Cardiopulmonary resuscitation within the last 10 days

2. Major nonvascular surgery or trauma within the last 10 days

3. Uncontrolled hypertension: >180 mm Hg systolic or >110 mm Hg diastolic

4. Puncture of noncompressible vessel

5. Intracranial tumor

6. Recent eye surgery

Relative minor contraindications:

1. Hepatic failure, particularly those with coagulopathy

2. Bacterial endocarditis

3. Pregnancy

4. Diabetic hemorrhagic retinopathy

patients with class I and class IIA ALI who can tolerate a slow restoration of blood flow. Because of the relatively longer time required to restore tissue perfusion, CDT is typically not recommended for patients classified as Rutherford class IIb. Complete or partial thrombus resolution with a satisfactory clinical outcome is achieved in up to 75% to 92% of cases.[24–26] The adjunctive use of glycoprotein IIb/IIIa receptor antagonists may improve reperfusion and reduce distal embolization, but the addition of these agents does not improve overall outcomes.[27] Several trials have compared CDT with surgical revascularization and established the efficacy and safety of CDT for ALI (Table 2).[28–31]

The available devices for CDT include side holes along their length (eg, UniFuse, Angiodynamics; Cragg-McNamara, Ev3), designed to elute low-dose thrombolytics over several hours, and ultrasound-enhanced thrombolysis catheters (USAT) (eg, EKOS) which emit ultrasonic pulses during thrombolysis, which may improve

clot penetration and dissolution. Initial retrospective reports showed higher success and low complication rates with USAT over a short-term follow-up period.[32] The Duet randomized controlled trial compared the safety and efficacy of USAT compared with standard CDT in treating thromboembolic infra-inguinal arterial occlusions, and showed significantly reduced thrombolysis time in the USAT group but high bleeding events in both treatment groups.[33] Nevertheless, the applicability of these results is limited due to the small sample size, short-term follow-up period.[34] Future trials comparing both modalities are encouraged.

Percutaneous Mechanical Thrombectomy

The development of percutaneous mechanical thrombectomy (PMT) techniques for thrombus extraction was prompted by the limitations of CDT, including protracted infusion times and bleeding complications. PMT involves endovascular thrombus fragmentation and removal using specialized devices. It is primarily indicated for Rutherford class IIb due to the significantly shorter reperfusion time compared with in situ thrombolysis alone. Additionally, patients with contraindications to thrombolysis and those at higher surgical risk are potential candidates for PMT. PMT can be used to debulk the thrombus before using CDT in patients with a higher risk of bleeding, since it can shorten the treatment time and the dose of the thrombolytic agent used.[35] Mechanical thrombectomy can also be used as an adjunctive procedure for incomplete thrombolysis or to address distal embolic complications following in situ thrombolysis. PMT is most effective when the thrombus burden is low, the thrombotic material is relatively fresh, and the anatomic characteristics (such as vessel size and location) are favorable.[36,37]

Several devices have been developed to perform mechanical thrombectomy using suction, rotational infusion, ultrasound, or a high-velocity rheolytic jet. Pharmaco-mechanical thrombolysis combines thrombolytic therapy with mechanical thrombectomy for enhanced efficacy. The AngioJet Thrombectomy System (Boston Scientific, Marlborough, MA, USA) is commonly used in this setting. Thrombolytic agent is sprayed through the catheter into the thrombus and allowed to dwell. The liquefied thrombus is then removed by circumferentially oriented pressurized saline jets, which creates a Venturi effect at the catheter tip, resulting in the fragmentation and aspiration of the thrombus.[36,37] The Trellis Peripheral Infusion System features an over-the-wire device

Table 2
Summary of the clinical trials comparing catheter-directed thrombolysis to surgical revascularization

	Comerota et al,[28] 1996	Topas Study (1998)	Stile Trial (1994)	Ouriel et al,[31] 1994
Patient population	243 patients with occluded lower extremity bypass grafts. 70% of the patients were categorized within Rutherford class II	544 patients with ALI. Patients were categorized within Rutherford class II–III	393 patients with ALI. Patients were categorized within Rutherford class II–III	116 patients with acute ALI. All patients were categorized within Rutherford class II
Primary endpoints	Graft patency, limb salvage, 30-d mortality	Limb salvage at 6 mo, survival, amputation-free survival	Limb salvage, amputation-free survival, 1-y mortality	Limb salvage, 30-day mortality, reintervention rates
Treatment methodology	Thrombolysis with urokinase vs surgical thrombectomy	Urokinase infusion via catheter vs surgical revascularization	Thrombolysis with streptokinase or urokinase vs surgical revascularization	Intra-arterial thrombolysis (urokinase) vs surgical bypass or thrombectomy
Key findings	• Surgery showed better long-term patency (60% vs 30%). • Thrombolysis had more early reocclusions and interventions. • Limb salvage rates were similar.	• Urokinase was noninferior in early ischemia. • Surgery was more effective in severe occlusions. • Thrombolysis increased bleeding risk but reduced need for surgery.	• Thrombolysis achieved better limb salvage in early ischemia (75%). • Surgery was superior for advanced ischemia. • Thrombolysis had higher mortality due to bleeding.	• Thrombolysis was effective in early ischemia (~65% limb salvage). • Surgery had better long-term outcomes. • Thrombolysis was less effective in severe ischemia.
Reintervention and complications	• Thrombolysis had a higher reintervention rate (45% vs 21%). • Increased bleeding and embolization. • Surgery had fewer reinterventions but higher morbidity (infections).	• Urokinase had higher major bleeding (12.5% vs 6.9%). • Reocclusion was more common with urokinase (15% vs 10%). • Distal embolization required further procedures.	• Thrombolysis had a higher reintervention rate (26% vs 17%). • Bleeding was more frequent with thrombolysis (10% higher). • Surgery had fewer complications in the long-term.	• Thrombolysis had a higher reintervention rate (32% vs 18%). • Increased embolization and bleeding complications. • Surgery had a lower reintervention rate but risked wound infections and cardiac events.

equipped with 2 inflatable balloons designed to isolate the treatment area when inflated. Within this isolated segment, thrombolytic drugs can be administered, and an oscillation wire can be activated to mechanically break down and liquefy the thrombus. Once the distal balloon is deflated, the liquefied thrombus can be aspirated through the sheath.[36,37]

Aspiration mechanical thrombectomy devices are another modality for thrombus removal. These catheters are navigated over a guidewire and employ different techniques for aspirating the thrombus, such as manual and handheld methods, along with continuous vacuum suction used in devices like the Indigo, which uses vacuum suction to mechanically extract clots. Two single-center retrospective studies utilizing the Indigo aspiration catheter in ALI reported technical success rates of 51% to 53.3%.[36,37] These studies suggested that the catheter can obviate the necessity for CDT or open surgery.[36,37] The Clearlumen-II system is another thrombectomy device that performs both thrombus aspiration and pulse spray thrombolysis simultaneously, utilizing a high-pressure jet of saline solution.[38] Clinical studies supporting the use of PMT are mostly observational analyses of small sample sizes. Randomized clinical trials evaluating the efficacy and safety of these devices are lacking.[34,39]

Surgical Revascularization

Patients with an immediately threatened limb (Rutherford IIb), particularly those with contraindications to thrombolysis, might be candidates for open surgical revascularization. This approach is also preferred for patients with ischemic symptoms lasting more than 2 weeks.[40] Surgical approaches for treating ALI include thrombo-embolectomy using a balloon catheter (Fogarty), bypass surgery, and adjunct procedures such as endarterectomy, patch angioplasty, and intraoperative thrombolysis. The cause of ischemia (embolic vs thrombotic) and anatomic features guide the surgical strategy, and frequently, a combination approach is required. Patients with a suspected embolism and a lack of a femoral pulse ipsilateral to the ischemic limb should be treated by exposing the common femoral artery bifurcation and performing a balloon-catheter thrombo-embolectomy. A recent refinement for thrombo-embolectomy is the use of over-the-wire catheters, allowing for selective guidance into distal vessels. After clot removal, intraoperative angiography is performed to ensure that the thrombectomy is complete and to guide further treatment if there are any persistent inflow or

outflow obstructions.[41,42] ALI secondary to thrombosis of a popliteal artery aneurysm warrants special mention because major amputation occurs with high frequency in these patients.[41,42] Diffuse thromboembolic occlusion of all major runoff arteries below the knee is frequently observed. Intra-arterial thrombolysis or thrombectomy may be necessary to restore flow in a runoff artery before performing aneurysm exclusion and surgical bypass.[36,37,41,42] Compartment syndrome is a possible complication after percutaneous or surgical revascularization procedure for ALI necessitating therapeutic fasciotomy to prevent irreversible muscle loss. Prophylactic fasciotomy could be considered after the revascularization if compartment syndrome is anticipated.[43]

LONG-TERM PREVENTION

Most patients with ALI will likely require long-term systemic anticoagulation. Oral anticoagulation is an established therapy for patients with ALI of thromboembolic origin to reduce recurrent ischemic events and amputation rates.[44,45] Patients with ALI due to cardioembolic phenomenon benefit from direct oral anticoagulants.[13,46,47] Additionally, the COMPASS and VOYAGER PAD trials showed that in patients with peripheral arterial disease, low-dose rivaroxaban plus aspirin reduced major adverse limb events compated with aspirin alone.[48,49,50] While oral anticoagulants have been proven superior in a few specific situations as earlier, the utility of oral anticoagulation to improve patency after lower limb autogenous vein or prosthetic bypass has not been determined.[51–53]

Other secondary preventative measures for ALI include aggressive atherosclerotic risk factor modification measures such as: smoking cessation, physical activity, weight reduction, diabetes, and hypertension control.[54–61]

SUMMARY

ALI is a potentially life-threatening condition requiring rapid diagnosis and immediate management. The clinical presentation and diagnostic tools help determine the severity of ischemia and guide therapeutic options. The Rutherford Classification is a clinical framework for stratifying patients and directing appropriate interventions, whether via thrombolysis, thrombectomy, or surgery. Despite advancements in diagnostic imaging and therapeutic modalities, timely intervention remains the key determinant of patient outcomes. Early anticoagulation and appropriate use of revascularization techniques can prevent irreversible damage, reduce the need for amputation, and improve overall survival.

FUNDING

None.

CLINICS CARE POINTS

- Acute limb ischemia is a potentially-life threatening condition and requires prompt diagnosis and intervention.
- Early initiation of systemic anticoagulation and timely revascularization techniques (percutaneous or surgical) can reduce the risk of amputation and improve survival.

ACKNOWLEDGMENTS

The authors are grateful for the contributions of our authors, Dr Mohamed Salah Mohamed, MD and Dr Montaser Elkholy, MD, without whom this work would not have been possible. Mohamed Salah Mohamed, MD, Department of Cardiovascular Medicine, Alleghany Health, Pittsburgh, PA; Montaser Elkholy, MD, Department of Internal Medicine, Detroit Medical Center, MI.

DISCLOSURE

The authors have nothing to disclose.

REFERENCES

1. Creager MA, Kaufman JA, Conte MS. Clinical practice. Acute limb ischemia. N Engl J Med 2012;366(23):2198–206.
2. Olinic DM, Stanek A, Tătaru DA, et al. Acute limb ischemia: an update on diagnosis and management. J Clin Med 2019;8(8).
3. Obara H, Matsubara K, Kitagawa Y. Acute limb ischemia. Ann Vasc Dis 2018;11(4):443–8.
4. Rutherford RB, Baker JD, Ernst C, et al. Recommended standards for reports dealing with lower extremity ischemia: revised version. J Vasc Surg 1997;26(3):517–38.
5. Luís Foroni Casas A. Acute arterial embolism of the lower limb. London, UK: IntechOpen; 2020.
6. Howard DP, Banerjee A, Fairhead JF, et al. Population-based study of incidence, risk factors, outcome, and prognosis of ischemic peripheral arterial events: implications for prevention. Circulation 2015;132(19):1805–15.
7. Knowles M, Timaran CH. Epidemiology of acute critical limb ischemia. In: Dieter RS, et al, editors.

Critical limb ischemia: acute and chronic. Cham: Springer International Publishing; 2017. p. 1–7.
8. Stonebridge PA, Clason AE, Duncan AJ, et al. Acute ischaemia of the upper limb compared with acute lower limb ischaemia; a 5-year review. Br J Surg 1989;76(5):515–6.
9. Gilliland C, Shah J, Martin JG, et al. Acute limb ischemia. Tech Vasc Interv Radiol 2017;20(4):274–80.
10. Kulezic A, Acosta S. Epidemiology and prognostic factors in acute lower limb ischaemia: a population based study. Eur J Vasc Endovasc Surg 2022;63(2):296–303.
11. Collins R, Burch J, Cranny G, et al. Duplex ultrasonography, magnetic resonance angiography, and computed tomography angiography for diagnosis and assessment of symptomatic, lower limb peripheral arterial disease: systematic review. BMJ 2007;334(7606):1257.
12. Arató E, Kürthy M, Sínay L, et al. Pathology and diagnostic options of lower limb compartment syndrome. Clin Hemorheol Microcirc 2009;41(1):1–8.
13. Gerhard-Herman MD, Gornik HL, Barrett C, et al. 2016 AHA/ACC guideline on the management of patients with lower extremity peripheral artery disease: a report of the American college of cardiology/American heart association task force on clinical practice guidelines. Circulation 2017;135(12). CIR.000000000000.
14. Tang GL, Chang DS, Sarkar R, et al. The effect of gradual or acute arterial occlusion on skeletal muscle blood flow, arteriogenesis, and inflammation in rat hindlimb ischemia. J Vasc Surg 2005;41(2):312–20.
15. Callum K, Bradbury A. ABC of arterial and venous disease: acute limb ischaemia. BMJ 2000;320(7237):764–7.
16. Menke J, Lüthje L, Kastrup A, et al. Thromboembolism in atrial fibrillation. Am J Cardiol 2010;105(4):502–10.
17. Saric M, Kronzon I. Aortic atherosclerosis and embolic events. Curr Cardiol Rep 2012;14(3):342–9.
18. Simon F, Oberhuber A, Floros N, et al. Acute limb ischemia-much more than just a lack of oxygen. Int J Mol Sci 2018;19(2):374.
19. Suggested standards for reports dealing with lower extremity ischemia. Prepared by the Ad hoc Committee on reporting standards, Society for vascular surgery/North American chapter, international Society for cardiovascular surgery. J Vasc Surg 1986;4(1):80–94.
20. Linkins LA, Dans AL, Moores LK, et al. Treatment and prevention of heparin-induced thrombocytopenia: antithrombotic therapy and prevention of thrombosis, 9th ed: American college of chest physicians evidence-based clinical practice guidelines. Chest 2012;141(2 Suppl):e495S–530S.
21. Thrombolysis in the management of lower limb peripheral arterial occlusion–a consensus document.

Working Party on Thrombolysis in the Management of Limb Ischemia. Am J Cardiol 1998;81(2):207–18.

22. Lukasiewicz A. Treatment of acute lower limb ischaemia. Vasa 2016;45(3):213–21.

23. Blaisdell FW, Steele M, Allen RE. Management of acute lower extremity arterial ischemia due to embolism and thrombosis. Surgery 1978;84(6):822–34.

24. Ouriel K, Veith FJ. Acute lower limb ischemia: determinants of outcome. Surgery 1998;124(2):336–41 [discussion 341-2].

25. Earnshaw JJ, Whitman B, Foy C. National audit of thrombolysis for acute leg ischemia (NATALI): clinical factors associated with early outcome. J Vasc Surg 2004;39(5):1018–25.

26. Razavi MK, Lee DS, Hofmann LV. Catheter-directed thrombolytic therapy for limb ischemia: current status and controversies. J Vasc Interv Radiol 2004;15(1 Pt 1):13–23.

27. Drescher P, Crain MR, Rilling WS. Initial experience with the combination of reteplase and abciximab for thrombolytic therapy in peripheral arterial occlusive disease: a pilot study. J Vasc Interv Radiol 2002;13(1):37–43.

28. Comerota AJ, Weaver FA, Hosking JD, et al. Results of a prospective, randomized trial of surgery versus thrombolysis for occluded lower extremity bypass grafts. Am J Surg 1996;172(2):105–12.

29. Ouriel K, Veith FJ, Sasahara AA. A comparison of recombinant urokinase with vascular surgery as initial treatment for acute arterial occlusion of the legs. N Engl J Med 1998;338(16):1105–11.

30. Results of a prospective randomized trial evaluating surgery versus thrombolysis for ischemia of the lower extremity the STILE trial. Ann Surg 1994;220(3):251–68.

31. Ouriel K, Shortell CK, DeWeese JA, et al. A comparison of thrombolytic therapy with operative revascularization in the initial treatment of acute peripheral arterial ischemia. J Vasc Surg 1994;19(6):1021–30.

32. Schrijver A, Vos J, Hoksbergen AW, et al. Ultrasound-accelerated thrombolysis for lower extremity ischemia: multicenter experience and literature review. J Cardiovasc Surg (Torino) 2011;52(4):467–76.

33. Schrijver AM, van Leersum M, Fioole B, et al. Dutch randomized trial comparing standard catheter-directed thrombolysis and ultrasound-accelerated thrombolysis for arterial thromboembolic infrainguinal disease (DUET). J Endovasc Ther 2015;22(1):87–95.

34. Araujo ST, Moreno DH, Cacione DG. Percutaneous thrombectomy or ultrasound-accelerated thrombolysis for initial management of acute limb ischaemia. Cochrane Database Syst Rev 2022;1(1):Cd013486.

35. Patel NH, Krishnamurthy VN, Kim S, et al. Quality improvement guidelines for percutaneous management of acute lower-extremity ischemia. J Vasc Interv Radiol 2013;24(1):3–15.

36. Kwok CHR, Fleming S, Chan KKC, et al. Aspiration thrombectomy versus conventional catheter-directed thrombolysis as first-line treatment for noniatrogenic acute lower limb ischemia. J Vasc Interv Radiol 2018;29(5):607–13.

37. Lopez R, Yamashita TS, Neisen M, et al. Single-center experience with Indigo aspiration thrombectomy for acute lower limb ischemia. J Vasc Surg 2020;72(1):226–32.

38. Canyiğit M, Ateş ÖF, Sağlam MF, et al. Clearlumen-II thrombectomy system for treatment of acute lower limb ischemia with underlying chronic occlusive disease. Diagn Interv Radiol 2018;24(5):298–301.

39. de Athayde Soares R, Matielo MF, Brochado Neto FC, et al. Analysis of the safety and efficacy of the endovascular treatment for acute limb ischemia with percutaneous pharmacomechanical thrombectomy compared with catheter-directed thrombolysis. Ann Vasc Surg 2020;66:470–8.

40. Karnabatidis D, Spiliopoulos S, Tsetis D, et al. Quality improvement guidelines for percutaneous catheter-directed intra-arterial thrombolysis and mechanical thrombectomy for acute lower-limb ischemia. Cardiovasc Intervent Radiol 2011;34(6):1123–36.

41. Kropman RH, Schrijver AM, Kelder JC, et al. Clinical outcome of acute leg ischaemia due to thrombosed popliteal artery aneurysm: systematic review of 895 cases. Eur J Vasc Endovasc Surg 2010;39(4):452–7.

42. Robinson WP 3rd, Belkin M. Acute limb ischemia due to popliteal artery aneurysm: a continuing surgical challenge. Semin Vasc Surg 2009;22(1):17–24.

43. Karonen E, Wrede A, Acosta S. Risk factors for fasciotomy after revascularization for acute lower limb ischaemia. Front Surg 2021;8:662744.

44. De Haro J, Bleda S, Varela C, et al. Meta-analysis and adjusted indirect comparison of direct oral anticoagulants in prevention of acute limb ischemia in patients with atrial fibrillation. Curr Med Res Opin 2016;32(6):1167–73.

45. Campbell WB, Ridler BM, Szymanska TH. Two-year follow-up after acute thromboembolic limb ischaemia: the importance of anticoagulation. Eur J Vasc Endovasc Surg 2000;19(2):169–73.

46. Lee HF, Chan YH, Li PR, et al. Oral anticoagulants and antiplatelet agents in patients with atrial fibrillation and concomitant critical limb ischemia: a nationwide cohort study. Can J Cardiol 2021;37(1):113–21.

47. Ruff CT, Giugliano RP, Braunwald E, et al. Comparison of the efficacy and safety of new oral anticoagulants with warfarin in patients with atrial fibrillation: a meta-analysis of randomised trials. Lancet 2014;383(9921):955–62.

48. Rockhold M, Kunkel L, Lacoste JL, et al. Comparison of direct oral anticoagulants and warfarin in

chronic limb-threatening ischemia. J Vasc Surg 2024;79(6):1466–72.e1.

49. Anand SS, Bosch J, Eikelboom JW, et al. Rivaroxaban with or without aspirin in patients with stable peripheral or carotid artery disease: an international, randomised, double-blind, placebo-controlled trial. Lancet 2018;391(10117):219–29.

50. Bonaca MP, Bauersachs RM, Anand SS, et al. Rivaroxaban in peripheral artery disease after revascularization. N Engl J Med 2020;382(21):1994–2004.

51. Efficacy of oral anticoagulants compared with aspirin after infrainguinal bypass surgery (The Dutch Bypass Oral Anticoagulants or Aspirin Study): a randomised trial. Lancet 2000;355(9201):346–51.

52. Bedenis R, Lethaby A, Maxwell H, et al. Antiplatelet agents for preventing thrombosis after peripheral arterial bypass surgery. Cochrane Database Syst Rev 2015;2015(2):Cd000535.

53. Sarac TP, Huber TS, Back MR, et al. Warfarin improves the outcome of infrainguinal vein bypass grafting at high risk for failure. J Vasc Surg 1998;28(3):446–57.

54. Clark D, Cain LR, Blaha MJ, et al. Cigarette smoking and subclinical peripheral arterial disease in blacks of the jackson heart study. J Am Heart Assoc 2019;8(3):e010674.

55. Ding N, Sang Y, Chen J, et al. Cigarette smoking, smoking cessation, and long-term risk of 3 major atherosclerotic diseases. J Am Coll Cardiol 2019; 74(4):498–507.

56. Hicks CW, Yang C, Ndumele CE, et al. Associations of obesity with incident hospitalization related to peripheral artery disease and critical limb ischemia in the ARIC study. J Am Heart Assoc 2018;7(16): e008644.

57. Lu Y, Ballew SH, Kwak L, et al. Physical activity and subsequent risk of hospitalization with peripheral artery disease and critical limb ischemia in the ARIC study. J Am Heart Assoc 2019;8(21):e013534.

58. Treat-Jacobson D, McDermott MM, Bronas UG, et al. Optimal exercise programs for patients with peripheral artery disease: a scientific statement from the American heart association. Circulation 2019;139(4):e10–33.

59. Yusuf S, Yusuf S, Teo KK, et al. Telmisartan, ramipril, or both in patients at high risk for vascular events. N Engl J Med 2008;358(15):1547–59.

60. Verma S, Mazer CD, Al-Omran M, et al. Cardiovascular outcomes and safety of empagliflozin in patients with type 2 diabetes mellitus and peripheral artery disease: a subanalysis of EMPA-REG outcome. Circulation 2018;137(4):405–7.

61. Ference BA, Ginsberg HN, Graham I, et al. Low-density lipoproteins cause atherosclerotic cardiovascular disease. 1. Evidence from genetic, epidemiologic, and clinical studies. A consensus statement from the European Atherosclerosis Society Consensus Panel. Eur Heart J 2017;38(32):2459–72.

Chronic Venous Insufficiency and Management

Robert R. Attaran, MD, FSCAI[a],*, Golsa Babapour, MD[a],
Carlos Mena-Hurtado, MD, FSCAI, RPVI[a],
Cassius Iyad Ochoa Chaar, MD, MPH, MS, RPVI[b]

KEYWORDS

- Chronic venous insufficiency • Chronic venous disease • Varicose veins
- Saphenous vein ablation • May-thurner syndrome • Postthrombotic syndrome

KEY POINTS

- Chronic venous disease of the lower extremities can be due to venous reflux, obstruction, or a combination of both.
- Compression therapy is still a fundamental part of therapy for chronic venous disease, particularly for venous leg ulcers.
- Over the past decades significant advances have been made in minimally invasive therapies for venous reflux and obstruction.

INTRODUCTION

Chronic venous insufficiency of the lower extremities is common and can be associated with progressive leg discomfort, heaviness, edema, discoloration and ulceration.[1–5] Prevalence increases with age and can adversely impact quality of life.[6,7] Venous insufficiency and varicose veins are widespread throughout the globe and are common in Western countries.[7–9] More advanced manifestations of the disease, such as edema and ulcers are more common above the age of 65.[2] Venous leg ulcer prevalence can be as high as 2% of the population.[10,11]

Risk factors for chronic venous disease include age, female gender, positive family history, pregnancy and parity, obesity, prolonged standing and history of deep vein thrombosis (DVT).[9,12,13]

A retrospective analysis found a positive correlation between body mass index (BMI) and severity of chronic venous insufficiency (CVI) symptoms. This correlation appeared to be exclusive of venous reflux severity.[14] Obesity is associated with increased intra-abdominal pressure which, in turn, is associated with increased deep (femoral) vein pressure.[15–17]

Chronic venous disease is also the leading etiology of leg ulcers, which are typically found in the gaiter zone of the leg (particularly at the medial and lateral malleoli and pretibial regions).[18] Venous ulcers can secrete exudate, be painful, malodorous, and take months to heal.[7,19,20] Not surprisingly, they are associated with poor quality of life.[21]

In the United States, an estimated 2.2% of Medicare beneficiaries have venous leg ulcers with an annual cost of nearly $15 billion dollars.[22]

PATHOPHYSIOLOGY

Chronic venous insufficiency is associated with venous obstruction, reflux, or both, resulting in

[a] Section of Cardiovascular Medicine, Yale School of Medicine, 333 Cedar Street, New Haven, CT 06519, USA;
[b] Division of Vascular Surgery and Endovascular Therapy, Department of Surgery, Yale School of Medicine, 333 Cedar Street, New Haven, CT 06519, USA
* Corresponding author.
E-mail address: Robert.attaran@yale.edu

Intervent Cardiol Clin 14 (2025) 283–296
https://doi.org/10.1016/j.iccl.2024.11.013

Abbreviations	
CAC	cyanoacrylate adhesive closure
CEAP	Clinical, etiology, anatomy, pathology
DVT	deep vein thrombosis
EVLA	endovenous laser ablation
GSV	great saphenous vein
MOCA	mechanochemical ablation
MPFF	micronized purified flavonoid fraction
MTS	May-Thurner syndrome
PTS	postthrombotic syndrome
RFA	radiofrequency ablation
SSV	small saphenous vein
STS	sodium tetradecyl sulfate
VCSS	venous clinical severity score

ambulatory venous hypertension.[23] This can lead to inflammation.[24,25] Having thinner media than arteries, veins are more distensible and possess unidirectional valves to facilitate antegrade flow. The calf muscles act as pumps to assist in venous return during walking.[26,27] Elevated venous pressure can lead to venous wall remodeling and varicose veins.[28] Ambulatory venous hypertension is associated with skin damage and ulceration.[29,30]

Elastin and laminin are decreased in varicose veins, which may play a role in weakening the venous wall.[31–33] Vascular smooth muscles can lose their contractility.[34,35] Saphenous veins in humans with venous insufficiency and varicose veins demonstrate lower contractility.[36]

There is increased endothelial permeability resulting in red blood cell extravasation. One breakdown product of these red blood cells is ferric iron, which potentially leads to hemosiderin deposition and hyperpigmentation.[37,38]

Blood collected from varicose veins carries higher levels of inflammatory markers such as C-reactive protein and interleukin-6.[39,40]

SYMPTOM SCORES AND CLASSIFICATION SYSTEMS IN CHRONIC VENOUS DISEASE

The CEAP classification (clinical, etiology, anatomy, pathology) was developed in 1993 and most recently revised in 2020.[41] Though not designed to be used as a symptom score, the C (clinical) class, ranging from 1 to 6, is often used alone to describe the severity of disease

(Table 1). Ulceration (C6 disease) is the most advanced (Figs. 1 and 2). The E (etiology) class can be designated as primary, secondary, congenital or as no cause identified. The A (anatomy) class refers to site of pathology: deep, superficial, or perforator veins. The P (pathology) class includes reflux, obstruction, both or none.

The most commonly used grading for severity of symptoms is the Venous Clinical Severity Score (VCSS). It is a validated tool[42] to measure the severity of venous disease and the response to treatment.[43,44] The VCSS has been frequently used in venous intervention trials. A number of other venous quality of life or symptom severity scores exist such as EuroQol-5D (EQ-5D)[45] and VEINES-QoL.[46] The VVSym Q (HASTI) score incorporates 5 symptoms (Heavy, Aching, Swelling, Throbbing, Itching legs).

The score has been the most frequently used tool for diagnosing postthrombotic syndrome (PTS) and quantifying its severity.[47–49] It incorporates 5 patient reported symptoms and 6 physician-reported findings into a single total score (5–9: mild; 10–14: moderate; $\geq$15, or presence of venous ulcer: severe).

COMPRESSION THERAPY

Compression therapy is a fundamental tool in the treatment of chronic venous disease.[50,51] The increased lower limb venous pressure in

Table 1
The C classes from the clinical, etiology, anatomy, pathology classification system for chronic venous disease

C Class	Description
C_0	No visible or palpable signs of venous disease
C_1	Telangiectasias or reticular veins
C_2	Varicose veins
C_{2r}	Recurrent varicose veins
C_3	Edema
C_4	Changes in skin or subcutaneous tissue secondary to chronic venous disease
C_{4a}	Pigmentation or eczema
C_{4b}	Lipodermatosclerosis or atrophie blanche
C_{4c}	Corona phlebectatica
C_5	Healed
C_6	Active venous ulcer
C_{6r}	Recurrent active venous ulcer

Abbreviation: r, recurrent.

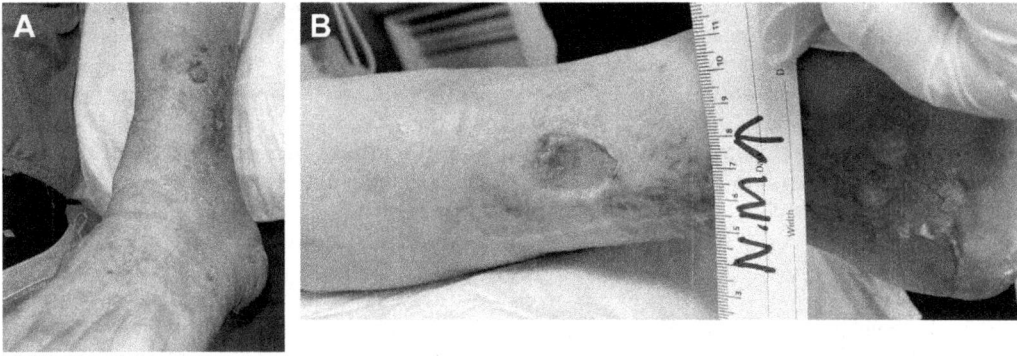

Fig. 1. (A, B) Venous ulcers, with periulcer inflammation.

CVI can drive fluid into the interstitial spaces.[52,53] Compression can reduce interstitial pooling and as a result decrease edema and inflammation.[54] Inflammatory cytokines levels within venous ulcers decrease with compression therapy.[55]

Grades of compression as measured at the ankle, can be divided into light (<20 mm Hg), class I (21–30 mm Hg), class II (31–40 mm Hg) and class III (>40 mm Hg), though other grading systems exist.[56]

Compression garments for the legs can take many forms such as stockings, bandages, velcro devices and pumps.[56–58]

In lower severity venous disease compression can decrease discomfort and edema.[59]

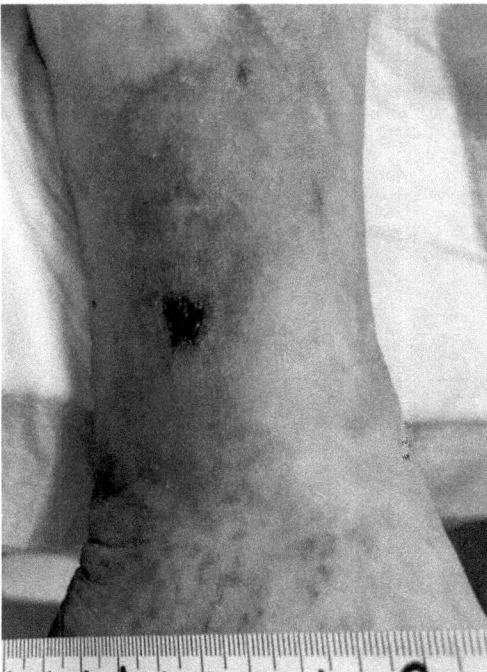

Fig. 2. Venous ulceration, inflammation, and corona phlebectatica.

Particularly when higher pressures (30–40 mm Hg+) are used, compression has been shown to improve venous ulcer healing and decrease ulcer recurrence.[56,58] Following vein ablation or sclerotherapy compression can lower postprocedural discomfort and edema.[60,61]

There is mixed data on the use of compression therapy in the prevention of PTS after acute lower limb DVT. A prospective control study did demonstrate lower rates of PTS at 24 months with 30-40 mm Hg knee-high compression stockings.[62] In the SOX trial no benefit was seen. As a differentiator between the 2 studies, in the SOX trial, participants were mailed the stockings 2 weeks following DVT and appeared to have lower compliance with compression.[63]

Chronic edema of the legs is a known risk factor for recurrent cellulitis and compression therapy has been shown in a prospective randomized control trial (RCT) to significantly reduce recurrent cellulitis.[64]

A frequent challenge with compression therapy is patient noncompliance due to discomfort and inability to apply (don) and remove (doff).[65,66] Joint disease, obesity, frailty, and lack of flexibility may all contribute. In an analysis of 58 clinical studies (median follow-up of 12 months), good compliance, defined as wearing compression greater than 50% of the time, was reported in only two-thirds of patients.[67] Compliance was lower with higher pressure (>25 mm Hg) stockings.

PHARMACOLOGIC THERAPY FOR CHRONIC VENOUS DISEASE

A number of pharmaceutical agents (venotonics) have been evaluated for the treatment of chronic venous disease symptoms. The list includes diosmin, hesperidin, rutosides, pine bark extract (pycnogenol), horse chestnut extract (escin), and micronized purified flavonoid fraction (MPFF).[68–70] These agents[71] may reduce some symptoms including edema and leg cramping. Their mechanisms of action are not entirely clear.[69,72] Rutosides may reduce capillary permeability.[73] Flavonoids may lower venous inflammation and enhance venous tone.[71] Pentoxifylline decreases blood viscosity and thrombus formation and may have efficacy as an adjunct in venous ulcer therapy.[74–78]

SUPERFICIAL VENOUS REFLUX

Superficial valvular incompetence has been frequently found in individuals with CVI and venous ulcers.[79] The great saphenous vein (GSV) is easily identifiable on duplex and can be evaluated (preferably whilst the patient stands), to demonstrate reflux (Fig. 3). Surgical techniques for treating varicose veins have existed in various forms for the past century. A common approach has historically been the flush ligation of the saphenofemoral junction accompanied by stripping of the (GSV).[80,81] Stab phlebectomy of varicose veins and tributaries can also be performed. The small saphenous vein (SSV) can be stripped in a similar manner. Complications include infection (<6%), DVT (<5%) and rarely saphenous or sural nerve injury.

Particularly in western countries, surgical stripping of the saphenous veins has largely been replaced by ultrasound-guided percutaneous ablation. Endovenous laser ablation (EVLA) and radiofrequency ablation (RFA) are 2 modes of thermal ablation. Both devices employ a low-profile intravenous catheter, directly delivering heat energy to the venous endothelium leading to injury and eventual fibrosis and occlusion of the vein. Before deploying the thermal ablation, tumescent anesthesia (typically a solution of lidocaine, epinephrine, bicarbonate and saline) is percutaneously injected around the target vein.

The EVLA devices currently in the US market include VenaCure (AngioDynamics, NY) and Vari-Lase (Teleflex, PA). The laser wavelength can target water or hemoglobin.[82] One year saphenous vein occlusion rates can exceed 90% with EVLA.[83]

The RFA devices currently available in the United States are ClosureFast (Medtronic, MN) and Venclose (Becton Dickinson, NJ). Five-year follow-up post-RFA reveal occlusion rates of 92%.[84] EVLA results in probably greater postprocedural pain compared to RFA.[85]

Both EVLA and RFA of the saphenous veins can be complicated by endothermal heat-induced thrombosis where thrombus may propagate into the deep system (<1% of cases).[86] The risk of pulmonary embolism is very low.[87]

Several nonthermal methods have also been introduced to ablate or seal the saphenous veins. These include cyanoacrylate adhesive closure (CAC), mechanochemical ablation (MOCA) and foam sclerotherapy. These nontumescent nonthermal techniques have several advantages. Without the need for injection of tumescent anesthesia they are often less painful.

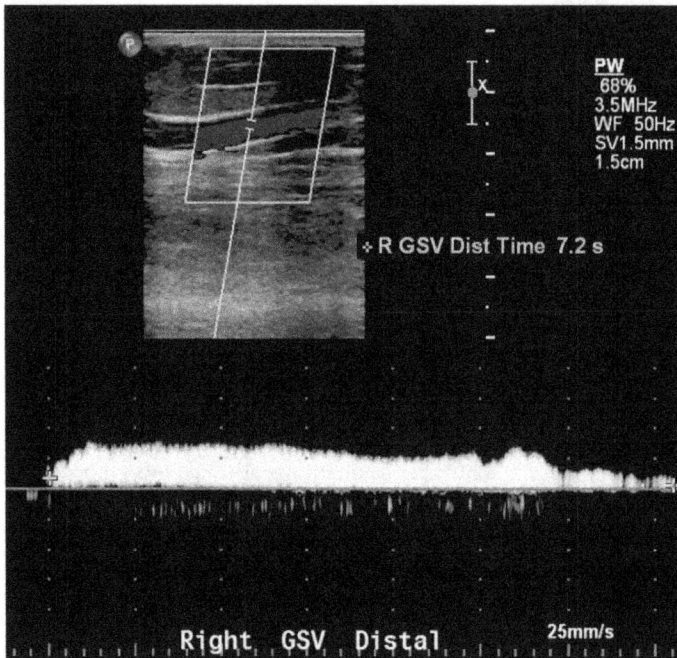

Fig. 3. Demonstration of great saphenous vein reflux using pulsed-wave Doppler.

They will not cause thermal injury to adjacent structures (eg nerves and skin).

The cyanoacrylate adhesive is delivered to the target vein through a catheter and rapidly polymerizes leading to closure and eventual fibrosis.

Sclerotherapy uses an agent that once injected into a target vein denatures surface proteins, resulting in eventual luminal fibrosis and obstruction.[88] Sclerosants have been used for elimination of telangiectasis, reticular, and varicose veins.[89] Sclerotherapy improves the cosmetic appearance of varicose veins and possibly quality of life.[90] In larger veins (eg, 3 mm or greater), the sclerosing agent can be injected as a foam to displace more blood, maintain sclerosant concentrations, and enhance sclerosant contact with the venous endothelium.[91–93] Both air and CO_2 have been used to generate the foam.

In the United States, sodium tetradecyl sulfate (STS) and polidocanol are approved for use as sclerotherapy agents. Both are detergents. Hyperpigmentation and telangiectatic matting can occur. Hyperpigmentation is probably more common with STS.

There is little evidence to suggest clinically significant right-to-left shunting of sclerosant.[94] There are rare reports of transient visual disturbance following sclerotherapy.[95] DVT or ulceration is also rare. Caution should be exercised with sclerosing agents because intra-arterial injection can lead to tissue necrosis.[96]

In the United States, a proprietary formulation of 1% polidocanol named Varithena (Boston Scientific, MA)[97] is available and is predominantly used for the treatment of saphenous vein reflux or large varicose tributaries. The efficacy of Varithena in the reduction of venous reflux symptoms was demonstrated in the Vanish-II trial.[98] Proximal DVT occurred in 2.6%.[99]

In the MOCA (ClariVein, Merit Medical, UT) procedure, the saphenous vein endothelium is scraped by a rotating metallic tip (3500 RPM) with simultaneous sclerosant injection and slow withdrawal of the rotating tip. This leads to eventual endothelial fibrosis and vein occlusion.[100] At 1-year follow-up, MOCA demonstrated 88% GSV occlusion and significant improvement in venous symptoms.[100] Complications include hematoma, phlebitis and rarely, DVT.[101] An RCT comparing MOCA to thermal ablation found lower GSV saphenous occlusion rates with MOCA but equivalent symptom score improvements at 1 year.[102]

VenaSeal CAC (Medtronic, MN) is the third nonthermal technology discussed here. Using ultrasound, a sheath is advanced into the saphenous vein, through which cyanoacrylate is delivered. In an RCT, at 5-year CAC demonstrated equivalent GSV occlusion rates and symptoms relief, compared to RFA.[103] In both arms of the study, approximately two-third of participants received adjunctive sclerotherapy at 6 months ($P = .77$).[104] A local hypersensitivity reaction has been seen in up to 23% of CAC cases, postprocedure[105,106] and some operators use corticosteroid and antihistamine therapy.

A Cochrane review of GSV reflux found equivalent technical success (GSV closure) up to 5 years and probably similar recurrence rates between RFA and EVLA.[107] EVLA and high ligation with stripping were superior to (ultrasound-guided) foam sclerotherapy with respect to closure of the saphenous vein. A multicenter randomized trial found RFA to be superior to foam sclerotherapy for small saphenous vein reflux. A recent prospective randomized trial (n = 248) compared RFA to CAC in symptomatic GSV reflux.[108] There were higher rates of thermal injury including paresthesia in the RFA group, not surprisingly, and higher satisfaction in the CAC group.[109]

The EVRA–RCT compared compression therapy alone to compression plus early endovenous ablation in venous ulcer patients with superficial reflux. There was faster ulcer healing (median 56 vs 82 days) and lower ulcer recurrence rates in the compression plus early ablation group.[110,111]

Recurrence of varicose veins after ablation is not uncommon. In 1 study there was varicose vein recurrence in approximately 22% of cases at 2-year following endovenous ablation. The most common underlying etiology was GSV recanalization followed by development of reflux in the anterior accessory GSV.[112] Additional factors can be SSV and perforator reflux.[113] In a retrospective study (n = 259 patients) an independent risk factor for delayed venous ulcer healing after saphenous vein ablation ($\pm$ sclerotherapy) was persistent reflux postablation.[114] The potential contribution of suprainguinal venous disease to ulcer formation or recurrence has not been well characterized.

There are limited data on the role of perforator ablation. Ablation of incompetent perforator veins may also be considered in the setting of venous ulcer disease.[115] Thermal ablation and sclerotherapy have both shown efficacy in occluding perforator vein,.[116,117] Ultrasound-guided foam sclerotherapy appears to result in lower perforator closure rates than thermal ablation.[117] In 1 study of ultrasound-guided perforator vein foam sclerotherapy resulted in calf DVT in 3%.[118]

Overall, the rate of postsaphenous vein ablation DVT is very low and the cost effectiveness of routine ultrasound studies after ablation following thermal or adhesive ablation of the saphenous veins has been challenged in the literature.

DEEP VENOUS REFLUX

Deep vein reflux can coexist with superficial reflux and is likely associated with symptom severity.[119] Thrombotic and nonthrombotic iliac vein obstruction may be associated with deep venous reflux.[120,121] Following a DVT, deep vein reflux which can contribute to symptoms of PTS.[122]

Several surgical techniques have been attempted to restore deep valvular function including transposition, transplantation, valvuloplasty, and neovalve formation, but are invasive, technically challenging and rarely used.[123–127] Trials of catheter-based techniques to fashion venous valves from the vein wall or to insert stent valves have been disappointing to date.[128] An ongoing trial looking at open surgical placement of a bioprosthetic valve in the femoral vein has shown promising results with 91% ulcer healing or improvement at 12 months in patients treated for C6 disease (manuscript submitted).

Currently, the mainstay treatment of deep vein reflux is compression therapy along with treatment of coincident superficial reflux and/ or deep vein obstruction.

NONTHROMBOTIC DEEP VENOUS OBSTRUCTION

In May-Thurner syndrome (MTS) the left common iliac vein is compressed by the adjacent right common iliac artery against the lumbar vertebrae, though multiple other areas of potential compression can exist.[129,130] In the literature, the term nonthrombotic iliac vein lesion has been used to encompass other segments of compression. Some additional mechanisms of compression have been reported such as those from iliac artery stents[131] and tumors.[132,133]

The prevalence of MTS in the general population is around 25%[134] and higher amongst symptomatic individuals.[120,134] It may lead to unilateral edema and even thrombosis of the ipsilateral limb, though it is often clinically silent.[135] Diagnostic modalities include MRI, computed tomography venography and invasive venography with intravascular ultrasound. A percentage stenosis of approximately 50% by lumen area has been proposed as *significant*.[136–138]

Endovenous stenting has become the invasive treatment of choice in symptomatic patients (Fig. 4).[139–141] Stents are deployed to overcome extrinsic compression, recoil and reobstruction.[142] Ideally, venous stents must be flexible, possess radial strength and conform to the vessel curvature. Undersizing of stents (in terms of diameter) can result in stent migration,[143] impede venous flow, and lower patency rates in the long-term.[144]

A number of dedicated self-expanding venous stents have been Food and Drug Administration (FDA)-approved and available on the US market, including Abre[145] (Medtronic, MN), Venovo[146] (Bard, NJ), Zilver Vena (Cook Medical, IN).[147] Unlike the Wallstent (Boston Scientific, MA), these stents do not shorten significantly during deployment and have more precise positioning.

A 2015 systematic review reported iliofemoral stent primary and secondary patency rates of 96% and 99% at 1 year.[148] However, it is not yet known which patient subsets may benefit from venous stenting. As one case in point, the VIDIO trial enrolled 100 patients with C4-C6 venous disease. Sixty-eight were stented based on imaging findings of stenosis. Clinical outcomes to stenting, however, were mixed. At 6 months 41% had VCSS improvements of greater than 4 points, 7.3% had no change, and 13.2% had worsening of VCSS.[149] Patient selection will be key for stenting and there is more to be learned in terms of which patient subsets will benefit.

In approximately 25% of individuals the popliteal vein can become compressed by the

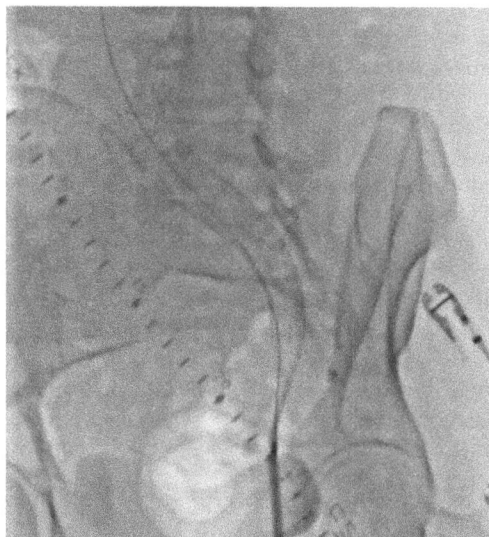

Fig. 4. Fluoroscopy of Liliac vein stent, postdeployment.

gastrocnemius muscles during knee extension.[150] Though normally asymptomatic, this can lead to popliteal vein entrapment syndrome.[151,152] It can present with edema[153] and rarely DVT[154] of the affected limb. Treatment of popliteal vein entrapment syndrome includes compression stockings, with gastrocnemius muscle botox injections[155] and surgical decompression reserved for more severe cases.[156]

THROMBOTIC DEEP VENOUS OBSTRUCTION

Acute DVT of the lower extremities can, in some instances, lead to PTS, a chronic condition associated with chronic obstruction, with or without reflux, limb venous hypertension and inflammation.[121,157] The affected vein can be left with permanent luminal scarring and obstruction associated with postthrombotic synechiae. PTS typically develops well after 3 months postacute DVT. The frequency of PTS has been estimated to range from 20% to 40%+.[158–160] Long-term sequelae are pain, edema, discoloration, weeping, and ulceration.[161,162] Individuals with more proximal location of DVT (common femoral vein or above) and recurrent DVT are at greater risk for PTS.[163,164]

Several endovascular recanalization techniques have been described to relieve postthrombotic venous outflow obstruction.[141] Recanalization can be combined with thrombolysis devices.[165]

Postthrombotic chronic total venous occlusions can be very difficult to traverse due to the hard texture of the occluded lumen and poor visualization of the true lumen and the large collaterals that often develop. Support catheters and even sharp recanalization techniques have been used.[166–168] Published primary and secondary patency rates for postthrombotic iliac vein stents at 1 year have been around 79% and 94%, respectively.[148] In postthrombotic stenotic disease involving the common femoral vein endophlebectomy can be performed combined with arteriovenous fistula formation (to improve flow and theoretically maintain patency). Compared to stenting alone this can lead to more complications and a longer hospital stay.[169]

There are currently no published RCTs to demonstrate the efficacy of deep vein interventions on the symptoms of PTS, although there is predominantly retrospective or case series data.[141,170–172] A systematic review of iliocaval stenting studies in 2020 found no reports of periprocedural mortality or pulmonary embolism.[171]

Complication rates were 3% and included access site hematoma, stent thrombosis, and bleeding. Primary and secondary patency rates (median follow-up 33 months) were 64% and 85%. In a retrospective analysis, predictors of stent occlusion (mean follow-up 41 months) included the presence of postthrombotic changes like synechiae, distal stent extension into the common femoral vein, and lower common femoral vein peak flow velocity.[173] The ongoing C-TRACT trial (NCT03250247) seeks to evaluate the effect of iliac vein stenting with or without superficial vein ablation on PTS outcomes.

There is currently limited data on optimal anticoagulation or antiplatelet therapy after iliocaval stenting.[174] In most studies, patients undergoing stenting for postthrombotic disease were placed on anticoagulation.[171]

SUMMARY

Chronic venous disease of the lower extremities is common. It is associated with venous obstruction, reflux, or both and often leads to chronic inflammation and debilitating symptoms. In addition to compression and pharmacologic therapy, several catheter-based techniques have shown promise for deep vein recanalization, closure of incompetent superficial veins and elimination of varicose veins. Further, quality clinical trials and training in comprehensive venous disease care are critical to enhance patient care and advance the field.

CLINICS CARE POINTS

- Chronic venous disease is a chronic and progressive condition. Patients should be followed longitudinally.
- Consider deep venous obstruction in patients with advanced forms of venous disease, in particular, those who have not responded to treatment for superficial venous insufficiency.
- There is currently no quality evidence to support incompetent perforator vein ablation, outside the setting of associated ulcer disease.

DISCLOSURES

R.R. Attaran and G. Babapour: None; C. Mena-Hurtado is Consultant for Cook, Terumo and BD Research grants: Shockwave, Abbott, Merck; C.I. Ochoa Chaar is consultant for EnVVeno Medical, has IP of patent

U.S.S.N. 10,524,89, and has received research support from Yale Department of Surgery, SVS, AVF, CT Innovation, VSGNE, NIH, EnVVeno, Boston Scientific, Medtronic, EnVVeno Medical, Inari Medical, United States.

REFERENCES

1. Pannier F, Rabe E. Progression in venous pathology. Phlebology 2015;30(1 Suppl):95–7.
2. Pappas PJ, Lakhanpal S, Nguyen KQ, et al. The center for vein restoration study on presenting symptoms, treatment modalities, and outcomes in Medicare-eligible patients with chronic venous disorders. J Vasc Surg Venous Lymphat Disord 2018;6(1):13–24.
3. Wrona M, Jockel KH, Pannier F, et al. Association of venous disorders with leg symptoms: results from the bonn vein study 1. Eur J Vasc Endovasc Surg 2015;50(3):360–7.
4. Evans CJ, Fowkes FG, Ruckley CV, et al. Prevalence of varicose veins and chronic venous insufficiency in men and women in the general population: Edinburgh Vein Study. J Epidemiol Community Health 1999;53(3):149–53.
5. Criqui MH, Jamosmos M, Fronek A, et al. Chronic venous disease in an ethnically diverse population: the San Diego Population Study. Am J Epidemiol 2003;158(5):448–56. Available at: https://www.ncbi.nlm.nih.gov/pubmed/12936900.
6. Carradice D, Mazari FA, Samuel N, et al. Modelling the effect of venous disease on quality of life. Br J Surg 2011;98(8):1089–98.
7. Beebe-Dimmer JL, Pfeifer JR, Engle JS, et al. The epidemiology of chronic venous insufficiency and varicose veins. Ann Epidemiol 2005; 15(3):175–84.
8. Moore HM, Lane TR, Thapar A, et al. The European burden of primary varicose veins. Phlebology 2013;28(Suppl 1):141–7.
9. Salim S, Machin M, Patterson BO, et al. Global epidemiology of chronic venous disease: a systematic review with pooled prevalence analysis. Ann Surg 2021;274(6):971–6.
10. Eberhardt RT, Raffetto JD. Chronic venous insufficiency. Circulation 2014;130(4):333–46.
11. Chi YW, Raffetto JD. Venous leg ulceration pathophysiology and evidence based treatment. Vasc Med 2015;20(2):168–81.
12. Robertson L, Evans C, Fowkes FG. Epidemiology of chronic venous disease. Phlebology 2008;23(3):103–11.
13. Robertson LA, Evans CJ, Lee AJ, et al. Incidence and risk factors for venous reflux in the general population: Edinburgh Vein Study. Eur J Vasc Endovasc Surg 2014;48(2):208–14.
14. Danielsson G, Eklof B, Grandinetti A, et al. The influence of obesity on chronic venous disease. Vasc Endovasc Surg 2002;36(4):271–6.
15. Arfvidsson B, Eklof B, Balfour J. Iliofemoral venous pressure correlates with intraabdominal pressure in morbidly obese patients. Vasc Endovasc Surg 2005;39(6):505–9.
16. Willenberg T, Clemens R, Haegeli LM, et al. The influence of abdominal pressure on lower extremity venous pressure and hemodynamics: a human in-vivo model simulating the effect of abdominal obesity. Eur J Vasc Endovasc Surg 2011;41(6):849–55.
17. Willenberg T, Schumacher A, Amann-Vesti B, et al. Impact of obesity on venous hemodynamics of the lower limbs. J Vasc Surg 2010;52(3):664–8.
18. Nelzen O, Bergqvist D, Lindhagen A. Venous and non-venous leg ulcers: clinical history and appearance in a population study. Br J Surg 1994;81(2):182–7.
19. Margolis DJ, Bilker W, Santanna J, et al. Venous leg ulcer: incidence and prevalence in the elderly. J Am Acad Dermatol 2002;46(3):381–6.
20. Couzan S, Leizorovicz A, Laporte S, et al. A randomized double-blind trial of upward progressive versus degressive compressive stockings in patients with moderate to severe chronic venous insufficiency. J Vasc Surg 2012;56(5):1344–1350 e1.
21. Maddox D. Effects of venous leg ulceration on patients' quality of life. Nurs Stand 2012;26(38):42–9.
22. Rice JB, Desai U, Cummings AK, et al. Burden of venous leg ulcers in the United States. J Med Econ 2014;17(5):347–56.
23. Meissner MH, Gloviczki P, Bergan J, et al. Primary chronic venous disorders. J Vasc Surg 2007;46(Suppl S):54S–67S.
24. Pocock ES, Alsaigh T, Mazor R, et al. Cellular and molecular basis of Venous insufficiency. Vasc Cell 2014;6(1):24.
25. Mansilha A, Sousa J. Pathophysiological mechanisms of chronic venous disease and implications for venoactive drug therapy. Int J Mol Sci 2018;19(6). https://doi.org/10.3390/ijms19061669.
26. Uhl JF, Gillot C. Anatomy of the foot venous pump: physiology and influence on chronic venous disease. Phlebology 2012;27(5):219–30.
27. Ludbrook J. The musculovenous pumps of the human lower limb. Am Heart J 1966;71(5):635–41. Available at: https://www.ncbi.nlm.nih.gov/pubmed/5935855.
28. Pfisterer L, Konig G, Hecker M, et al. Pathogenesis of varicose veins - lessons from biomechanics. Vasa 2014;43(2):88–99.
29. Payne SP, London NJ, Newland CJ, et al. Ambulatory venous pressure: correlation with skin condition and role in identifying surgically correctible disease. Eur J Vasc Endovasc Surg 1996;11(2):195–200.

30. Nicolaides AN, Hussein MK, Szendro G, et al. The relation of venous ulceration with ambulatory venous pressure measurements. J Vasc Surg 1993;17(2):414–9.
31. Sansilvestri-Morel P, Rupin A, Badier-Commander C, et al. Imbalance in the synthesis of collagen type I and collagen type III in smooth muscle cells derived from human varicose veins. J Vasc Res 2001;38(6):560–8. Available at: https://www.ncbi.nlm.nih.gov/pubmed/11740155.
32. Sansilvestri-Morel P, Fioretti F, Rupin A, et al. Comparison of extracellular matrix in skin and saphenous veins from patients with varicose veins: does the skin reflect venous matrix changes? Clin Sci (Lond) 2007;112(4):229–39.
33. Kirsch D, Dienes HP, Kuchle R, et al. Changes in the extracellular matrix of the vein wall–the cause of primary varicosis? Vasa 2000;29(3):173–7.
34. Xiao Y, Huang Z, Yin H, et al. In vitro differences between smooth muscle cells derived from varicose veins and normal veins. J Vasc Surg 2009;50(5):1149–54.
35. Badier-Commander C, Couvelard A, Henin D, et al. Smooth muscle cell modulation and cytokine overproduction in varicose veins. An in situ study. J Pathol 2001;193(3):398–407.
36. Rizzi A, Quaglio D, Vasquez G, et al. Effects of vasoactive agents in healthy and diseased human saphenous veins. J Vasc Surg 1998;28(5):855–61. Available at: https://www.ncbi.nlm.nih.gov/pubmed/9808853.
37. Wlaschek M, Singh K, Sindrilaru A, et al. Iron and iron-dependent reactive oxygen species in the regulation of macrophages and fibroblasts in non-healing chronic wounds. Free Radic Biol Med 2019;133:262–75.
38. Caggiati A, Rosi C, Casini A, et al. Skin iron deposition characterises lipodermatosclerosis and leg ulcer. Eur J Vasc Endovasc Surg 2010;40(6):777–82.
39. Lattimer CR, Kalodiki E, Geroulakos G, et al. Are inflammatory biomarkers increased in varicose vein blood? Clin Appl Thromb Hemost 2016;22(7):656–64.
40. Lattimer CR, Kalodiki E, Geroulakos G, et al. d-Dimer levels are significantly increased in blood taken from varicose veins compared with antecubital blood from the same patient. Angiology 2015;66(9):882–8.
41. Lurie F, Passman M, Meisner M, et al. The 2020 update of the CEAP classification system and reporting standards. J Vasc Surg Venous Lymphat Disord 2020;8(3):342–52.
42. Kakkos SK, Rivera MA, Matsagas MI, et al. Validation of the new venous severity scoring system in varicose vein surgery. J Vasc Surg 2003;38(2):224–8.
43. Rutherford RB, Padberg FT Jr, Comerota AJ, et al. Venous severity scoring: an adjunct to venous outcome assessment. J Vasc Surg 2000;31(6):1307–12.
44. Meissner MH, Natiello C, Nicholls SC. Performance characteristics of the venous clinical severity score. J Vasc Surg 2002;36(5):889–95.
45. Iglesias CP, Birks Y, Nelson EA, et al. Quality of life of people with venous leg ulcers: a comparison of the discriminative and responsive characteristics of two generic and a disease specific instruments. Qual Life Res 2005;14(7):1705–18.
46. Lamping DL, Schroter S, Kurz X, et al. Evaluation of outcomes in chronic venous disorders of the leg: development of a scientifically rigorous, patient-reported measure of symptoms and quality of life. J Vasc Surg 2003;37(2):410–9.
47. Lattimer CR, Kalodiki E, Azzam M, et al. Validation of the villalta scale in assessing post-thrombotic syndrome using clinical, duplex, and hemodynamic comparators. J Vasc Surg Venous Lymphat Disord 2013;1(1):104–5.
48.. Prandoni P, Villalta S, Polistena P, et al. Symptomatic deep-vein thrombosis and the post-thrombotic syndrome. Haematologica 1995;80(2 Suppl):42–8.
49. S V. Assessment of validity and reproducibility of a clinical scale for the post-thrombotic syndrome. Haemostasis 1994;24:158a (Abstract).
50. Lurie F, Lal BK, Antignani PL, et al. Compression therapy after invasive treatment of superficial veins of the lower extremities: clinical practice guidelines of the American venous forum, society for vascular surgery, American college of phlebology, society for vascular medicine, and international union of phlebology. J Vasc Surg Venous Lymphat Disord 2019;7(1):17–28.
51. Masuda E, Ozsvath K, Vossler J, et al. The 2020 appropriate use criteria for chronic lower extremity venous disease of the American venous forum, the society for vascular surgery, the American vein and lymphatic society, and the society of interventional radiology. J Vasc Surg Venous Lymphat Disord 2020;8(4):505–525 e4.
52. Beaconsfield P, Ginsburg J. Effect of changes in limb posture on peripheral blood flow. Circ Res 1955;3(5):478–82. Available at: https://www.ncbi.nlm.nih.gov/pubmed/13250716.
53. Mellander S, Oberg B, Odelram H. Vascular adjustments to increased transmural pressure in cat and man with special reference to shifts in capillary fluid transfer. Acta Physiol Scand 1964;61:34–48.
54. Abu-Own A, Shami SK, Chittenden SJ, et al. Microangiopathy of the skin and the effect of leg compression in patients with chronic venous insufficiency. J Vasc Surg 1994;19(6):1074–83.

Available at: https://www.ncbi.nlm.nih.gov/pubmed/8201709.

55. Beidler SK, Douillet CD, Berndt DF, et al. Inflammatory cytokine levels in chronic venous insufficiency ulcer tissue before and after compression therapy. J Vasc Surg 2009;49(4):1013–20.

56. Attaran RR, Ochoa Chaar CI. Compression therapy for venous disease. Phlebology 2017;32(2):81–8.

57. Stout N, Partsch H, Szolnoky G, et al. Chronic edema of the lower extremities: international consensus recommendations for compression therapy clinical research trials. Int Angiol 2012;31(4):316–29. Available at: https://www.ncbi.nlm.nih.gov/pubmed/22801397.

58. Partsch H, Flour M, Smith PC, et al. Indications for compression therapy in venous and lymphatic disease consensus based on experimental data and scientific evidence. Under the auspices of the IUP. Int Angiol 2008;27(3):193–219. Available at: https://www.ncbi.nlm.nih.gov/pubmed/18506124.

59. Motykie GD, Caprini JA, Arcelus JI, et al. Evaluation of therapeutic compression stockings in the treatment of chronic venous insufficiency. Dermatol Surg 1999;25(2):116–20. Available at: https://www.ncbi.nlm.nih.gov/pubmed/10037516.

60. Bakker NA, Schieven LW, Bruins RM, et al. Compression stockings after endovenous laser ablation of the great saphenous vein: a prospective randomized controlled trial. Eur J Vasc Endovasc Surg 2013;46(5):588–92.

61. Belramman A, Bootun R, Lane TRA, et al. COmpressioN following endovenous TreatmenT of Incompetent varicose veins by sclerotherapy (CONFETTI). J Vasc Surg Venous Lymphat Disord 2024;12(2):101729.

62. Yang X, Zhang X, Yin M, et al. Elastic compression stockings to prevent post-thrombotic syndrome in proximal deep venous thrombosis patients without thrombus removal. J Vasc Surg Venous Lymphat Disord 2022;10(2):293–9.

63. Kahn SR, Shapiro S, Wells PS, et al. Compression stockings to prevent post-thrombotic syndrome: a randomised placebo-controlled trial. Lancet 2014;383(9920):880–8.

64. Webb E, Neeman T, Bowden FJ, et al. Compression therapy to prevent recurrent cellulitis of the leg. N Engl J Med 2020;383(7):630–9.

65. Mayberry JC, Moneta GL, Taylor LM Jr. Porter JM. Fifteen-year results of ambulatory compression therapy for chronic venous ulcers. Surgery 1991;109(5):575–81. Available at: https://www.ncbi.nlm.nih.gov/pubmed/2020902.

66. Uhl JF, Benigni JP, Chahim M, et al. Prospective randomized controlled study of patient compliance in using a compression stocking: importance of recommendations of the practitioner as a factor for better compliance. Phlebology 2018;33(1):36–43.

67. Kankam HKN, Lim CS, Fiorentino F, et al. A summation analysis of compliance and complications of compression hosiery for patients with chronic venous disease or post-thrombotic syndrome. Eur J Vasc Endovasc Surg 2018;55(3):406–16.

68. Carpentier P, van Bellen B, Karetova D, et al. Clinical efficacy and safety of a new 1000-mg suspension versus twice-daily 500-mg tablets of MPFF in patients with symptomatic chronic venous disorders: a randomized controlled trial. Int Angiol 2017;36(5):402–9.

69. Martinez-Zapata MJ, Vernooij RW, Uriona Tuma SM, et al. Phlebotonics for venous insufficiency. Cochrane Database Syst Rev 2016;4:CD003229.

70. Belcaro G, Cesarone MR, Cox D, et al. Improvements in edema and microcirculation in chronic venous insufficiency with Pycnogenol(R) or elastic compression. Minerva Surg 2024;79(4):448–54.

71. Kakkos SK, Nicolaides AN. Efficacy of micronized purified flavonoid fraction (Daflon(R)) on improving individual symptoms, signs and quality of life in patients with chronic venous disease: a systematic review and meta-analysis of randomized double-blind placebo-controlled trials. Int Angiol 2018;37(2):143–54.

72. Rabinovich A, Kahn SR. How I treat the postthrombotic syndrome. Blood 2018;131(20):2215–22.

73. de Jongste AB, Jonker JJ, Huisman MV, et al. A double blind three center clinical trial on the short-term efficacy of 0-(beta-hydroxyethyl)-rutosides in patients with post-thrombotic syndrome. Thromb Haemost 1989;62(3):826–9. Available at: https://www.ncbi.nlm.nih.gov/pubmed/2688186.

74. Varatharajan L, Thapar A, Lane T, et al. Pharmacological adjuncts for chronic venous ulcer healing: a systematic review. Phlebology 2016;31(5):356–65.

75. Jull AB, Arroll B, Parag V, et al. Pentoxifylline for treating venous leg ulcers. Cochrane Database Syst Rev 2012;12:CD001733.

76. Colgan MP, Dormandy JA, Jones PW, et al. Oxpentifylline treatment of venous ulcers of the leg. BMJ 1990;300(6730):972–5.

77. Brenner MA. Nonhealing venous stasis ulcers. Pentoxifylline as adjunctive therapy. J Am Podiatr Med Assoc 1987;77(11):586–8.

78. Stellin GP, Waxman K. Current and potential therapeutic effects of pentoxifylline. Compr Ther 1989;15(5):11–3. Available at: https://www.ncbi.nlm.nih.gov/pubmed/2659249.

79. Labropoulos N, Leon M, Nicolaides AN, et al. Superficial venous insufficiency: correlation of anatomic extent of reflux with clinical symptoms and signs. J Vasc Surg 1994;20(6):953–8.

80. Dwerryhouse S, Davies B, Harradine K, et al. Stripping the long saphenous vein reduces the rate of reoperation for recurrent varicose veins: five-year results of a randomized trial. J Vasc Surg 1999; 29(4):589–92.

81. Keith LM Jr, Smead WL. Saphenous vein stripping and its complications. Surg Clin North Am 1983; 63(6):1303–12.

82. Kabnick LS. Outcome of different endovenous laser wavelengths for great saphenous vein ablation. J Vasc Surg 2006;43(1):88–93.

83. Spreafico G, Kabnick L, Berland TL, et al. Laser saphenous ablations in more than 1,000 limbs with long-term duplex examination follow-up. Ann Vasc Surg 2011;25(1):71–8.

84. Proebstle TM, Alm BJ, Gockeritz O, et al. Five-year results from the prospective European multicentre cohort study on radiofrequency segmental thermal ablation for incompetent great saphenous veins. Br J Surg 2015;102(3):212–8.

85. Goode SD, Chowdhury A, Crockett M, et al. Laser and radiofrequency ablation study (LARA study): a randomised study comparing radiofrequency ablation and endovenous laser ablation (810 nm). Eur J Vasc Endovasc Surg 2010;40(2):246–53.

86. Dermody M, Schul MW, O'Donnell TF. Thromboembolic complications of endovenous thermal ablation and foam sclerotherapy in the treatment of great saphenous vein insufficiency. Phlebology 2015;30(5):357–64.

87. Kane K, Fisher T, Bennett M, et al. The incidence and outcome of endothermal heat-induced thrombosis after endovenous laser ablation. Ann Vasc Surg 2014;28(7):1744–50.

88. Bergan J, Cheng V. Foam sclerotherapy for the treatment of varicose veins. Vascular 2007;15(5): 269–72.

89. Fegan WG. Continuous compression technique of injecting varicose veins. Lancet 1963;2(7299): 109–12.

90. de Avila Oliveira R, Riera R, Vasconcelos V, et al. Injection sclerotherapy for varicose veins. Cochrane Database Syst Rev 2021;12:CD001732.

91. Alder G, Lees T. Foam sclerotherapy. Phlebology 2015;30(2 Suppl):18–23.

92. Orbach EJ. Clinical evaluation of a new technic in the sclerotherapy of varicose veins. J Int Coll Surg 1948;11(4):396–402. Available at: https://www.ncbi.nlm.nih.gov/pubmed/18874792.

93. Tessari L, Cavezzi A, Frullini A. Preliminary experience with a new sclerosing foam in the treatment of varicose veins. Dermatol Surg 2001;27(1):58–60. Available at: https://www.ncbi.nlm.nih.gov/pubmed/11231246.

94. Guex JJ, Allaert FA, Gillet JL, et al. Immediate and midterm complications of sclerotherapy: report of a prospective multicenter registry of 12,173 sclerotherapy sessions. Dermatol Surg 2005; 31(2):123–8 [discussion: 128] Available at: https://www.ncbi.nlm.nih.gov/pubmed/15762201.

95. Willenberg T, Smith PC, Shepherd A, et al. Visual disturbance following sclerotherapy for varicose veins, reticular veins and telangiectasias: a systematic literature review. Phlebology 2013;28(3): 123–31.

96. Hafner F, Froehlich H, Gary T, et al. Intra-arterial injection, a rare but serious complication of sclerotherapy. Phlebology 2013;28(2):64–73.

97. Todd KL 3rd, Wright DI, Group V-I. Durability of treatment effect with polidocanol endovenous microfoam on varicose vein symptoms and appearance (VANISH-2). J Vasc Surg Venous Lymphat Disord 2015;3(3):258–264 e1.

98. King JT, O'Byrne M, Vasquez M, et al. Treatment of truncal incompetence and varicose veins with a single administration of a new polidocanol endovenous microfoam preparation improves symptoms and appearance. Eur J Vasc Endovasc Surg 2015;50(6):784–93.

99. Todd KL 3rd, Wright DI, Group V-I. The VANISH-2 study: a randomized, blinded, multicenter study to evaluate the efficacy and safety of polidocanol endovenous microfoam 0.5% and 1.0% compared with placebo for the treatment of saphenofemoral junction incompetence. Phlebology 2014;29(9): 608–18.

100. van Eekeren RR, Boersma D, Holewijn S, et al. Mechanochemical endovenous ablation for the treatment of great saphenous vein insufficiency. J Vasc Surg Venous Lymphat Disord 2014;2(3): 282–8.

101. Deijen CL, Schreve MA, Bosma J, et al. Clarivein mechanochemical ablation of the great and small saphenous vein: early treatment outcomes of two hospitals. Phlebology 2016;31(3):192–7.

102. Vahaaho S, Mahmoud O, Halmesmaki K, et al. Randomized clinical trial of mechanochemical and endovenous thermal ablation of great saphenous varicose veins. Br J Surg 2019;106(5):548–54.

103. Morrison N, Gibson K, Vasquez M, et al. Five-year extension study of patients from a randomized clinical trial (VeClose) comparing cyanoacrylate closure versus radiofrequency ablation for the treatment of incompetent great saphenous veins. J Vasc Surg Venous Lymphat Disord 2020;8(6): 978–89.

104. Morrison N, Kolluri R, Vasquez M, et al. Comparison of cyanoacrylate closure and radiofrequency ablation for the treatment of incompetent great saphenous veins: 36-Month outcomes of the VeClose randomized controlled trial. Phlebology 2019;34(6):380–90.

105. Park I. Initial outcomes of cyanoacrylate closure, venaseal system, for the treatment of the

incompetent great and small saphenous veins. Vasc Endovasc Surg 2017;51(8):545–9.

106. Proebstle TM, Alm J, Dimitri S, et al. The European multicenter cohort study on cyanoacrylate embolization of refluxing great saphenous veins. J Vasc Surg Venous Lymphat Disord 2015;3(1):2–7.

107. Whing J, Nandhra S, Nesbitt C, et al. Interventions for great saphenous vein incompetence. Cochrane Database Syst Rev 2021;8:CD005624.

108. Hamel-Desnos C, Nyamekye I, Chauzat B, et al. FOVELASS: a randomised trial of endovenous laser ablation versus polidocanol foam for small saphenous vein incompetence. Eur J Vasc Endovasc Surg 2023;65(3):415–23.

109. Alhewy MA, Abdo EM, Ghazala EAE, et al. Outcomes of cyanoacrylate closure versus radiofrequency ablation for the treatment of incompetent great saphenous veins. Ann Vasc Surg 2024;98:309–16.

110. Gohel MS, Heatley F, Liu X, et al. A randomized trial of early endovenous ablation in venous ulceration. N Engl J Med 2018;378(22):2105–14.

111. Gohel MS, Mora MJ, Szigeti M, et al. Long-term clinical and cost-effectiveness of early endovenous ablation in venous ulceration: a randomized clinical trial. JAMA Surg 2020;155(12):1113–21.

112. O'Donnell TF, Balk EM, Dermody M, et al. Recurrence of varicose veins after endovenous ablation of the great saphenous vein in randomized trials. J Vasc Surg Venous Lymphat Disord 2016;4(1): 97–105.

113. Bush RG, Bush P, Flanagan J, et al. Factors associated with recurrence of varicose veins after thermal ablation: results of the recurrent veins after thermal ablation study. Sci World J 2014;2014: 505843.

114. Pihlaja T, Vanttila LM, Ohtonen P, et al. Factors associated with delayed venous ulcer healing after endovenous intervention for superficial venous insufficiency. J Vasc Surg Venous Lymphat Disord 2022;10(6):1238–44.

115. Lawrence PF, Hager ES, Harlander-Locke MP, et al. Treatment of superficial and perforator reflux and deep venous stenosis improves healing of chronic venous leg ulcers. J Vasc Surg Venous Lymphat Disord 2020;8(4):601–9.

116. Reitz KM, Salem K, Mohapatra A, et al. Complete venous ulceration healing after perforator ablation does not depend on treatment modality. Ann Vasc Surg 2021;70:109–15.

117. Hager ES, Washington C, Steinmetz A, et al. Factors that influence perforator vein closure rates using radiofrequency ablation, laser ablation, or foam sclerotherapy. J Vasc Surg Venous Lymphat Disord 2016;4(1):51–6.

118. Kiguchi MM, Hager ES, Winger DG, et al. Factors that influence perforator thrombosis and predict

healing with perforator sclerotherapy for venous ulceration without axial reflux. J Vasc Surg 2014; 59(5):1368–76.

119. Danielsson G, Eklof B, Grandinetti A, et al. Deep axial reflux, an important contributor to skin changes or ulcer in chronic venous disease. J Vasc Surg 2003;38(6):1336–41.

120. Raju S, Neglen P. High prevalence of nonthrombotic iliac vein lesions in chronic venous disease: a permissive role in pathogenicity. J Vasc Surg 2006;44(1):136–43 [discussion: 144].

121. Johnson BF, Manzo RA, Bergelin RO, et al. The site of residual abnormalities in the leg veins in long-term follow-up after deep vein thrombosis and their relationship to the development of the post-thrombotic syndrome. Int Angiol 1996;15(1): 14–9. Available at: https://www.ncbi.nlm.nih.gov/pubmed/8739531.

122. Kahn SR, Comerota AJ, Cushman M, et al. The postthrombotic syndrome: evidence-based prevention, diagnosis, and treatment strategies: a scientific statement from the American Heart Association. Circulation 2014;130(18):1636–61.

123. Queral LA, Whitehouse WM Jr, Flinn WR, et al. Surgical correction of chronic deep venous insufficiency by valvular transposition. Surgery 1980; 87(6):688–95. Available at: https://www.ncbi.nlm.nih.gov/pubmed/7376079.

124. Raju S, Neglen P, Doolittle J, et al. Axillary vein transfer in trabeculated postthrombotic veins. J Vasc Surg 1999;29(6):1050–62 [discussion: 1062-4]. Available at: https://www.ncbi.nlm.nih.gov/pubmed/10359939.

125. Taheri SA, Lazar L, Elias S, et al. Surgical treatment of postphlebitic syndrome with vein valve transplant. Am J Surg 1982;144(2):221–4. Available at: https://www.ncbi.nlm.nih.gov/pubmed/7102929.

126. Lugli M, Guerzoni S, Garofalo M, et al. Neovalve construction in deep venous incompetence. J Vasc Surg 2009;49(1):156–62, 162 e1-2; [discussion: 162].

127. Camilli S, Guarnera G. External banding valvuloplasty of the superficial femoral vein in the treatment of primary deep valvular incompetence. Int Angiol 1994;13(3):218–22. Available at: https://www.ncbi.nlm.nih.gov/pubmed/7822897.

128. Vasudevan T, Robinson DA, Hill AA, et al. Safety and feasibility report on nonimplantable endovenous valve formation for the treatment of deep vein reflux. J Vasc Surg Venous Lymphat Disord 2021;9(5):1200–8.

129. May R, Thurner J. The cause of the predominantly sinistral occurrence of thrombosis of the pelvic veins. Angiology 1957;8(5):419–27.

130. May R, Thurner J. [A vascular spur in the vena iliaca communis sinistra as a cause of predominantly left-sided thrombosis of the pelvic veins].

Z Kreislaufforsch 1956;45(23–24):912–22. Available at: https://www.ncbi.nlm.nih.gov/pubmed/13402032.

131. Hermany PL, Badheka AO, Mena-Hurtado CI, et al. A Unique case of may-thurner syndrome: extrinsic compression of the common iliac vein after iliac artery stenting. JACC Cardiovasc Interv 2016;9(5):e39–41.

132. Hermus L, Tielliu IF, Zeebregts CJ, et al. B-cell lymphoma related iliac vein occlusion treated by endovenous stent placement. Minerva Chir 2012;67(3):277–82. Available at: https://www.ncbi.nlm.nih.gov/pubmed/22691832.

133. Liao TY, Hsu HC, Wen MS, et al. Iliofemoral venous thrombosis mainly related to iliofemoral venous obstruction by external tumor compression in cancer patients. Case Rep Oncol 2016;9(3):760–71.

134. Kibbe MR, Ujiki M, Goodwin AL, et al. Iliac vein compression in an asymptomatic patient population. J Vasc Surg 2004;39(5):937–43.

135. Negus D, Fletcher EW, Cockett FB, et al. Compression and band formation at the mouth of the left common iliac vein. Br J Surg 1968;55(5):369–74. Available at: https://www.ncbi.nlm.nih.gov/pubmed/5648014.

136. Jayaraj A, Crim W, Knight A, et al. Characteristics and outcomes of stent occlusion after iliocaval stenting. J Vasc Surg Venous Lymphat Disord 2019;7(1):56–64.

137. Raju S, Kirk O, Davis M, et al. Hemodynamics of "critical" venous stenosis and stent treatment. J Vasc Surg Venous Lymphat Disord 2014;2(1):52–9.

138. Raju S. Long-term outcomes of stent placement for symptomatic nonthrombotic iliac vein compression lesions in chronic venous disease. J Vasc Intervent Radiol 2012;23(4):502–3.

139. Raju S, Darcey R, Neglen P. Unexpected major role for venous stenting in deep reflux disease. J Vasc Surg 2010;51(2):401–8 [discussion: 408].

140. Raju S. Best management options for chronic iliac vein stenosis and occlusion. J Vasc Surg 2013;57(4):1163–9.

141. Neglen P, Hollis KC, Olivier J, et al. Stenting of the venous outflow in chronic venous disease: long-term stent-related outcome, clinical, and hemodynamic result. J Vasc Surg 2007;46(5):979–90.

142. Nazarian GK, Austin WR, Wegryn SA, et al. Venous recanalization by metallic stents after failure of balloon angioplasty or surgery: four-year experience. Cardiovasc Intervent Radiol 1996;19(4):227–33.

143. Sayed MH, Salem M, Desai KR, et al. A review of the incidence, outcome, and management of venous stent migration. J Vasc Surg Venous Lymphat Disord 2022;10(2):482–90.

144. Attaran RR, Ozdemir D, Lin IH, et al. Evaluation of anticoagulant and antiplatelet therapy after iliocaval stenting: factors associated with stent occlusion. J Vasc Surg Venous Lymphat Disord 2019;7(4):527–34.

145. Murphy E, Gibson K, Sapoval M, et al. Pivotal study evaluating the safety and effectiveness of the abre venous self-expanding stent system in patients with symptomatic iliofemoral venous outflow obstruction. Circ Cardiovasc Interv 2022;15(2):e010960.

146. Dake MD, O'Sullivan G, Shammas NW, et al. Three-year results from the venovo venous stent study for the treatment of iliac and femoral vein obstruction. Cardiovasc Intervent Radiol 2021;44(12):1918–29.

147. Hofmann LR, Gagne P, Brown JA, et al. Twelve-month end point results from the evaluation of the Zilver Vena venous stent in the treatment of symptomatic iliofemoral venous outflow obstruction (VIVO clinical study). J Vasc Surg Venous Lymphat Disord 2023;11(3):532–541 e4.

148. Razavi MK, Jaff MR, Miller LE. Safety and effectiveness of stent placement for iliofemoral venous outflow obstruction: systematic review and meta-analysis. Circ Cardiovasc Interv 2015;8(10):e002772.

149. Gagne PJ, Gasparis A, Black S, et al. Analysis of threshold stenosis by multiplanar venogram and intravascular ultrasound examination for predicting clinical improvement after iliofemoral vein stenting in the VIDIO trial. J Vasc Surg Venous Lymphat Disord 2018;6(1):48–56 e1.

150. Leon M, Volteas N, Labropoulos N, et al. Popliteal vein entrapment in the normal population. Eur J Vasc Surg 1992;6(6):623–7.

151. Raju S, Neglen P. Popliteal vein entrapment: a benign venographic feature or a pathologic entity? J Vasc Surg 2000;31(4):631–41.

152. Love JW, Whelan TJ. Popliteal artery entrapment syndrome. Am J Surg 1965;109:620–4.

153. Sinha S, Houghton J, Holt PJ, et al. Popliteal entrapment syndrome. J Vasc Surg 2012;55(1):252–262 e30.

154. White JM, Comerota AJ. Venous compression syndromes. Vasc Endovasc Surg 2017;51(3):155–68.

155. Hislop M, Brideaux A, Dhupelia S. Functional popliteal artery entrapment syndrome: use of ultrasound guided Botox injection as a non-surgical treatment option. Skeletal Radiol 2017;46(9):1241–8.

156. Igari K, Sugano N, Kudo T, et al. Surgical treatment for popliteal artery entrapment syndrome. Ann Vasc Dis 2014;7(1):28–33.

157. Johnson BF, Manzo RA, Bergelin RO, et al. Relationship between changes in the deep venous

system and the development of the postthrombotic syndrome after an acute episode of lower limb deep vein thrombosis: a one- to six-year follow-up. J Vasc Surg 1995;21(2):307–12 [discussion: 313].

158. Kahn SR, Galanaud JP, Vedantham S, et al. Guidance for the prevention and treatment of the postthrombotic syndrome. J Thromb Thrombolysis 2016;41(1):144–53.

159. Kahn SR, Shrier I, Julian JA, et al. Determinants and time course of the postthrombotic syndrome after acute deep venous thrombosis. Ann Intern Med 2008;149(10):698–707.

160. Vedantham S, Goldhaber SZ, Julian JA, et al. Pharmacomechanical catheter-directed thrombolysis for deep-vein thrombosis. N Engl J Med 2017; 377(23):2240–52.

161. Kahn SR, Shbaklo H, Lamping DL, et al. Determinants of health-related quality of life during the 2 years following deep vein thrombosis. J Thromb Haemostasis 2008;6(7):1105–12.

162. Kahn SR, Hirsch A, Shrier I. Effect of postthrombotic syndrome on health-related quality of life after deep venous thrombosis. Arch Intern Med 2002;162(10):1144–8.

163. Douketis JD, Crowther MA, Foster GA, et al. Does the location of thrombosis determine the risk of disease recurrence in patients with proximal deep vein thrombosis? Am J Med 2001;110(7): 515–9. Available at: https://www.ncbi.nlm.nih.gov/pubmed/11343664.

164. Tick LW, Doggen CJ, Rosendaal FR, et al. Predictors of the post-thrombotic syndrome with non-invasive venous examinations in patients 6 weeks after a first episode of deep vein thrombosis. J Thromb Haemostasis 2010;8(12): 2685–92.

165. Garcia MJ, Sterling KM, Kahn SR, et al. Ultrasound-accelerated thrombolysis and venoplasty for the treatment of the postthrombotic syndrome: results of the ACCESS PTS study. J Am Heart Assoc 2020;9(3):e013398.

166. Raju S. Treatment of iliac-caval outflow obstruction. Semin Vasc Surg 2015;28(1):47–53.

167. Neglen P, Berry MA, Raju S. Endovascular surgery in the treatment of chronic primary and postthrombotic iliac vein obstruction. Eur J Vasc Endovasc Surg 2000;20(6):560–71.

168. McDevitt JL, Srinivasa RN, Gemmete JJ, et al. Approach, technical success, complications, and stent patency of sharp recanalization for the treatment of chronic venous occlusive disease: experience in 123 patients. Cardiovasc Intervent Radiol 2019;42(2):205–12.

169. Alhewy MA, Abdelhafez AA, Metwally MH, et al. Femoral vein stenting versus endovenectomy as adjuncts to iliofemoral venous stenting in extensive chronic iliofemoral venous obstruction. Phlebology 2024;39(6):393–402.

170. Raju S, Neglen P. Percutaneous recanalization of total occlusions of the iliac vein. J Vasc Surg 2009;50(2):360–8.

171. Williams ZF, Dillavou ED. A systematic review of venous stents for iliac and venacaval occlusive disease. J Vasc Surg Venous Lymphat Disord 2020; 8(1):145–53.

172. Yin M, Shi H, Ye K, et al. Clinical assessment of endovascular stenting compared with compression therapy alone in post-thrombotic patients with iliofemoral obstruction. Eur J Vasc Endovasc Surg 2015;50(1):101–7.

173. Hugel U, Khatami F, Muka T, et al. Criteria to predict midterm outcome after stenting of chronic iliac vein obstructions (PROMISE trial). J Vasc Surg Venous Lymphat Disord 2023;11(1):91–99 e1.

174. Notten P, Ten Cate H, Ten Cate-Hoek AJ. Postinterventional antithrombotic management after venous stenting of the iliofemoral tract in acute and chronic thrombosis: a systematic review. J Thromb Haemostasis 2021;19(3):753–96.

Iliofemoral Acute Deep Venous Thrombosis, Chronic Deep Venous Thrombosis, and May-Thurner Syndrome

Anthony Teta, MD[a], Jay Mohan, DO, FSCAI, RPVI[b],
Vincent Varghese, DO[c], Jon C. George, MD, FSCAI[c,d],
Jacqueline Powers, BS[e],
Ehrin J. Armstrong, MD, MSc, MAS, FSCAI, FSVM[e,f],
Yulanka Castro-Dominguez, MD, FSCAI, FSVM, RPVI[g,*]

KEYWORDS

- Iliofemoral acute deep venous thrombosis • Chronic deep venous thrombosis
- And may-thurner syndrome • Iliac vein stenting • Venous thrombectomy

KEY POINTS

- Iliofemoral deep venous thrombosis (DVT) carries a significant risk of severe acute symptoms, recurrence, and chronic post-thrombotic symptoms compared to distal DVTs.
- Post-thrombotic syndrome (PTS), reported in 20-50% of chronic DVT, represents a collection of symptoms including leg edema, skin changes, vein dilation, pain, fatigue, and ulcer formation.
- May-Thurner syndrome is defined as an iliofemoral DVT associated with compression of the left iliac vein by the right common iliac artery.

ILIOFEMORAL ACUTE DEEP VENOUS THROMBOSIS

Iliofemoral deep vein thrombosis (DVT) involves thrombosis in the iliac and femoral veins, accounting for a substantial portion of venous thromboembolic (VTE) events. This condition is associated with significant risks, including the potential for pulmonary embolism (PE) and the development of long-term complications like post thrombotic syndrome (PTS). In 2020, there were an estimated over 600,000 cases of DVT in the United States in inpatient settings. This number underestimates the actual occurrence of DVT as over a third of DVT cases are treated in outpatient settings.[1] Acute iliofemoral DVT refers to complete or partial thrombosis of the iliac vein or common femoral vein, with or without involvement of the lower

a Department of Cardiovascular Medicine, McLaren Macomb Medical Center, Mount Clemens, MI, USA; b Department of Cardiovascular Medicine, Michigan State University McLaren Macomb-Oakland Medical Center, Mount Clemens, MI, USA; c Interventional Cardiology and Endovascular Medicine; ReVascMedProfessionals, Philadelphia, PA, USA; d Thomas Jefferson University Hospital, Philadelphia, PA, USA; e Advanced Heart and Vein Center, Denver, CO, USA; f Interventional Cardiology and Vascular Intervention; g Harrington Heart & Vascular Institute, University Hospitals, Case Western Reserve University School of Medicine, Cleveland, OH, USA
* Corresponding author. 29101 Health Campus Drive, Building 2 Suite 320, Westlake, OH 44145.
E-mail address: yulankacastro@gmail.com
Twitter: @DrAnthonyTeta (A.T.); @DrJayMohan (J.M.); @jcgeorgemd (J.C.G.); @ehrin_armstrong (E.J.A.); @YSCastroMD (Y.C.-D.)

Intervent Cardiol Clin 14 (2025) 297–310
https://doi.org/10.1016/j.iccl.2024.11.014
2211-7458/25/© 2024 Elsevier Inc. All rights reserved, including those for text and data mining, AI training, and similar technologies.

Abbreviations	
CaVENT	Catheter-Directed Thrombolysis for Deep Vein Thrombosis
CDT	catheter-directed thrombolysis
C-DVT	chronic deep vein thrombosis
CEAP	Clinical, Etiology, Anatomic Pathophysiology score
CT	computed tomography
CTV	computed tomography venography
DOAC	direct oral anticoagulant
DUS	duplex ultrasound
DVT	deep vein thrombosis
IV	intravenous
IVC	inferior vena cava
IVUS	intravascular ultrasound
LMWH	low-molecular-weight heparin
MRV	magnetic resonance venography
NIVL	non-thrombotic iliac vein lesion
PCDT	pharmacomechanical catheter-directed thrombolysis
PE	pulmonary embolism
PTS	post-thrombotic syndrome
UFH	unfractionated heparin
VCSS	Venous Clinical Severity Score
VTE	venous thromboembolic

extremity veins.[2] Iliac or common femoral involvement has been reported in 1-quarter of all lower extremity DVT cases and iliac involvement is seen in about 9% of cases.[3,4] Iliofemoral DVT is associated with a higher risk of adverse outcomes compared to DVT in other locations, with a higher likelihood of severe acute symptoms, recurrent events, and late disability.[5,6]

Given its association with worse clinical outcomes, accurate and early identification of iliofemoral DVT is paramount. Compared to other lower extremity DVT, the management of iliofemoral DVT may need to be modified. This is due to the potential benefits of endovascular intervention and the need for closer clinical follow-up, as there is a greater likelihood of late and long-term clinical complications. If left unresolved, residual obstruction leads to increased ambulatory venous pressure, which impairs venous return, increased tissue permeability at the microvasculature and leads to chronic venous

hypertension.[7] Long-term venous hypertension may eventually lead to PTS, an important complication of iliofemoral DVT. Even with anticoagulation, PTS can occur in up to 70% of patients at a 5-year follow-up.[1]

Clinical Presentation

Patients commonly present with sudden onset swelling, pain, warmth, and erythema in the affected lower extremity. Symptoms are usually unilateral but can be bilateral, particularly in those with hypercoagulability syndromes or in those with iliocaval thrombosis, typically associated with inferior vena cava (IVC) filter thrombosis or malignancy.[8] In rare cases, patients may display signs of impaired limb perfusion due to significant venous outflow obstruction from extensive DVT that subsequently results in diminished arterial flow. This can lead to stages of phlegmasia starting with alba dolens where the affected limb will be swollen and appear pale. As perfusion continues to decline an emergent venous condition can developed termed phlegmasia cerulea dolens where the limb appears cyanotic, with violaceous discoloration, severe persistent pain, and ultimately frank venous gangrene. This condition is associated with significant post-thrombotic morbidity and recurrence. In cases of progression to frank venous gangrene, there is a 20% to 50% risk of amputation and mortality of 20% to 40%.[9,10]

Diagnosis

Iliofemoral DVT should be suspected when patients present with massive swelling of the proximal part of the leg and buttock pain. The diagnosis of iliofemoral DVT involves a combination of clinical assessment and imaging studies.

- *Duplex ultrasonography:* The first-line imaging modality for suspected DVT, providing real-time assessment of venous flow and thrombus visualization. Visualization of thrombus, lack of vein compressibility, and lack of venous augmentation with compression or respiratory variation is diagnostic of DVT (Fig. 1). Evaluation of pelvic veins is often limited; however, pulsed doppler of the visualized iliac or common femoral veins can be used to assess for presence of abnormal venous waveforms. An abnormal waveform, such as a flat or continuous waveform identified in an otherwise patent common femoral vein by color doppler can reflect upstream obstruction, especially if different compared to contralateral extremity.[7]

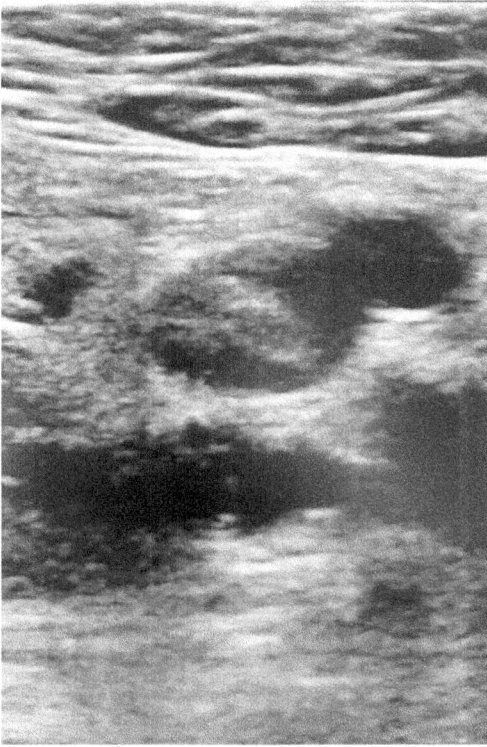

Fig. 1. Femoral DVT visualized with the use of ultrasound.

- *Contrast-enhanced computed tomography (CT) venography (CTV):* Offers detailed imaging of the iliofemoral veins and evaluation of any potential anatomic variations and abnormalities. CTV is not needed for diagnosis but is particularly useful in cases where ultrasound findings in the iliac veins are inconclusive and for procedural planning especially in the setting of previous device implants (ie, stents or IVC filter).[3]
- *Magnetic Resonance Venography (MRV):* Provides high-resolution imaging of the venous system without ionizing radiation and is useful in patients with contraindications to CT.[3] Both CTV and MRV are particularly helpful when identifying potential anatomic causes for iliofemoral DVT. These include May-Thurner syndrome, as well as masses, tumors or devices that can cause compression of the iliac veins.

Medical Management
Anticoagulation
Parenteral anticoagulation. Depending on the clinical presentation and need for potential intervention, most patients hospitalized with iliofemoral DVT are managed initially with parenteral anticoagulation. This includes intravenous (IV) unfractionated heparin (UFH), subcutaneous low-molecular-weight heparin (LMWH), and subcutaneous fondaparinaux. IV UFH is more often used due to its rapid clearance from circulation upon discontinuation; however, it does require frequent monitoring to ensure therapeutic levels. LMWH, on the other hand, has a more predictable dose response and longer half-life, making routine monitoring unnecessary.[11] LMWH requires dose reductions in patients with impaired renal function, and its therapeutic dosing is less predictable in patients with severe obesity. Fondaparinaux, like LMWH, has a long half-life, does not require routine monitoring, and is contraindicated when creatinine clearance is less than 30 mL/minute, but it can potentially be more reliably used in patients with obesity.[12] Direct thrombin inhibitors, such as bivalirudin, are used in cases of patients with heparin-induced thrombocytopenia.[7]

Oral anticoagulation. Direct oral anticoagulants (DOACs) have become the most used anticoagulants for the management of DVT. Compared with warfarin, DOACs have shown to have similar efficacy with superior safety, particularly in the reduction of major bleeding events. They should be avoided in patients with a creatinine clearance less than 30 mL/minute, since these patients were excluded from their pivotal clinical trials. Rivaroxaban and apixaban can be used as the sole initial anticoagulant with an initial higher *loading* dose for the initial weeks of treatment followed by a maintenance dose, while dabigatran and edoxaban have been studied only with a preceding course of 5 days of parenteral heparin and are not used as initial sole monotherapy.[13,14]

Compression therapy
Graduated compression stockings providing 30 to 40 mm Hg of ankle pressure have traditionally been recommended in the treatment of proximal VTE after starting anticoagulation therapy to prevent PTS. However, evidence to support their efficacy has been conflicting. While smaller studies suggested a benefit, a larger randomized trial of graduated compression stockings versus placebo stockings for 2 years showed no significant reduction in the incidence of PTS.[15,16] While some patients with moderate to severe symptoms may find symptomatic improvement when wearing compression stockings, many patients are not

adherent to their use due to cost, inconvenience, and discomfort.

Invasive Management

Over 40% of patients with proximal DVT progress to developing chronic venous insufficiency, leg ulceration, and venous claudication despite treatment with anticoagulation.[1] Several trials have tried to address whether a strategy of early thrombus removal is effective at minimizing the incidence and severity of these venous congestion symptoms.

The Post-Thrombotic Syndrome After Catheter-Directed Thrombolysis for Deep Vein Thrombosis (CaVenT) trial randomized 209 patients with iliofemoral DVT to standard therapy with anticoagulation and compression stockings versus standard therapy plus catheter-directed thrombolysis (CDT). Patients in the CDT group had greater rates of iliofemoral patency at 6 months (65.9% vs 47.4%, P = .012) and lower rates of PTS at 2 years (41% vs 55.6%, P = .047) compared with those in the standard therapy group. Overall, this study found an absolute risk reduction in the development of PTS of 14.4% at 2 years and 28% at 5 years.[17]

The Acute Venous Thrombosis: Thrombus Removal with Adjunctive Catheter-Directed Thrombolysis (ATTRACT) trial randomized 692 patients with iliofemoral or femoropopliteal DVT to conventional therapy with anticoagulation alone versus conventional therapy plus pharmacomechanical CDT (PCDT), which integrates aspiration or reolytic thrombectomy in addition to lytic therapy. This trial failed to demonstrate a significant reduction in the rates of PTS at 6 and 24 months in the PCDT group compared with standard therapy, with higher bleeding events in the intervention group. However, subgroup analysis in patients with iliofemoral DVT showed a lower incidence of moderate and severe PTS symptoms, faster pain relief, and improved quality-of-life.[18,19]

The Dutch Catheter-Directed Thrombolysis Versus Anticoagulation trial randomized 184 patients with acute iliofemoral DVT to ultrasound-assisted CDT versus standard anticoagulation therapy and found no differences in rates of PTS or quality-of-life at 1 year.[20] Considering the findings of the multiple clinical trials and observational studies, most recent society guidelines have recommended the use of CDT in selected cases of patients with limb-threatening DVT and for ambulatory patients with symptomatic iliofemoral DVT at low risk of bleeding and with long life expectancy.[21–23]

The ClotTriever outcomes registry prospectively enrolled 500 patients with DVT treated with thrombectomy using ClotTreiver device, where 67% had iliofemoral segment involvement. Complete or near complete resolution of thrombus was achieved in most patients (91.2%), nearly all in a single session of treatment, and without need for subsequent intensive care unit monitoring. In this registry, health status outcomes such as self-reported pain and circumferential measurement of limb edema significantly improved at discharge.[24] The upcoming ClotTriever System Versus Anticoagulation in Deep Vein Thrombosis randomized control trial will provide further insights on the use and effectiveness of this technology in iliofemoral DVT.

Endovascular Techniques
Catheter-directed thrombolysis

CDT refers to the infusion of a thrombolytic drug directly into the location of the DVT via a multisidehole catheter. Access can be obtained in the popliteal, common femoral, posterior tibial or internal jugular vein, and should be obtained under ultrasound guidance. There are multiple catheters available designed for this purpose such as the Cragg-McNamara (Medtronic) infusion catheter for simple direct infusion. The Ekos system (Boston Scientific Corporation) combines high-frequency, low-power ultrasound with simultaneous CDT to accelerate clot dissolution. The ultrasound waves loosen the fibrin mesh to make more surface area of the fibers available to the lytic agent.

Mechanical thrombectomy

Mechanical thrombectomy techniques encompass different modalities for thrombus removal including aspiration (Indigo [Penumbra], FlowTriever [Inari Medical], Jeti [Abbot]), rheolytic thrombectomy (with or without lytics) (Angiojet [Boston Scientific Corporation]), and direct mechanical maceration using a coring element (ClotTriever [Inari Medical]). Aspiration thrombectomy devices are typically medium to large bore and employ different mechanisms for aspiration such as manual syringe suction, vacuum assisted, or saline jets to break the thrombus before aspiration. Rheolytic thrombectomy devices (Angiojet) use the Bernoulli effect to aspirate thrombus into the device and can be used with or without adjunctive lytic infusion. While devices such as the ClotTriever utilize an atraumatic nitinol coring element and mesh collection bag to dislodge and collect the thrombus as it is retracted through the area with the DVT, without need for lytic infusion. Mechanical thrombectomy represents a fast-growing market in the treatment of acute DVT due to emerging data and improved training and experience with the technology. A summary of thrombectomy devices can be reviewed in Table 1. Acute proximal DVT on digital subtraction angiography (DSA) with acute clot specimens from mechanical thrombectomy using the ClotTriever (Inari Medical) device can be seen in Fig. 2.

Intravascular ultrasound
Venography alone has poor diagnostic sensitivity in identifying obstructive lesions. Intravascular Ultrasound (IVUS) provides a fundamental

tool used during diagnostic and endovascular procedures to provide a detailed assessment of the vein lumen, thrombus burden, degree of stenosis, and stent placement. An example of an acute femoral DVT identified on IVUS can be seen in Fig. 3. IVUS serves as an essential complementary tool for procedural planning and post-procedural assessment.

Stent placement
For patients where IVUS confirms the presence of a stenotic or compressive iliac vein lesion, venoplasty and stenting is typically recommended.[25] A single center trial found that venous stenting in patients with residual iliac vein

Table 1
The table summarizes various percutaneous mechanical thrombectomy devices, highlighting their sheath sizes, unique features, and mechanisms of thrombosis removal

Device Name/Company	Characteristics	Description	Potential Caveats
AngioJet/Boston Scientific	• Sheath size: 6–8 F • Over-the-wire system (0.035-inch)	Rheolytic thrombectomy using the Bernoulli effect. Effective without the need for thrombolytic infusion.	Risk of hemolysis and renal complications due to the high-velocity saline jet.
AngioVac/ AngioDynamics	• Cannula: 22 F with straight or funneled tip • Venous blood return catheter: 16 F	Large-bore suction device with a recirculation circuit for thrombus removal from large vessels, like the inferior vena cava.	Requires large sheath size, which may increase risk of vessel trauma or bleeding, especially in smaller vessels.
Cleaner/Argon Medical Devices	• 6 F with 9-mm sinusoidal wave, or 7 F with 15-mm sinusoidal wave • Non-over-the-wire device	Rotational sinusoidal design enables effective thrombus release within the vessel lumen for enhanced clearance.	Limited use in larger thrombi due to smaller diameter; risk of vessel injury from rotational motion in fragile vessels.
ClotTriever/Inari Medical	• Sheath size: 13 F with side port for aspiration - Self-expanding nitinol mesh funnel • Nitinol coring catheter with collection bag	Designed to mechanically core and capture thrombus from vessel walls using a 0.035-inch wire-guided system.	May be less effective in highly calcified thrombi; larger sheath size increases risk of access site complications.
Indigo/Penumbra, Inc.	• Sheath size: 6–16 F • Proprietary separator wire paired with catheter	Small- to large- bore device for aspiration mechanical thrombectomy, suitable for targeted thrombus extraction.	Limited effectiveness for large thrombus burden for smaller devices.
Jeti/Walk Vascular, LLC	• Sheath size: 8 F • Integrated catheter with aspiration	Aspiration device with saline jet technology to dislodge thrombus with minimal hemolysis risk.	Potential for incomplete thrombus removal in extensive clot burden; risk of vessel wall damage with repeated use.

These devices range from rheolytic and aspiration systems to rotational and recirculation techniques, allowing targeted thrombus clearance in different vascular settings without or with minimal lytic use.

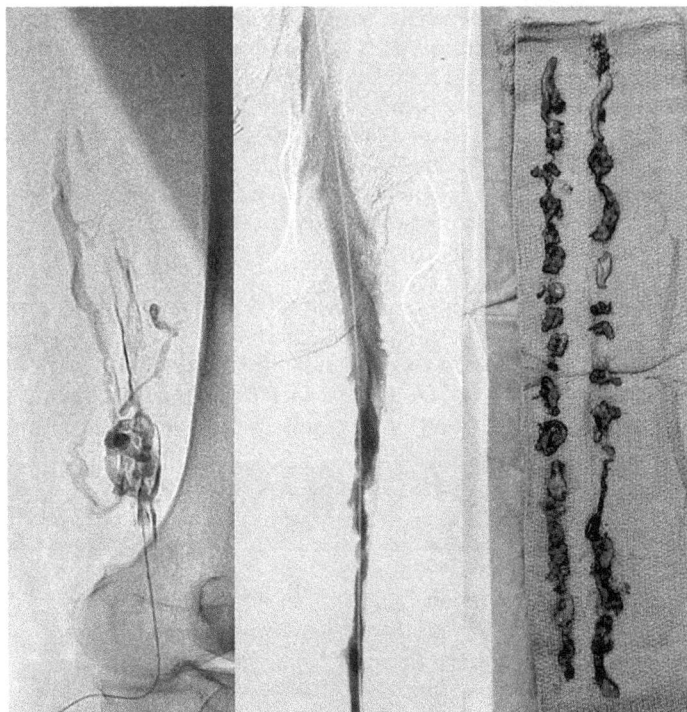

Fig. 2. Acute proximal DVT with acute clot extracted by mechanical thrombectomy using ClotTriever (Inari).

stenosis (>50% diameter narrowing) after CDT led to superior 1-year patency and reduced venous clinical severity compared with CDT alone.[26] Dedicated venous stents have recently been developed and currently available in the market such as the Venovo (Bard), Vena (Cook), and Abre stents (Medtronic). These stents made from nitinol are constructed to adapt to the large deformations and movements of the iliac veins. Use of IVUS for proper sizing of reference areas and landing in healthy zones is a key when performing venous stenting. Complications from venous stenting include device related back pain, thrombosis, fractures, and stent migration and embolization.

Follow-up
After intervention, patients should be maintained on uninterrupted anticoagulation. Depending on the clinical presentation surveillance imaging is often considered during index hospitalization, as well as followed closely in the outpatient center to assess for recurrence and procedure success. Monitoring for thrombosis recurrence, adherence to anticoagulation, and bleeding risk are important aspects of immediate post-procedure management.

CHRONIC DEEP VEIN THROMBOSIS
Background
Patients with acute DVT may progress to chronic DVT (C-DVT) despite the use of anticoagulation.[27] A DVT present for greater than 4 weeks is categorized as C-DVT and, contingent on

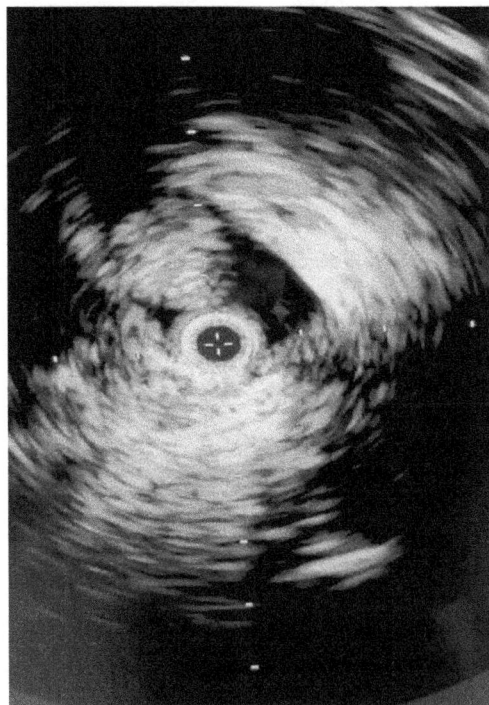

Fig. 3. Acute femoral DVT visualized using IVUS.

thrombus location and severity, may lead to PTS.[27,28] PTS, reported in 20% to 50% of patients with C-DVT, represents a collection of symptoms including lower extremity edema, skin changes, vein dilation, pain, fatigue, and ulcer formation.[27,28] Deep vein valvular structure and function are compromised by thrombotic damage, leading to deep vein insufficiency and the physical manifestations of PTS.[29] Severe PTS can be debilitating and may include up to 5% to 10% of patients with the condition.[30]

Therapeutic options for PTS include chronic oral anticoagulation, primarily with DOACs and supportive care. The daily use of compression socks is controversial with disparate evidence suggesting minor clinical benefit.[31] Prevention of PTS with catheter-based interventions is also disputed owing to the overall negative results of the ATTRACT trial, which studied acute iliofemoral DVT patients randomized to oral anticoagulation or CDT.[32] There were no significant differences in the primary endpoint, which included PTS development, noted between the 2 arms; however, the subset of iliocaval DVT patients showed benefit when treated with thrombolytics. PTS was also reduced in the CAVENT trial when patients were treated with catheter-directed thrombolytics and anticoagulation compared to anticoagulation alone.[33]

Device and technology development
There have been significant advances in chronic iliocaval DVT intervention over the past several years, most notably with the development of dedicated venous stents. These stents are composed primarily of nickel-titanium alloy with strong outward radial force, compressive resistance, and longitudinal flexibility. There are currently 4 Food and Drug Administration (FDA)-approved venous stents in the United States. The Venovo stent (Becton Dickinson Company, Franklin Lakes NJ) was the first FDA-approved venous stent in 2019. In the VERNACULAR trial, 156 patients were enrolled in a multi-center, prospective, single arm study with 84 PTS patients, and 72 non-thrombotic iliac vein lesion (NIVL) patients. 12-month primary patency was reported at 88.3%, superior to a performance goal of 74% (P-value<.0001), with freedom from major adverse events at 93.5% at 30 days. There were no stent fractures noted at 12 months and Venous Clinical Severity Score (VCSS) improved from 2.3 to 0.6.[34] The Vici stent (Boston Scientific Corporation, Malborough MA) was the next venous stent approved in 2019. In the prospective, single arm, multi-center VIRTUS trial, 170 patients were studied with a 12-month primary patency of 84%, exceeding the predetermined performance goal of 72.1% (P-value<.0001). Venographic patency of thrombotic and NIVL lesions were 79.8% and 96.2%, respectively. VCSS decreased from 10 to 5.6 with a 98.9% freedom from major adverse events at 30 days.[35] This stent has since been taken off the market from the manufacturer due to an FDA recall out of concerns for stent migration. The Zilver Vena stent (COOK Medical, Bloomington IN), FDA-approved in 2020, was studied in the VIVO trial. This was a prospective,

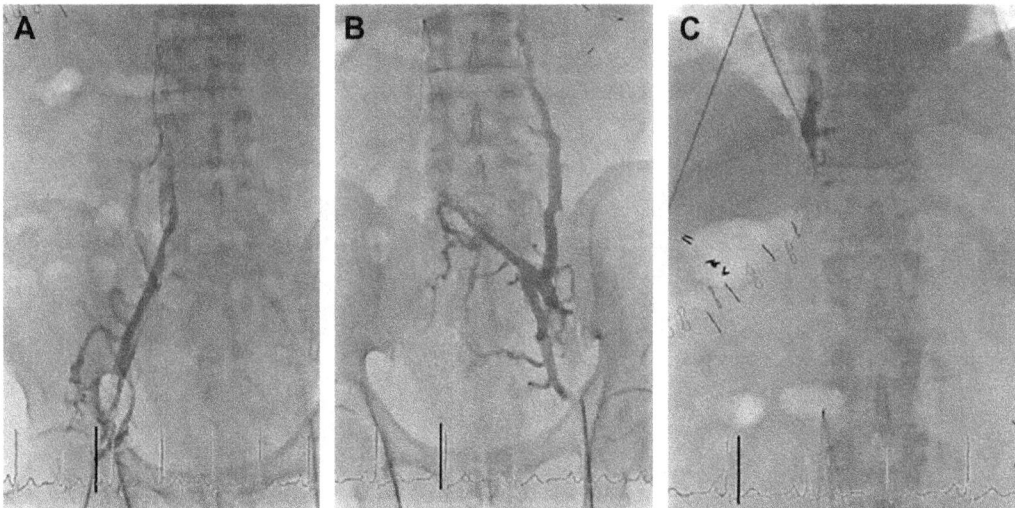

Fig. 4. (A) Right external iliac venogram demonstrating right common iliac vein occlusion with collateralization (B) Left external iliac venogram demonstrating left common iliac vein occlusion and extensive collateralization. (C) Right internal jugular vein access for inferior vena cavagram demonstrating occlusion of the IVC.

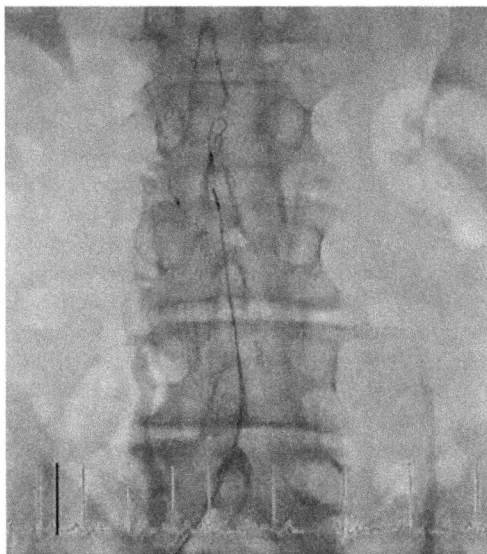

Fig. 5. Complex IVC occlusion involving an occluded IVC filter requiring the use of tunneled sheaths and catheters for support and crossing.

multi-center, single arm study, which enrolled 243 patients, 191 patients with NIVL and 52 patients with thrombotic disease. The 12-month primary patency was reported at 89.9%, exceeding the predetermined performance goal of 76% (P-value<.0001). Freedom from major adverse events at 30 days was 96.7%, with a VCSS reduction of 4.2 at 12 months.[36] The ABRE venous stent (Medtronic, Minneapolis MN), receiving FDA approval in 2020, was studied in the ABRE clinical trial. This prospective, multi-center, single arm study enrolled 200 patients, with 33 patients having acute DVT, 95 patients with post-thrombotic disease, and 72 patients with NIVL. The 12-month primary patency rate was 88% with a freedom from major adverse events of 98% at 30 days. Patients

VCSS decreased from 8.8 at baseline to 4.3 at 12 month follow-up.[37]

A recently released device, the RevCore thrombectomy catheter (Inari Medical, Irvine CA) FDA-cleared in 2023, can be used to debulk chronic thrombus associated with in-stent thrombosis. RevCore is a rotational device with an expandable coring element that can be used to break up and liberate thrombus in the iliocaval circulation. It is used in tandem with a sheath, which is inserted via internal jugular access and a basket filter from the distal end of the sheath positioned in the IVC to capture any embolized thrombus. The Venacore device (Inari Medical, Irvine CA), which also uses a rotational debulking element is indicated for de novo chronic venous thrombotic disease. In a retrospective, multi-center study of 65 thrombosed iliocaval stents in 44 patients, patency was reported at 95.8% at 40 day follow-up.[38]

Procedural considerations

Complex C-DVT interventions can be a challenging subset of patients to treat due to the presence of well-formed, dense, and thrombotic obstruction. These patients often have (IVC) or bilateral iliac vein involvement, and successful guidewire passage may be arduous or challenging (Fig. 4A, B]. Multiple venous access sites may be required to engage occlusive disease from both antegrade and retrograde approaches (Fig. 4C). Additionally, the presence of an IVC filter may increase the development of a thrombotic occlusion. With an estimated risk of 0.6% to 8% using contemporary filters, this syndrome may lead to further complications related to PTS.[39] Advancement, in these complex occlusions, may require the use of multiple tunneled sheaths and catheters utilizing *mother-in-child* techniques for adequate support with wire escalation to facilitate crossing (Fig. 5).

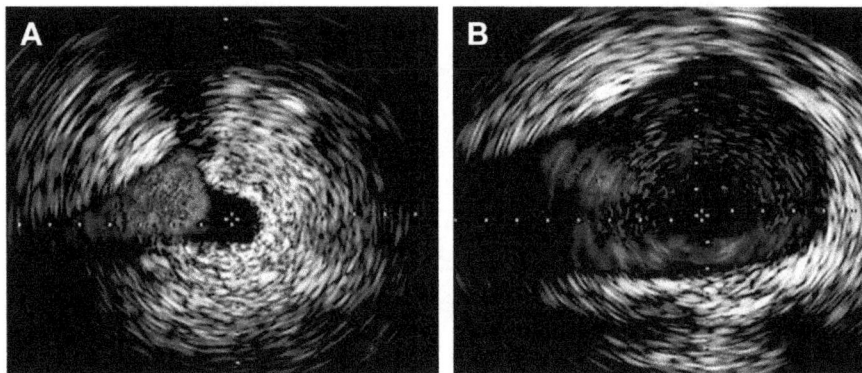

Fig. 6. IVUS imaging confirming lumen loss with chronic fibrosis (A) in comparison to the reference vessel size (B).

The use of IVUS is essential in properly sizing the vein and assessing lesion morphology to optimize definitive therapy (Fig. 6A, B). Based on chronicity and morphology of thrombotic occlusion, debulking with thrombectomy devices could further accentuate luminal gain (Fig. 7). The majority of C-DVT is ultimately treated with stent deployment (Fig. 8); however, up to 20% of patients will develop in-stent thrombosis within 2 to 3 years.[38] Re-crossing occlusive in-stent lesions can be challenging, but often still require repeat stenting for optimal results.

Recent therapeutic advancements within the field of venous intervention have demonstrated potential in addressing the need for revascularization in C-DVT patients. Improved stent design and innovation for chronic thrombus removal have bolstered clinical success; yet there remains opportunity to optimize treatment of the complex C-DVT patient.

MAY-THURNER SYNDROME

Within the pelvis, the major circulatory vessels include the descending aorta branching into the right and left common iliac arteries, as well as the IVC, which arises from the confluence of the right and left common iliac veins. The descending

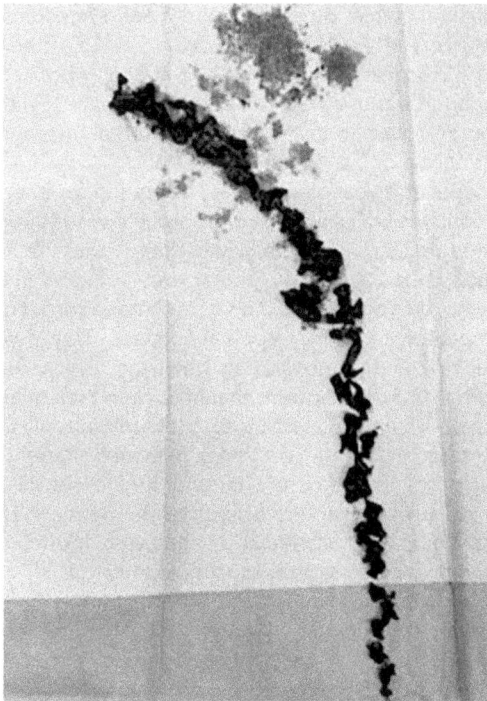

Fig. 8. Final venogram demonstrating successful revascularization of chronic IVC and iliac vein occlusion after stenting with dedicated venous stents.

Fig. 7. Use of adjunctive thrombectomy allows retrieval of subacute and chronic thrombus in complex venous occlusions.

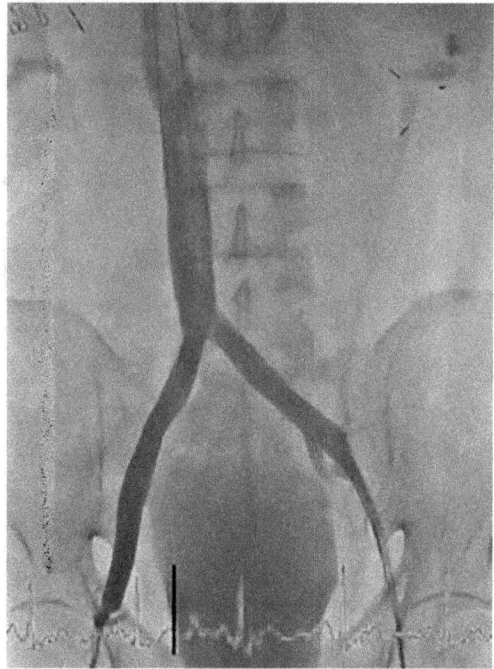

aorta and the IVC run parallel to one another with the former on the left, resulting in the right common iliac artery anteriorly crossing the proximal left common iliac vein.[41] This crossing can lead to compression of the left common iliac vein against the anterior spine and results in dynamic compression, scarring, and potential predisposition to thrombus (Fig. 9).[42] While this anatomy has been more frequently described in the left common iliac vein, compression can also occur in the right common iliac vein and in other pelvic locations, especially in cases of extrinsic compression.

NIVL is defined as the external compression of the left common iliac vein without the presence of a DVT.[42] May-Thurner syndrome is the presence of DVT most associated in the left lower extremity as a result of the compression of the left iliac vein by the right common iliac artery.[43] While both May Thurner syndrome and NIVL are a result of compression of iliac vein, the primary difference between these 2 terms is that May-Thurner includes the presence of a DVT.

Patients who are symptomatic with NIVL may present with leg edema, leg pain, paresthesia, leg heaviness, varicose veins, venous dermatitis, and/or venous ulcers. Clinical objective symptoms can be classified with a Clinical, Etiology,

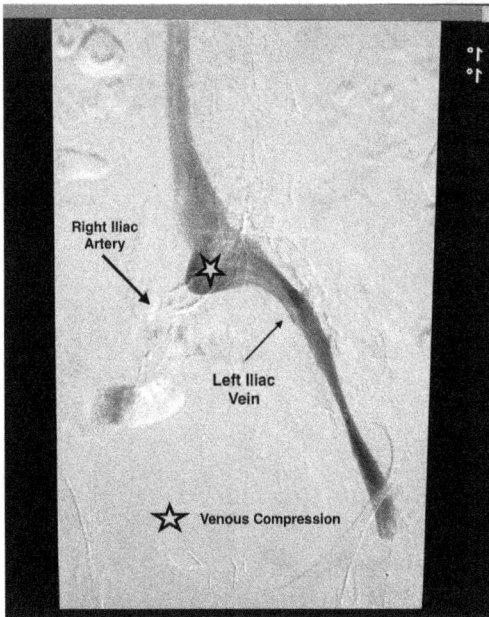

Fig. 9. Venogram of left iliac vein and inferior vena cava with overlying right iliac artery causing venous compression.

Anatomic Pathophysiology (CEAP) score and subjective symptoms can be quantified using VCSS.[42] Using the CEAP classification system patients with CEAP level 4 to 6 should be evaluated for presence of a NIVL[40]

Due to anatomic differences in women of having a narrower pelvic space between the iliac artery and anterior spine, they are more predisposed to iliac vein compression than men.[44] Patients who have history of DVT or familial history of DVT also have an increased prevalence of a NIVL.[45] Approximately 25% of people with venous ulcers have NIVL.[44] Patients with severe symptoms may present with venous stasis ulcers. Venous ulcers are associated with significant pain and increased risk of morbidity.[44]

Evaluation to determine which patients would benefit from treatment starts initially with non-invasive testing with a lower extremity venous duplex ultrasound (DUS) to provide axial images of the venous system. Ultrasound findings of venous insufficiency in the common femoral vein are an indicator of potential iliac vein compression and further evaluation is indicated.[46] The limitations of duplex US include the inability to accurately assess the iliac veins themselves because of their deep location in the pelvis.[47] Another form of testing includes abdominal CTV for visualization of vascular system, with the limitation being exposure to radiation and contrast dye.[48] MRV is a radiation free

alternative to CTV and allows for assessment of both the magnitude and direction of venous flow.[47] The decision to perform CVT versus MRV may be dependent on local image protocols, as timing of the contrast can make these tests technically difficult to interpret.[48]

The gold standard in determining compression of the iliac vein is done with a venogram using IVUS.[48] IVUS provides information of the vein diameter, cross-sectional area to allow for calculations of vein stenosis, as well as provide critical information for stent sizing.[42] A venogram is a low-risk procedure that can typically be performed in less than 15 minutes. Popliteal vein access is commonly used to evaluate both the inflow and outflow.

Not all patients who have demonstrated compression of the iliac veins are symptomatic. In the absence of symptoms, NIVL may be considered a normal anatomic variant and occurs in up to 24% of patients.[48] Therefore, patients who demonstrate the presence of NIVL without symptoms do not have an indication for treatment.[42] Patients who are symptomatic should be evaluated to rule out comorbid diagnoses of heart failure, compartment syndrome, superficial venous reflux, lymphedema, medication induced edema, and other metabolic causes of edema.[40,42]

The goal of treatment is to improve overall quality of life by reducing patient symptoms, which is measured by a decrease in CEAP and VCSS scores. For example, patients who had been diagnosed with NIVL and treated with venous-specific stents demonstrated an average decrease of 1.8 in VCSS scores and 1.4 in CEAP scores at 1 year.[49] The exact indication for intervention remains an area of ongoing investigation though it is generally accepted that IVUS measured stenosis of greater than 50% and in a symptomatic patient meets the criteria for stent implantation.[4] For optimal patient care, we recommend incorporating both the clinical assessments of symptoms that impact on their quality of life and IVUS stenosis measurement when determining if intervention is indicated. Patients who do not meet the criteria for intervention and are symptomatic are recommended to continue with conservative therapies including compression and possible anticoagulation.[50]

Upon determining that intervention is indicated, the process of determining the optimal type of stent, as well as proper sizing is critical. We recommend adhering to each manufacturer's specific sizing instructions, which range from oversizing of the reference vessel from 1 to 4 mm using IVUS.[40] Under sizing of stents can

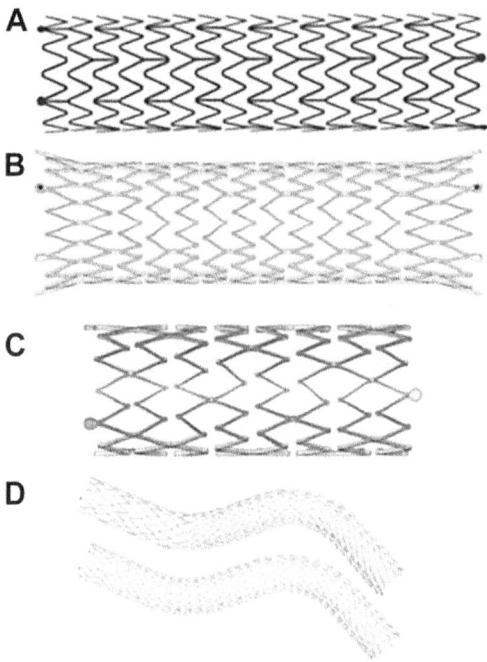

Fig. 10. Images of Venous purpose-built stents (A) Zilver Vena, (B) Venovo, (C) Abre, (D) Duo venous system.

lead to residual symptoms, stent occlusion, or migration.[51] In a review of studies on stent migration, 82.6% of stents were shorter than 60 mm, 44 of 47 had diameters measuring 14 mm or smaller, and 56% migrated to the heart.[40]

Given the anatomic differences in size, compliance, and radial force between the venous and arterial system, the use of arterial stents is contraindicated in veins.[52] Historically treatments included Wallstents, which are composed of self-expanding Eligioly alloy braided structure.[52] The Wallstent demonstrates weak radial force at its ends allowing for possible migration and poor blood flow in segments, as well as a tendency to shorten due to braided structure.[52] More recently, a number of purpose-built venous

stents have been developed for the treatment of NIVL. These include the Venovo, Abre, Zilver Vena, and Duo stents, which are all nitinol self-expanding stents (Fig. 10A–D). The Venovo stent has flared ends to aid in anchoring and is designed for the largest range in diameter of veins (52,49). The ABRE stent is a self-expanding stent made of high-purity nitinol designed for maximum flexibility.[52] Zilver Vena Venous is a nitinol self-expanding stent purpose-designed to endure external compression and resistance while accommodating bending.[53] The Duo venous stent system includes both Duo Hybrid and Duo Extend stents that accommodate a range of anatomic variations and mechanical requirements.[54] In general, these stents all have greater crush resistance, predictable deployment, and simplified sizing relative to the reference vein diameter.[52]

VCSS allows for a quantifiable measure to the burden of chronic venous disease on a patient's quality of life. As seen in Table 2, treatment of NIVL with venous stents is associated with significant reduction in VCSS at 1 year. The decline in VCSS values demonstrates the improvement in patients' symptoms and enhancement in their quality-of-life following treatment.

Patency values can be maximized with accurate preoperative evaluations, appropriate stent sizing, optimal postoperative antithrombic therapy and diligent post-operation follow-up. Table 2 demonstrates successful intervention with the newly purpose-build venous stents Venovo, ABRE, and Zilver demonstrating comparable patency at 1 year of approximately 88%.

The optimal pharmacologic strategy following venous stenting remains controversial, especially in NIVL patients. The objective of using antithrombotic therapy is to ensure long-term stent patency and mitigate risk of future thrombus.[55] According to an International Delphi Consensus, the recommended treatment includes anticoagulation in the initial 6 to 12 months following

	Patency at 1 Year	Average Lesion Length per Treated Limb	Number of Patients in the Study	Changes in VCSS
Stent Type				
Wallstent[52]	81.8%	Not available	81	Not available
Zilver Vena Venous[53]	89.8%	98.6 mm	243	−4.2
Venovo[49]	88.6%	67.8 mm	170	−1.8
ABRE[45]	88%	112.4 mm	200	−4.5
Duo Venous stent system[54]	90.2%	Not available	162	Not available

Table 2
Venous purpose-built stent comparison

Comparison of venous stent types measuring patency at 1-year, average lesion length, and changes in VCSS.

venous stenting.[56] However, NIVL patients post stent with additional thrombotic risk factors should tailor their antithrombotic therapy to align with standard-of-care based on risk factor profile.[40] We recommend proceeding with imaging to evaluate stent patency and placement as ongoing surveillance treatment.[40] Given the excellent patency of venous stents, patients can generally be followed from a symptomatic perspective and reimage only in the setting of recurrent symptoms.

DISCLOSURES

Dr A. Teta has nothing to disclose. Dr J. Mohan is a consultant for Inari Medical. Dr Y. Castro-Dominguez is a consultant for Medtronic and Boston Scientific. Dr V. Varghese has nothing to disclose. Dr J.C. George is a consultant for Abbott Vascular, Boston Scientific, Medtronic, Philips. Ms J. Powers has nothing to disclose. Dr E.J. Armstrong has nothing to disclose.

REFERENCES

1. Martin SS, Aday AW, Almarzooq ZI, et al. 2024 Heart disease and stroke statistics: a report of US and global data from the American heart association. Circulation 2024;149(8):e347–913.
2. Jaff MR, McMurtry MS, Archer SL, et al. Management of massive and submassive pulmonary embolism, iliofemoral deep vein thrombosis, and chronic thromboembolic pulmonary hypertension: a scientific statement from the American Heart Association. Circulation 2011;123(16):1788–830.
3. Crisostomo PR, Cho J, Feliciano B, et al. Period frequency of iliofemoral venous occlusive disease by Doppler ultrasound and corresponding treatment in a tertiary care facility. J Vasc Surg 2010;52(5):1272–7.
4. Kahn SR, Shrier I, Julian JA, et al. Determinants and time course of the postthrombotic syndrome after acute deep venous thrombosis. Ann Intern Med 2008;149(10):698–707.
5. Douketis JD, Crowther MA, Foster GA, et al. Does the location of thrombosis determine the risk of disease recurrence in patients with proximal deep vein thrombosis? Am J Med 2001;110(7):515–9.
6. Vedantham S, Sista AK, Klein SJ, et al. Quality improvement guidelines for the treatment of lower-extremity deep vein thrombosis with use of endovascular thrombus removal. J Vasc Intervent Radiol 2014;25(9):1317–25.
7. Creager M, Beckman J, Loscalzo J, et al. Vascular medicine: a companion to braunwald's heart disease. 3rd edition. USA: Elsevier; 2019.
8. Goldhaber SZ, Tapson VF, Committee DFS. A prospective registry of 5,451 patients with ultrasound-confirmed deep vein thrombosis. Am J Cardiol 2004;93(2):259–62.
9. Mumoli N, Invernizzi C, Luschi R, et al. Phlegmasia cerulea dolens. Circulation 2012;125(8):1056–7.
10. Gardella L, Faulk J. Phlegmasia alba and cerulea dolens. Treasure island (FL): StatPearls; 2024. Disclosure: JimBob Faulk declares no relevant financial relationships with ineligible companies.
11. van Den Belt AG, Prins MH, Lensing AW, et al. Fixed dose subcutaneous low molecular weight heparins versus adjusted dose unfractionated heparin for venous thromboembolism. Cochrane Database Syst Rev 2000;2:CD001100.
12. Davidson BL, Buller HR, Decousus H, et al. Effect of obesity on outcomes after fondaparinux, enoxaparin, or heparin treatment for acute venous thromboembolism in the Matisse trials. J Thromb Haemost 2007;5(6):1191–4.
13. Agnelli G, Buller HR, Cohen A, et al. Oral apixaban for the treatment of acute venous thromboembolism. N Engl J Med 2013;369(9):799–808.
14. Investigators E, Bauersachs R, Berkowitz SD, et al. Oral rivaroxaban for symptomatic venous thromboembolism. N Engl J Med 2010;363(26):2499–510.
15. Appelen D, van Loo E, Prins MH, et al. Compression therapy for prevention of post-thrombotic syndrome. Cochrane Database Syst Rev 2017;9(9):CD004174.
16. Kahn SR, Shapiro S, Wells PS, et al. Compression stockings to prevent post-thrombotic syndrome: a randomised placebo-controlled trial. Lancet (London, England) 2014;383(9920):880–8.
17. Enden T, Haig Y, Klow NE, et al. Long-term outcome after additional catheter-directed thrombolysis versus standard treatment for acute iliofemoral deep vein thrombosis (the CaVenT study): a randomised controlled trial. Lancet (London, England) 2012;379(9810):31–8.
18. Vedantham S, Goldhaber SZ, Julian JA, et al. Pharmacomechanical catheter-directed thrombolysis for deep-vein thrombosis. N Engl J Med 2017;377(23):2240–52.
19. Comerota AJ, Kearon C, Gu CS, et al. Endovascular thrombus removal for acute iliofemoral deep vein thrombosis. Circulation 2019;139(9):1162–73.
20. Notten P, Ten Cate-Hoek AJ, Arnoldussen C, et al. Ultrasound-accelerated catheter-directed thrombolysis versus anticoagulation for the prevention of post-thrombotic syndrome (CAVA): a single-blind, multicentre, randomised trial. Lancet Haematol 2020;7(1):e40–9.
21. Kakkos SK, Gohel M, Baekgaard N, et al. Editor's choice - European society for vascular surgery (ESVS) 2021 clinical practice guidelines on the management of venous thrombosis. Eur J Vasc Endovasc Surg 2021;61(1):9–82.

22. Ortel TL, Neumann I, Ageno W, et al. American Society of Hematology 2020 guidelines for management of venous thromboembolism: treatment of deep vein thrombosis and pulmonary embolism. Blood Adv 2020;4(19):4693–738.

23. Vedantham S, Desai KR, Weinberg I, et al. Society of interventional radiology position statement on the endovascular management of acute iliofemoral deep vein thrombosis. J Vasc Intervent Radiol 2023; 34(2):284–299 e7.

24. Kolluri R, Berlet T, Zafar M, et al. Safety and effectiveness of mechanical thrombectomy from the fully enrolled multicenter, prospective CLOUT registry. JSCAI 2024;3(2).

25. Razavi MK, Jaff MR, Miller LE. Safety and effectiveness of stent placement for iliofemoral venous outflow obstruction: systematic review and meta-analysis. Circ Cardiovasc Interv 2015;8(10):e002772.

26. Jiang K, Li XQ, Sang HF, et al. Mid-term outcome of endovascular treatment for acute lower extremity deep venous thrombosis. Phlebology 2017; 32(3):200–6.

27. Chopard R, Albertsen IE, Piazza G. Diagnosis and treatment of lower extremity venous thromboembolism: a review. JAMA 2020;324(17):1765–76.

28. Cucuruz B, Kopp R, Pfister K, Noppenev J, Tripal K, Korff T, Zeman F, Koller M, Noppenev T. Risk and protective factors for post-thrombotic syndrome after deep venous thrombosis. J Vasc Surg Venous Lymphat Disord 2020;8:390–5.

29. Galanaud JP, Monreal M, Kahn SR. Epidemiology of the post-thrombotic syndrome. Thromb Res 2018;164:100–9.

30. Kahn SR. The post-thrombotic syndrome: the forgotten morbidity of deep venous thrombosis. J Thromb Thrombolysis 2006;21:41–8.

31. Subbiah R, Aggarwal V, Zhao H, et al. Effect of compression stockings on post thrombotic syndrome in patients with deep vein thrombosis: a meta-analysis of randomised controlled trial. Lancet Haematology 2016;3(6):e293–300.

32. Vedantham S, Goldhaber S, Julian J, et al. Catheter-directed thrombolysis for deep-vein thrombosis. N Engl J Med 2017;377:2240–52.

33. Haig Y, Enden T, Grotta O, et al. Post-thrombotic syndrome after catheter-directed thrombolysis for deep vein thrombosis (CaVenT): 5-year follow-up results of an open-label, randomised controlled trial. Lancet Haematology 2016;3(2):e64–71.

34. Dake MD, O'Sullivan G, Shammas NW, et al. Three-year results from the Venovo venous stent study for the treatment iliac and femoral vein obstruction. Cardiovasc Intervent Radiol 2021;44:1918–29.

35. Razavi MK, Gagne P, Black S, et al. Mid- and long term outcomes following dedicated venous nitinol stent placement for symptomatic ileofemoral venous obstruction: 3-5 year results of the VIRTUS

study. J Vasc Intervent Radiol 2022. https://doi.org/10.1016/j.jvir.2022.08.028.

36. Comerota AJ, Gagne P, Brown JA, et al. Final 3-year study outcomes from the evaluation of the zilver vena venous stent for the treatment of symptomatic iliofemoral venous outflow obstruction (the VIVO clinical study). J Vasc Intervent Radiol 2024; 35(6):834–45.

37. Erin M, Kathleen G, Marc S, et al. Pivotal study evaluating the safety and effectiveness of the Abre venous self-expanding stent system in patients with symptomatic iliofemoral venous outflow obstruction. Circ Cardiovasc Interv 2022;15:e010960.

38. Abramowitz SD, Choi M, Marino AG, et al. A multicenter and retrospective study of 65 thrombosed stents treated with the new RevCore thrombectomy catheter. J Vasc Surg 2024;79(6):e298–9.

39. Andreoli JM, Thornburg BG, Hickey RM. Inferior vena cava filter-related thrombus/deep vein thrombosis: data and management. Semin Intervent Radiol 2016;33(2):101–4.

40. Ibrahim W, Al Safran Z, Hasan H, et al. Endovascular management of may-thurner syndrome. Ann Vasc Dis 2012;5(2):217–21.

41. Raju S, Neglen P. High prevalence of nonthrombotic iliac vein lesions in chronic venous disease: a permissive role in pathogenicity. J Vasc Surg 2006;44(1):136–44.

42. Joh M, Desai KR. Treatment of nonthrombotic iliac vein lesions. Semin Intervent Radiol 2021;38(2):155–9.

43. Marston W, Fish D, Unger J, et al. Incidence of and risk factors for iliocaval venous obstruction in patients with active or healed venous leg ulcers. J Vasc Surg 2011;53(5):1303–8.

44. Desai KR, Sabri SS, Elias S, et al. Consensus statement on the management of nonthrombotic iliac vein lesions from the VIVA foundation, the American venous forum, and the American vein and lymphatic society. Circ Cardiovasc Interv 2024; 17(8):e014160 [published correction appears in Circ Cardiovasc Interv 2024:e000093. doi: 10.1161/HCV.0000000000000093].

45. Murphy E, Gibson K, Sapoval M, et al. Pivotal study evaluating the safety and effectiveness of the Abre venous self-expanding stent system in patients with symptomatic iliofemoral venous outflow obstruction. Circ Cardiovasc Interv 2022;15(2):e010960.

46. Necas M. Duplex ultrasound in the assessment of lower extremity venous insufficiency. Australas J Ultrasound Med 2010;13(4):37–45.

47. Zucker EJ, Ganguli S, Ghoshhajra BB, et al. Imaging of venous compression syndromes. Cardiovasc Diagn Ther 2016;6(6):519–32.

48. Radaideh Q, Patel NM, Shammas NW. Iliac vein compression: epidemiology, diagnosis and treatment. Vasc Health Risk Manag 2019;15:115–22. Published 2019 May 9.

49. Dake MD, O'Sullivan G, Shammas NW, et al. Three-year results from the Venovo venous stent study for the treatment of iliac and femoral vein obstruction. Cardiovasc Intervent Radiol 2021;44(12):1918–29 [published correction appears in Cardiovasc Intervent Radiol 2021;44(12):2027].

50. Rognoni C, Lugli M, Maleti O, et al. Venous stenting for patients with outflow obstruction and leg ulcers: cost-effectiveness and budget impact analyses. J Comp Eff Res 2020;9(10):705–20.

51. Saleem T. An overview of specific considerations in chronic venous disease and iliofemoral venous stenting. J Pers Med 2023;13(2):331. Published 2023 Feb 15.

52. Salimi J, Chinisaz F, Yazdi SAM. A comprehensive study on venous endovascular management and stenting in deep veins occlusion and stenosis: a review study. Surg Open Sci 2024;19:131–40. Published 2024 Apr 16.

53. Hofmann LR, Gagne P, Brown JA, et al. Twelve-month end point results from the evaluation of the Zilver Vena venous stent in the treatment of symptomatic iliofemoral venous outflow obstruction (VIVO clinical study). J Vasc Surg Venous Lymphat Disord 2023;11(3):532–41.e4 [published correction appears in J Vasc Surg Venous Lymphat Disord 2023;11(6):1292].

54. VIVID in. Philips Duo Venous Stent System for Iliofemoral Occlusive Disease Evaluated in VIVID Trial. Endovascular Today 2023. Available at: https://evtoday.com/news/philips-duo-venous-stent-system-for-the-iliofemoral-occlusive-disease-evaluated-in-vivid-trial. Accessed August 28, 2024.

55. Guo B, Chen C, Li Y, et al. Principles of optimal antithrombotic therapy for iliac VEnous stenting (POATIVES): a national expert based Delphi Consensus study. J Vasc Surg Venous Lymphat Disord 2024;101739.

56. Milinis K, Thapar A, Shalhoub J, et al. Antithrombotic therapy following venous stenting: international Delphi Consensus. Eur J Vasc Endovasc Surg 2018;55(4):537–44.

Moving?

Make sure your subscription moves with you!

To notify us of your new address, find your **Clinics Account Number** (located on your mailing label above your name), and contact customer service at:

Email: journalscustomerservice-usa@elsevier.com

800-654-2452 (subscribers in the U.S. & Canada)
314-447-8871 (subscribers outside of the U.S. & Canada)

Fax number: 314-447-8029

Elsevier Health Sciences Division
Subscription Customer Service
3251 Riverport Lane
Maryland Heights, MO 63043

*To ensure uninterrupted delivery of your subscription, please notify us at least 4 weeks in advance of move.

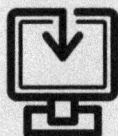

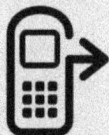

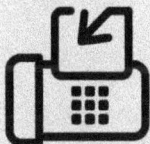

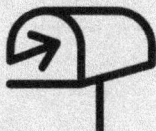

ELSEVIER

www.ingramcontent.com/pod-product-compliance
Lightning Source LLC
Chambersburg PA
CBHW082007190326
41458CB00010B/3103